Handbook of Vitamin D

Handbook of Vitamin D

Editor: John Edwards

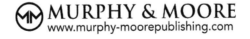

MURPHY & MOORE
www.murphy-moorepublishing.com

www.murphy-moorepublishing.com

ⓂMURPHY & MOORE

Cataloging-in-Publication Data

Handbook of vitamin D / edited by John Edwards.
    p. cm.
Includes bibliographical references and index.
ISBN 978-1-63987-796-6
1. Vitamin D. 2. Calcium regulating hormones. 3. Vitamins, Fat-soluble.
4. Steroid hormones. I. Edwards, John.
QP772.V53 H36 2023
612.399--dc23

Murphy & Moore Publishing
1 Rockefeller Plaza,
New York City,
NY 10020, USA

ISBN 978-1-63987-796-6 (Hardback)

Contents

Preface

It is often said that books are a boon to mankind. They document every progress and pass on the knowledge from one generation to the other. They play a crucial role in our lives. Thus I was both excited and nervous while editing this book. I was pleased by the thought of being able to make a mark but I was also nervous to do it right because the future of students depends upon it. Hence, I took a few months to research further into the discipline, revise my knowledge and also explore some more aspects. Post this process, I begun with the editing of this book.

Vitamin D refers to a group of fat-soluble secosteroids which are responsible for improving intestinal absorption of phosphate, calcium and magnesium and several others biological effects. It plays a crucial role in metabolism and calcium homeostasis. The most significant compounds of vitamin D in human beings are vitamin D2 and vitamin D3. The main source of vitamin D found in nature is the synthesis of cholecalciferol in the lower layers of epidermis of the skin by a chemical reaction which relies on sun exposure. Foods such as the flesh of fatty fish also comprises major amounts of vitamin D. The mushrooms which are exposed to ultraviolet light contains a useful amount of vitamin D2. The lack of vitamin D can cause severe diseases including rickets, osteomalacia and osteoporosis. Vitamin D supplements are helpful in preventing or treating rickets and osteomalacia. This book unravels the recent studies in the research and clinical application of Vitamin D. It combines key researches focused on promoting role of vitamin D in health. The readers would gain knowledge that would broaden their perspective in this area.

I thank my publisher with all my heart for considering me worthy of this unparalleled opportunity and for showing unwavering faith in my skills. I would also like to thank the editorial team who worked closely with me at every step and contributed immensely towards the successful completion of this book. Last but not the least, I wish to thank my friends and colleagues for their support.

Editor

Total Vitamin D Assay Comparison of the Roche Diagnostics "Vitamin D Total" Electrochemiluminescence Protein Binding Assay with the Chromsystems HPLC Method in a Population with both D2 and D3 forms of Vitamin D

Laila Abdel-Wareth [1,*], Afrozul Haq [1], Andrew Turner [1], Shoukat Khan [2], Arwa Salem [1], Faten Mustafa [1], Nafiz Hussein [1], Fasila Pallinalakam [1], Louisa Grundy [1], Gemma Patras [1] and Jaishen Rajah [3]

[1] Pathology & Laboratory Medicine Institute, Sheikh Khalifa Medical City, Abu Dhabi 51900, UAE;
E-Mails: haq2000@gmail.com (A.H.); aturner@skmc.ae (A.T.); asalem@skmc.ae (A.S.);
fmostafa@skmc.ae (F.M.); nnimer@skmc.ae (N.H.); fpallinalakam@skmc.ae (F.P.);
lgrundy@skmc.ae (L.G.); gpatras@skmc.ae (G.P.)

[2] Pathology & Laboratory Medicine Department, Military Hospital, Riyadh 11159,
Kingdom of Saudi Arabia; E-Mail: sakhan@rmh.med.sa

[3] Pediatric Institute, Sheikh Khalifa Medical City, Abu Dhabi 51900, UAE; E-Mail: jrajah@skmc.ae

* Author to whom correspondence should be addressed; E-Mail: labdelwareth@skmc.ae;

Abstract: This study compared two methods of assaying the 25-hydroxylated metabolites of cholecalciferol (vitamin D3) and ergocalciferol (vitamin D2). A fully automated electrochemiluminescence assay from Roche Diagnostics and an HPLC based method from Chromsystems were used to measure vitamin D levels in surplus sera from 96 individuals, where the majority has the D2 form of the vitamin. Deming regression, concordance rate, correlation and Altman Bland agreement were performed. Seventy two subjects (75%) had a D2 concentration >10 nmol/L while the remaining twenty four subjects had vitamin D2 concentration of less than 10 nmol/L by HPLC. Overall, the Roche Diagnostics method showed a negative bias of -2.59 ± 4.11 nmol/L on the e602 as compared to the HPLC with a concordance rate of 84%. The concordance rate was 91% in samples with D2 of less than 10 nmol/L and 82% in those with D2 concentration >10 nmol/L. The overall correlation had an r value of 0.77. The r value was higher in samples with D2 levels of less than 10 nmol/L, $r = 0.96$, as compared to those with D2 values of greater than 10 nmol/L,

$r = 0.74$. The observed bias had little impact on clinical decision and therefore is clinically acceptable.

Keywords: 25-hydroxyvitamin D; method evaluation; electrochemiluminescence; high performance liquid chromatography

---

1. Introduction

The last decade has witnessed a dramatic increase in both clinical and public awareness of the health implications associated with vitamin D status [1]. Consequently, clinical laboratories are receiving an increasing number of requests to measure vitamin D levels, which has led to the need for highly automated assays. A recent publication evaluated the performance of six routine 25-Hydroxyvitamin D assays in relation to variation in vitamin D binding protein concentration [2]. The majority of the study population had the D3 form of the vitamin (cholecalciferol). In contrast, our study evaluates the performance of one of those assays, the Roche Diagnostics "Vitamin D total" electrochemiluminescence protein binding assay, in a population where the majority have the D2 form of the vitamin (ergocalciferol). The technical performance of the Roche assay was evaluated by comparison to the Chromsystems HPLC-UV assay and the clinical performance was assessed in terms of classification of subjects as sufficient or deficient for the vitamin.

2. Material and Methods

2.1. Samples

Left over sera obtained from specimens analyzed at the SKMC Pathology & Laboratory Medicine Institute ($n = 96$) were used in this study. The use of this material was approved by the institutional ethics review board and is in accordance with the general consent signed by all patients prior to treatment at SKMC. Serum aliquots were given unique sample numbers, to conceal the identity of the patient from the staff performing the study. These aliquots were stored at 2–8 °C and analyzed within two days.

2.2. Analytical Platforms

2.2.1. Chromsystems HPLC Assay

The Chromsystems reagent kit used on the Waters HPLC 2695 allows the main metabolites of vitamin D3 and D2 to be determined in a simultaneous chromatographic manner by using a fully validated, modified high-performance liquid chromatography (HPLC) method [3]. The Waters HPLC 2695 analyzer uses a simple isocratic HPLC system, with a HPLC pump, injector and a UV detector. In summary, protein is precipitated, and through selective solid phase extraction, interfering components are removed and the analytes are concentrated. A stable vitamin D derivative is used as an internal standard in order to allow for accurate quantification. The chromatographic separation takes approximately 12 min (Chromsystems Instruments & Chemicals GmbH, Heimburgstrasse, Munich, Germany) [3]. The assay has within run imprecision of 3.0% and total (between days) imprecision of 4.6%.

2.2.2. Roche Diagnostics Vitamin D Total Assay

The Roche Diagnostics Vitamin D total assay is a competitive electrochemiluminescence protein binding assay intended for the quantitative determination of total 25-OH vitamin D in human serum and plasma. The assay employs a vitamin D binding protein (VDBP) as capture protein, which binds to both 25-OH D3 and 25-OH D2 (Roche Diagnostics, Mannheim , Germany) [4].

The assay utilizes a 3-step incubation process, which has a duration of 27 minutes. In step 1, the sample is incubated with pretreatment reagent, which releases bound 25-OH vitamin D from the VDBP. In step 2, the pretreated sample is incubated with ruthenium labeled VDBP creating a complex between the 25-OH vitamin D and the ruthenylated VDBP. The third incubation step sees the addition of streptavidin-coated microparticles and 25-OH vitamin D labeled with biotin. The free sites of the ruthenium labeled VDBP become occupied, forming a complex consisting of the ruthenium labeled vitamin D binding protein and the biotinylated 25-OH vitamin D. The entire complex becomes bound to the solid phase via interaction of biotin and streptavidin.

Between day precision was CV = 4.9% and 1.9% at mean concentrations of 43.3 and 105 nmol/L respectively using quality control material provides by Roche Diagnostics.

Both assays were validated in our laboratory following "Clinical Laboratory Standards Institute" (CLSI) protocols for validation of precision, linearity and accuracy.

Reference ranges used in this study were based upon the recommendations of the American Society for Bone and Mineral Research, 28th Annual Meeting 2006 and the Canadian consensus conference on osteoporosis, 2006 [5,6] and were defined as follows: Deficiency: <25 nmol/L, Optimal/Sufficiency: 75–200 nmol/L, Insufficiency: 25–75 nmol/L and Toxicity: >250 nmol/L. This study also considered the latest recommendations published by the Institute of Medicine (IOM) for dietary reference intake for calcium and vitamin D. According to the latest IOM recommendations, 25(OH) D levels corresponding to a serum 25(OH) D status of at least 50 nmol/L indicates sufficiency [1].

2.2.3. Statistical Analysis

All data points were included in the study. Results were classified into three groups; the entire population, those with vitamin D2 concentration of less than 10 nmol/L and those with vitamin D2 concentration greater than 10 nmol/L. Method comparison was performed by using Deming regression. Method agreement was analyzed by the mean difference method of Bland and Altman. Pearson correlation was also calculated for the three groups. In addition, linear regression for the difference between the Roche method and the HPLC method in relation to concentration of vitamin D2 and D3 was performed to determine the influence of increasing concentrations of each of the forms respectively. Analysis was performed using "Analyse-it" (The Tannery, 91 Kirkstall Road, Leeds, LS3 1HS, UK) and Microsoft Excel softwares (Thames Valley Park Reading, Berkshire, RG6 1WG, UK).

The concordance rate was calculated by classifying the results obtained on each platform as sufficient, insufficient or deficient using the criteria already established in our laboratory as stated earlier as well as those recently suggested by the Institute of Medicine (IOM) [1].

Secondary analysis was performed to determine the predicted bias as the data demonstrated a non-constant scatter. The data was classified into three groups (low, middle and high) in order of increasing values based on the HPLC results. Predicted bias was then calculated using partitioned residuals as described in CLSI guideline EP09-A2-IR Section 6.3. Polynomial regression analysis was performed to determine the polynomial fit equation for each group.

3. Results

Samples

A total of 96 samples were analyzed. Seventy two samples had D2 concentrations greater than 10 nmol/L as detected by the HPLC, while in the remaining twenty four the concentration of D2 was less than 10 nmol/L. None of the samples analyzed were hemolyzed or lipemic. The mean, standard deviation, median and the range were; mean 65.22 and 62.12 nmol/L ± 30.38 and 29.54, median 60.90 and 57.8 nmol/L, range 16.3–180.9 and 7.5–175.0 nmol/L, for the Chomsystem HPLC and Roche Diagnostics Cobas e602 respectively.

The Roche Diagnostics method demonstrated a negative bias of −2.59 nmol/L (95% CI = −6.7–1.52) when compared to the HPLC method using the Bland-Altman analysis (Figure 1).

Figure 1. Deming regression of total 25(OH) D comparison: Chromsystems HPLC as the reference method *vs.* Roche Diagnostics Vitamin D total method on the Cobas e602.

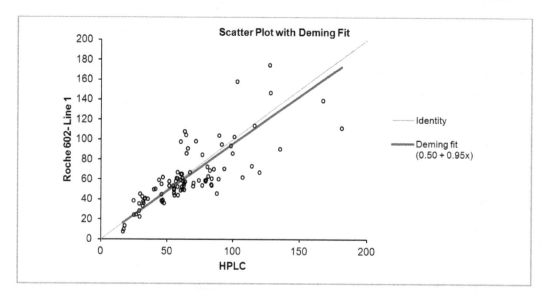

Deming regression result, correlation, slope and intercept for all samples, samples with D2 concentrations less than and greater than 10 nmol/L is summarized in Table 1. The difference between the two methods is dependent on the concentration of D2 and D3 with negative bias observed more with increasing D2 concentrations and positive bias with increasing D3 concentration (Figure 2). Linear regression analysis scatter plot of the difference in concentration between Roche Diagnostics total 25 (OH) and HPLC as a function of D2 and D3 concentrations is shown in Figure 3.

Table 1. Person correlation, bias as calculated by Bland—Altman comparison, slope and intercept according to Deming regression for all samples, samples with D2 concentration less and more than 10 nmol/L as determined by HPLC.

Sample Group	n	Concentration Range in nmol/L	r	Bias	Slope	Intercept
All samples	96	16.30–180.9	0.77	−2.59	0.95	0.5
D2 concentration <10 nmol/L	24	16.30–127.80	0.96	10.14	1.43	−11.81
D2 concentration >10 nmol/L	72	16.90–180.90	0.74	−6.63	0.79	8.07

Figure 2. Bland-Altman plot showing means of paired difference between the HPLC method and the Roche Diagnostics Cobas e602 in samples with D2 greater than and less than 10 nmol/L respectively.

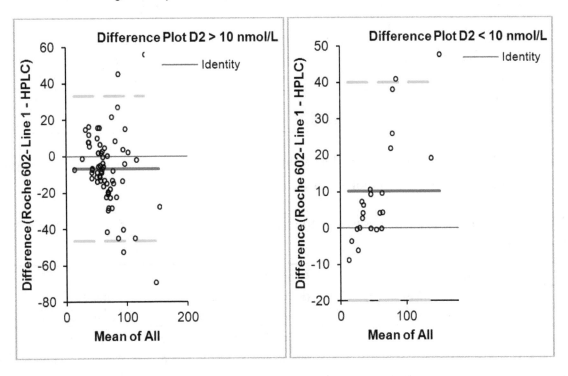

Figure 3. Linear regression analysis scatter plot of the difference in concentration between Roche Diagnostics total 25 (OH) and HPLC as a function of D2 and D3 concentrations.

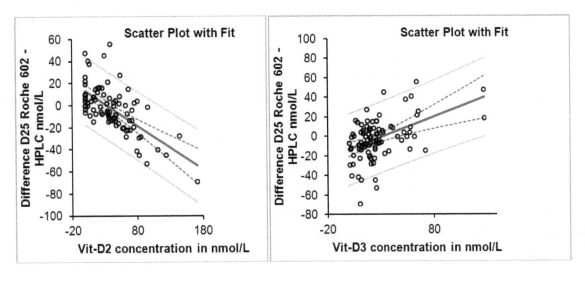

The concordance rate between the Cobas e602 and HPLC was 74% using the 75 nmol/L cutoff value as indication of vitamin D sufficiency. When applying the cutoff proposed by the IOM [1] the concordance rate increased to 84%. The concordance rate was 91% in samples with D2 of less than 10 nmol/L and 82% in those with D2 concentration >10 nmol/L. The majority of the disagreement was in the sufficient to insufficient range as the Roche method slightly underestimated at the higher concentrations (>50 nmol/L). There was no major discrepancy as to sufficiency *versus* deficiency noted. The detail of the sub classification is summarized in Table 2 for the two cutoffs respectively.

Table 2. Concordance of HPLC and Roche Diagnostics assays to 25 (OH) D based on 2 decision criteria.

	Concordance Based on the 75 nmol/L Cutoff				Concordance Based on the 50 nmol/L Cutoff		
Roche	70–25 Cutoff	HPLC		Roche	50–30 Cutoff	HPLC	
		Sufficient	Insufficient	Dificient			Sufficient	Insufficient	Dificient
	Sufficient	13	7	0		Sufficient	60	6	0
	Insufficient	17	53	1		Insufficient	7	15	2
	Dificient	0	0	5		Dificient	0	0	6

The calculated predicted biases as absolute values and percentages at four medical decision limits (25 and 75 nmol/L) and (30 and 50 nmol/L) are summarized in Table 3.

Table 3. Calculated predicted biases at four medical decision cutoffs for low, middle and high groups.

Medical Decision Cutoff	Group 1 (16.3–51.5 nmol/L) Predicted Bias (%)	Group 2 (54.2–69.6 nmol/L) Predicted Bias (%)	Group 3 (71.1–180.9 nmol/L) Predicted Bias (%)
25 nmol/L	2.6 (10.4%)	Not applicable for this group	Not applicable for this group
30 nmol/L	2.9 (9.6%)	Not applicable for this group	Not applicable for this group
50 nmol/L	Not applicable for this group	−4.0 (8%)	−1.57 (3%)
75 nmol/L	Not applicable for this group	11.27 (15%)	−7.7 (10.3%)

4. Discussion

Testing for vitamin D is required not only to screen for its deficiency, but also increasingly to adjust "therapeutic targets" and monitor efficacy of treatment. In addition to the skeletal effects, vitamin D may have a role in relation to diabetes, cancer and cardiovascular diseases [7–13]. Growing awareness of the clinical importance of vitamin D has resulted in clinical laboratories receiving a surge in requests for the assay. This has led to a need to migrate vitamin D testing from labor intensive methods, such as HPLC, to more highly automated testing platforms. Until recently the major challenge with vitamin D analysis has been the lack of standardization and the wide analytical variation between methods due to absence of reference standards [14]. The situation is further complicated by the discovery of C-3 epimers of vitamin D2 and D3 particularly in infants that might interfere with the accurate measurement and interpretation of vitamin D status in infants [15].

Recently, the National Institute of Standards and Technology (NIST) developed standard reference materials (SRMs) for 25(OH) D3/D2 in both human serum (SRM 972) and in solution (SRM 2972) [16]. This was supported by the recent introduction of reference measurement procedures using isotope—dilution liquid chromatography-tandem mass spectrometry [17].

The Roche Diagnostics Total Vitamin D kit has 80% cross reactivity to D2 and 100% cross reactivity to D3. This method was recently evaluated and its performance was deemed satisfactory in a population where D3 constituted the main form of total vitamin D [2]. In the United Arab Emirates, vitamin D deficiency is prevalent and the majority of the deficient population is receiving D2 supplementation [18]. In this study 75% of the participants had D2 levels >10 nmol/L. In this population, the Roche Diagnostics method had an overall negative bias, which was directly dependent on the increasing concentration of D2 as compared to the HPLC method. However, it was also observed that the method has positive bias, which was dependent on the concentration of D3 and therefore the overall negative bias was attenuated when both forms are present. More subjects were classified as "insufficient" by the Roche Diagnostics method. However, the clinical impact of the slight underestimation, one can argue, is of little clinical significance giving the wide range for the optimum level of vitamin D (50–150 nmol/L). The analytical quality goals for 25-vitamin D based on biological variation were a subject of a recent publication [19]. According to this publication, the desirable analytical bias goal is around 10% and 6% for the imprecision [20]. The calculated predicted bias using the was found to be within 10% when the IOM decision criteria of 30 and 50 nmol/L were applied and within 15% when the criteria of American Society for Bone and Mineral Research were applied. The method has an imprecision of less than 5%. We subscribe to the UK-based DEQAS vitamin D external quality assessment scheme. According to DEKAS 2012 review report, the Roche total vitamin D method had a mean % bias of less than 10% from all laboratory trimmed mean (ALTM) while the IDS RIA and IDS iSYS assays had a high positive bias which reached up to 21%. LC-MS method had positive bias according to this review of less than 10% while HPLC method had a positive bias slightly higher than 10% in one of the cycles [21]. Since both methods in this study used different standards, a clear cut 100% concordance on all samples might not be achievable. Adding to the lack of standardization are the inherent technical limitations of the protein binding assays relative to the direct chemical methods, the effect of vitamin D binding protein concentration of the results and the possible interferences from the C-3 epimers of D2 or D3 forms on the HPLC method [15].

5. Conclusions

In conclusion, Roche Diagnostics "Vitamin D total" assay performance in a population where the D2 component is negatively biased when compared to the HPLC Chromsystems method, and this is directly related the concentration of D2. The negative bias is less often observed when D3 is also present. The negative bias may impact classification of individuals receiving the test in terms of sufficiency or insufficiency for vitamin D and it should be taken in consideration when interpreting results of patients on D2 supplementation. The observed bias had little impact on clinical decision when the IOM criteria were applied and therefore is clinically acceptable.

Acknowledgement

We thank Bindu Madhavi and Aurora Mabini for their help in formatting this manuscript. We also thank Roche Diagnostics for donating the total Vitamin D kits used in this study.

Conflict of Interest

Competing interests: The authors have no competing interests to disclose.

Financial interests: The authors have none to declare.

Funding: This research was funded by Sheikh Khalifa Medical City. Roche diagnostics provided free kits for evaluation, and purchased from the College of American Pathologist vitamin D accuracy based survey material that was used in this study.

Ethical approval: This study was approved by the institution review board of Sheikh Khalifa Medical City (reference number: REC-04.08.2011 approval number RS:177).

Guarantor: LA-W.

Contribution: LA-W conceived the study, analyzed the data, submitted the research protocol to the institutional review board and wrote the manuscript. AH & SK, researched the literature and contributed to the introduction and discussion sections of the manuscript. AS, FM, NH & GP performed the actual analysis on both platforms. LG & FP wrote the methods section and provided technical supervision for the analytical part of study. AT assisted in the statistical analysis. JR was involved in the protocol development, review of the data, review of the results & conclusion and assisted in gaining ethical approval by providing guidelines.

References

1. Ross, C.; Manson, J.A.E.; Abrams, S.A.; Aloia, J.F.; Brannon, P.M.; Clinton, S.K.; Durazo-Arvizu, R.A.; Gallagher, J.C.; Gallo, R.L.; Jones, G.; *et al.* The 2011 report on dietary reference intakes for calcium and Vitamin D from the Institute of Medicine: What clinicians need to know. *J. Clin. Endocrinol. Metab.* **2011**, *96*, 53–58.

2. Heijboer, A.; Blankenstein, M.; Kema, I.P.; Buijs, M.M. Accuracy of 6 Routine 25-Hydroxyvitamin D assays: Influence of vitamin D binding protein concentration. *Clin. Chem.* **2012**, *58*, 543–548.

3. Haq, A.; Rajah, J.; Abdel-Wareth, L.O. Routine HPLC analysis of vitamin D3 and D2. *DIALOG (Ger.)* **2007**, *2*, 1–2.

4. Cobas E411 Vitamin D Total Reagent Insert (06268668001V1). Roche Diagnostics Web site. Available online: http://www.captodayonline.com/productguides/instruments/automated-immuno assay-analyzers-july-2012/roche-diagnostics-cobas-e411-immunoassay-analyzers-june-2011.html (accessed on 19 March 2013).

5. Brown, J.P.; Fortier, M.; Frame, H.; Lalonde, A.; Papaioannou, A.; Senikas, V.; Yuen, C.K. Canadian Consensus Conference on Osteoporosis, Update. *J. Gynecol. Canad.* **2006**, *172*, S95–S112.

6. Hollick, M.F. Vitamin D deficiency. *N. Engl. J. Med.* **2007**, *357*, 266–281.

7. Joergensen, C.; Hovind, P.; Schmedes, A.; Parving, H.H.; Rossing, P. Vitamin D Levels, microvascular cmplications and mortality in Type 1 Diabetes. *Diabetes Care* **2011**, *34*, 1081–1085.

8. Wang, T.J.; Pencina, M.J.; Booth, S.L.; Jacques, P.F.; Ingelsson, E.; Lanier, K.; Benjamin, E.J.; D'Agostino, R.B.; Wolf, M.; Vasan, R.S. Vitamin D deficiency and risk of cardiovascular disease. *Circulation* **2008**, *117*, 503–511.

9. Lappe, J.M.; Travers-Gustafson, D.; Davies, K.M.; Recker, R.R.; Heaney, R.P. Vitamin D and calcium supplementation reduces cancer risk: Results of a randomized trial. *Am. J. Clin. Nutr.* **2007**, *85*, 1586–1591.

10. Rosen, C.J. Vitamin D insufficiency. *N. Engl. J. Med.* **2011**, *364*, 248–254.

11. Hanley, D.A.; Cranney, A.; Jones, G.; Whiting, S.J.; Leslie, W.D.; Cole, D.E.C.; Atkinson, S.A.; Josse, R.G.; Feldman, S.; Kline, G.A.; *et al.* Vitamin D in adult health and disease: A review and guideline statement from osteoporosis Canada. *Can. Med. Assoc. J.* **2010**, *182*, E610–E618.

12. Norman, A.W.; Bouillon, R.; Whiting, S.J.; Veith, R.; Lips, P. 13th Workshop consensus for vitamin D nutritional guidelines. *J. Steroid Biochem. Mol. Biol.* **2007**, *103*, 204–205.

13. Manson, J.E.; Mayne, S.T.; Clinton, S.K. Vitamin D and prevention of cancer—Ready for prime time? *N. Engl. J. Med.* **2011**, *364*, 1385–1387.

14. Phinney, K.W. Development of a standard reference material for vitamin D in serum. *Am. J. Clin. Nutr.* **2008**, *88*, 511S–512S.

15. Singh, R.J.; Taylor, R.L.; Reddy, G.S.; Grebe, S.K.G. C-3 Epimers can account for a significant proportion of total circulating 25-Hydroxyvitamin D in infants, complicating accurate measurement and interpretation of Vitamin D status. *J. Clin. Endocrinol. Metab.* **2006**, *91*, 3055–3061.

16. May, W.; Parris, R.; Beck, C.; Fassett, J.; Greenberg, R.; Guenther, F.; Kramer, G.; Wise, S.; Gills, T.; Colbert, J.; *et al. Definitions of Terms and Modes Used at NIST for Value-Assignment of Reference Materials for Chemical Measurements*; National Institute of Standards and Technology: Gaithersburg, MD, USA, 2000; Available online: http://www.cstl.nist.gov/nist839/ NIST_special_publications.htm (accessed on 19 March 2013).

17. Gaithersburg. *Certificate of Analysis, Standard Reference Material 2972: 25-Hydroxivitamin D2 and D3 Calibration Solutions. Standard Reference Materials Program*; National Institute of Standards and Technology: Gaithersburg, MD, USA, 2009; Available online: http://www.nist. gov/srm/upload/March-2010-Spotlight-3.pdf (accessed on 19 March 2013).

18. Al Anouti, F.; Thomas, J.; Abdel-Wareth, L.; Rajah, J.; Grant, W.; Haq, A. Vitamin D deficiency and sun avoidance among university students at Abu Dhabi, United Arab Emirates. *Dermato-Endocrinology* **2011**, *3*, 235–239.

19. Stepman, H.C.M.; Vanderroost, A.; Uytfanghe, K.V.; Thienpont, L.M. Candidate reference measurement procedures for serum 25-Hydroxyvitamin D3 and 25-Hydroxyvitamin D2 by using isotope-dilution liquid chromatography-tandem mass spectrometry. *Clin. Chem.* **2011**, *57*, 441–448.

20. Viljoen, A.; Singh, D.; Farrington, K.; Twomey, P. Analytical quality goals for 25-vitamin D based on biological variation. *J. Clin. Lab. Anal.* **2011**, *25*, 130–133.

21. Knudsen, C.S.; Nexo, E.; Højskov, C.S.; Heickendorff, L. Analytical validation of the Roche 25-OH Vitamin D Total assay. *Clin. Chem. Lab. Med.* **2012**, *50*, 1965–1968.

Pharmacokinetics of High-Dose Weekly Oral Vitamin D3 Supplementation during the Third Trimester of Pregnancy in Dhaka, Bangladesh

Daniel E. Roth [1,†,*], **Abdullah Al Mahmud** [2], **Rubhana Raqib** [2], **Evana Akhtar** [2], **Robert E. Black** [1] **and Abdullah H. Baqui** [1,2]

[1] Department of International Health, The Johns Hopkins Bloomberg School of Public Health, 615 North Wolfe Street, Baltimore, MD 21205, USA; E-Mails: rblack@jhsph.edu (R.E.B.); abaqui@jhsph.edu (A.H.B.)

[2] International Center for Diarrhoeal Disease Research, Bangladesh (ICDDR,B), GPO Box 128, Dhaka 1000, Bangladesh; E-Mails: mahmud@icddrb.org (A.A.M.); rubhana@icddrb.org (R.R.); evana@icddrb.org (E.A.)

[†] Present Address: Division of Paediatric Medicine, The Hospital for Sick Children and University of Toronto, 555 University Avenue, Toronto, Ontario, M5G 1X8, Canada.

[*] Author to whom correspondence should be addressed; E-Mail: daniel.roth@sickkids.ca;

Abstract: A pharmacokinetic study was conducted to assess the biochemical dose-response and tolerability of high-dose prenatal vitamin D3 supplementation in Dhaka, Bangladesh (23°N). Pregnant women at 27–30 weeks gestation ($n = 28$) were randomized to 70,000 IU once + 35,000 IU/week vitamin D3 (group PH: pregnant, higher dose) or 14,000 IU/week vitamin D3 (PL: pregnant, lower dose) until delivery. A group of non-pregnant women ($n = 16$) was similarly administered 70,000 IU once + 35,000 IU/week for 10 weeks (NH: non-pregnant, higher-dose). Rise (Δ) in serum 25-hydroxyvitamin D concentration ([25(OH)D]) above baseline was the primary pharmacokinetic outcome. Baseline mean [25(OH)D] were similar in PH and PL (35 nmol/L *vs.* 31 nmol/L, $p = 0.34$). A dose-response effect was observed: Δ[25(OH)D] at modeled steady-state was 19 nmol/L (95% CI, 1 to 37) higher in PH *vs.* PL ($p = 0.044$). Δ[25(OH)D] at modeled steady-state was lower in PH *versus* NH but the difference was not significant (−15 nmol/L, 95% CI −34 to 5; $p = 0.13$). In PH, 100% attained [25(OH)D] $\geq$ 50 nmol/L and 90% attained

[25(OH)D] $\geq$ 80 nmol/L; in PL, 89% attained [25(OH)D] $\geq$ 50 nmol/L but 56% attained [25(OH)D] $\geq$ 80 nmol/L. Cord [25(OH)D] ($n = 23$) was slightly higher in PH *versus* PL (117 nmol/L *vs.* 98 nmol/L; $p = 0.07$). Vitamin D3 was well tolerated; there were no supplement-related serious adverse clinical events or hypercalcemia. In summary, a regimen of an initial dose of 70,000 IU and 35,000 IU/week vitamin D3 in the third trimester of pregnancy was non-hypercalcemic and attained [25(OH)D] $\geq$ 80 nmol/L in virtually all mothers and newborns. Further research is required to establish the safety of high-dose vitamin D3 in pregnancy and to determine if supplement-induced [25(OH)D] elevations lead to maternal-infant health benefits.

Keywords: vitamin D; Bangladesh; pregnancy; pharmacokinetics; hypercalcemia

---

1. Introduction

The maternal-infant health benefits of vitamin D supplementation during pregnancy remain uncertain [1,2]. However, observational studies have suggested associations between vitamin D status during pregnancy and postnatal infant health outcomes [3–5]. Serum 25-hydroxyvitamin D concentration ([25(OH)D]) $\geq$ 50 nmol/L is associated with skeletal health benefits [1], but some data suggest that improving vitamin D status to attain serum [25(OH)D] $\geq$ 80 nmol/L may enhance a range of vitamin D-related functions [6–8]. However, there have been relatively few published studies of vitamin D3 pharmacokinetics, safety and clinical effects during pregnancy [9].

The possible association between maternal-fetal vitamin D status and infant health outcomes may be particularly relevant to South Asian countries such as Bangladesh, where adverse perinatal outcomes and infant mortality are public health priorities [10], and where vitamin D deficiency has been observed among women of reproductive age [11] and young infants [12]. Therefore, to guide the design of clinical trials of antenatal vitamin D supplementation in Bangladesh, we conducted a randomized open-label pilot trial of two antenatal vitamin D3 supplementation doses that were several fold higher than those in typical prenatal supplements. The primary aims were to establish the biochemical dose-response in terms of the change in serum [25(OH)D], and to specifically assess whether the regimens achieved [25(OH)D] $\geq$ 80 nmol/L in most participants. The response to the higher-dose supplement regimen was also assessed in a cohort of non-pregnant participants that served as a separate comparison group. The present study builds on previously reported observations of single-dose vitamin D3 pharmacokinetics in the same setting [13].

2. Experimental Section

2.1. Participants

Pregnant women were enrolled at a maternal health clinic in inner-city Dhaka, Bangladesh (23°N) in February 2010 if they were: Aged 18 to <35 years; at 27 to <31 completed weeks of gestation based on the reported first day of the last menstrual period; held permanent residence in Dhaka at a fixed address; and, planned to stay in Dhaka for at least four months. Reasons for exclusion were:

preexisting medical condition; current vitamin D supplement use; anti-convulsant or anti-mycobacterial medications; severe anemia (hemoglobin concentration <70 g/L); hypertension at enrollment (systolic blood pressure ≥140 mmHg or diastolic blood pressure ≥90 mmHg on at least two measurements); major risk factors for preterm delivery or pregnancy complications; or previous delivery of an infant with a congenital anomaly or perinatal death. Healthy non-pregnant women attending the same clinic for health maintenance (e.g., contraception), or because they were accompanying pregnant women, were enrolled in August–September 2009 if they were non-lactating, had not missed a recent menses at the expected date, and had a negative urine pregnancy test (First Response Early Results, Church & Dwight Company, Inc., Princeton, NJ, USA). Otherwise, inclusion and exclusion criteria were similar to the pregnant participants.

The study was approved by the Institutional Review Board at The Johns Hopkins Bloomberg School of Public Health and the International Center for Diarrheal Disease Research, Bangladesh (ICDDR, B). All participants gave signed informed consent prior to participation. The trial was registered at ClinicalTrials.gov (NCT00938600).

2.2. Study Design and Interventions

Pregnant participants were randomized at enrollment to receive a single dose of vitamin D3 70,000 IU (1.75 mg, where 1 mg = 40,000 IU) on day 0 followed by vitamin D3 35,000 IU (0.875 mg) per week starting on day 7 and continuing until delivery (referred to as group "PH"; pregnant, higher dose), or to vitamin D3 14,000 IU (0.350 mg) per week starting on day 0 and continuing until delivery ("PL"; pregnant, lower dose). Participants in the non-pregnant cohort ("NH"; non-pregnant, higher dose) received the same higher-dose intervention as PH, *i.e.*, a single dose of vitamin D3 70,000 IU on day 0 followed by vitamin D3 35,000 IU per week starting on day 7 and continuing until the last dose on day 63 (total of 10 doses). Vitamin D3 was administered as Vigantol Oil (Merck KGaA, Germany), a liquid supplement (20,000 IU D3/mL) commercially available in Bangladesh (see Ref 13 for details regarding quality assurance). Participants were advised not to take other vitamin D-containing supplements during the study period. Pregnant participants were provided with standard prenatal supplemental iron (60 mg/day) and folic acid (400 mcg/day). NH was studied before enrolment of PH, to establish safety of the high-dose regimen in non-pregnant women prior to its use in pregnant women. As an additional safety measure, the response to a single initial dose vitamin D3 (70,000 IU) was observed in a separate cohort, prior to the initiation of enrollment of cohorts of participants who received weekly doses [13]. A preceding report of single-dose vitamin D3 pharmacokinetics included data from participants in weekly-dose groups PH and NH, but only from days 0 to 7 (*i.e.*, preceding the administration of a second vitamin D dose) [13]. Women who received only the single 70,000 IU dose are not included in any of the present analyses.

2.3. Data Collection Procedures

Pregnant women were assessed weekly until delivery. Non-pregnant participants had weekly follow-ups for 10 weeks (the last visit was on day 70, one week after the final D3 dose). Weekly assessments included a checklist of symptoms and blood pressure measurement. In NH and PH, participants provided up to six scheduled blood specimens and at least seven urine samples during a

10-week follow-up period beginning on the day of supplement administration (day 0), according to one of two randomly assigned sampling schedules, A or B (Figure 1). Specimens on days 65 and 67 were intended to measure inter-dose fluctuations in [25(OH)D] and serum calcium. Urine was collected at visits without scheduled blood collection up to day 70 (Figure 1). Participants in PL were asked to provide three blood specimens and four urine specimens (schedule C in Figure 1). From day 70, pregnant participants provided urine specimens on a weekly basis until delivery.

Figure 1. Blood and urine specimen collection schedules. Participants in groups PH and NH were randomly assigned to either scheduled "A" or "B". Participants in group PL all followed schedule "C".

	Day														
	0	2	4	7	14	21	28	35	42	49	56	63	65	67	70
A	O■		O	O	■	■	■	O	■	■	■	O		O	■
B	O■		O	■	■	O	■	■	■	O	■	■	O		O
C	O■					■	O		■			O■			

O   Blood collection

■   Urine collection

2.4. Specimen Collection and Biochemical Analyses

Maternal and cord serum samples were collected by standard techniques and maintained at 4 °C prior to same-day transfer to the laboratory. Spot urine specimens were collected in sterile plastic containers and maintained at 4 °C until same or next-day analysis of the calcium:creatinine ratio (ca:cr). Serum aliquots for the 25(OH)D assay were frozen at −20 °C for up to five months prior to shipment from Bangladesh to Toronto. Total serum [25(OH)D] was measured with the Diasorin Liaison Total assay in the laboratory of Reinhold Vieth in Toronto [14], which meets the International Vitamin D External Quality Assessment Scheme (DEQAS) performance targets [15]. Mean within-run coefficient of variation (CV%) was 7.8% (5.8% for specimens with values <150 nmol/L) and mean between-run CV% was 10.5% (9.0% for specimens <150 nmol/L). Serum calcium, serum albumin, and urine calcium:creatinine ratio (ca:cr) were routinely measured using the AU640 Olympus Autoanalyzer (Olympus Corporation, Japan) in the Clinical Biochemistry Laboratory at the International Center for Diarrheal Disease Research, Bangladesh (ICDDR, B) in Dhaka within 24–48 h of collection of serum or urine aliquots. Total serum calcium concentration ([Ca]) was adjusted for the serum albumin concentration by the following conventional formula: [Ca] + (0.02 × (40-albumin)). Intact parathyroid hormone (PTH) was measured using a chemiluminescent assay on the i1000SR Architect Autoanalyzer (Abbott Diagnostics, Lake Forest, IL, USA), with a reference range of 1.59–7.23 pmol/L (Clinical Biochemistry Lab, icddr,b).

2.5. Safety Monitoring

The adjusted [Ca] reference range was 2.10–2.60 mmol/L. Umbilical cord venous serum [Ca] was considered elevated if greater than 3.0 mmol/L [16]. Urine ca:cr were expressed as mmol Ca/mmol Cr, considering 1.0 as the upper limit of the reference range [17]. An albumin-adjusted serum calcium concentration >2.60 mmol/L prompted a repeat measurement on a new specimen as soon as possible. Confirmed hypercalcemia was *a priori* defined as albumin-adjusted serum calcium concentration >2.60 mmol/L on both specimens (since hypercalcemia caused by vitamin D intoxication would not be expected to resolve within a few days without intervention). Episodes of urinary calcium:creatinine ratio (ca:cr) >1.0 mmol/mmol prompted a repeat urine ca:cr measurement within one week. A ca:cr > 0.85 mmol/mmol that was also 2-fold or greater relative to the lowest previously observed value in the same participant prompted repeat urine assessment. Persistent hypercalciuria was defined as ca:cr > 1.0 mmol/mmol on two consecutive results, or on two non-consecutive measurements but in the presence of persistent symptoms suggestive of possible hypercalcemia. Persistent hypercalciuria or persistent ca:cr > 0.85 mmol/mmol that was also 2-fold or greater relative to the lowest previously observed value were indications for unscheduled measurement of serum calcium. Abnormal urinalyses, hypertension, reported severe symptoms, or persistence of any mild symptomatic complaints prompted referral to the study physician for further evaluation. Participants were referred to an antenatal care physician at the maternity clinic for treatment of urinary tract infections, hypertension, or other medical problems. Participants with obstetric complications were transported to a local tertiary-care hospital with advanced neonatal care facilities. All costs of medical and obstetric care were borne by the study.

2.6. Statistical Analysis

Pharmacokinetic outcomes were expressed as the attained maternal/cord [25(OH)D] and the rise in maternal [25(OH)D] above baseline (Δ[25(OH)D]). Distributions in each group and at specific time points were summarized as geometric mean [25(OH)D] and 95% confidence intervals (CI). Between-group differences were analyzed by linear regression of log-transformed [25(OH)D]. To facilitate comparisons to other studies, the Δ[25(OH)D] at days 63 and beyond was also expressed as a function of the equivalent daily dose administered to each group, in micrograms (*i.e.*, 125 mcg/day in groups NH and PH, and 50 mcg/day in group PL). To investigate inter-dose fluctuations, the mean [25(OH)D] at days 65, 67, and 70 were compared to day 63 in groups NH and PH. The proportion of participants and cord blood specimens with [25(OH)D] ≥ 50 nmol/L or ≥80 nmol/L were compared across groups using log-binomial regression. Mean changes in [25(OH)D] over time in each group were also modeled as continuous non-linear parametric functions (see Appendix). These analyses used all available individual participant-level data; standard errors were corrected to account for the within-subject correlation of repeated outcomes. Serum [Ca] and urine log-transformed ca:cr were each modeled as functions of time using fixed indicator variables for baseline, weeks 2 to 5 (days 4 to 34), and week 6 and later (day 35 and thereafter). Comparisons of PH to NH or PL were analyzed using group-by-time interaction terms. Serum [Ca] and urine ca:cr were also expressed in terms of the proportions of episodes above the references ranges. In all analyses, $p < 0.05$ was considered statistically significant; however, the Holm procedure was used for multiple pair-wise comparisons [18]. Where appropriate, generalized estimating equations (GEE) with robust error estimation were used to account for non-independence of repeated measures. Analyses were conducted using Stata versions 10.1 and 11.1 (Stata Corporation, College Station, TX, USA).

3. Results

3.1. Participant Characteristics and Retention.

Twenty-eight pregnant women were recruited and randomly assigned to one of two groups, PH ($n = 14$) and PL ($n = 14$). Sixteen non-pregnant women were enrolled (Figure 2).

Figure 2. Study flow diagram. Participant screening, enrollment, exclusions, and withdrawal over the course of the study.

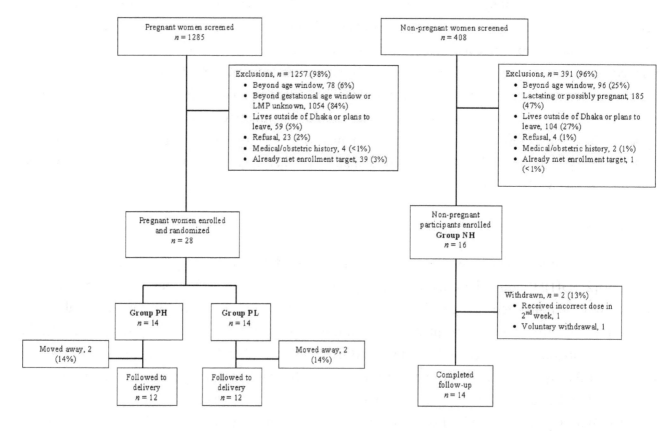

Of 28 randomized pregnant participants, 4 (14%) left the Dhaka area prior to completion of the study protocol (2 in PH and 2 in PL). Specimens in the 10th week were available in 10/14 women in PH and 9/14 in PL. Cord specimens were available in 23 (82%) of enrolled participants. PH and PL were generally similar with respect to baseline characteristics (Table 1) and [25(OH)D] (Table 2). However, NH enrollment occurred in the summer rather than mid-winter and NH participants had higher average baseline [25(OH)D] compared to the pregnant participants (Table 1).

Table 1. Participant characteristics at enrollment.

	NH	PH	PL	*p*
# Enrolled	16	14	14	
Age (years), Mean (±SD)	24.6 (±4.5)	22.2 (±3.1)	22.1 (±4.8)	0.190
Gestational age at enrollment (weeks)				
Mean (±SD)	-	28.4 (±1.2)	28.5 (±1.3)	0.760
Range	-	26.1–30.6	27–30.7	
Married	12 (75%)	14 (100%)	13 (93%)	0.110
Education level attained				
None	2 (13%)	4 (29%)	3 (21%)	0.285
Primary	10 (63%)	9 (64%)	11 (79%)	
Secondary or higher	4 (25%)	1 (7%)	0	
Height (cm), mean (±SD)	152.1 (±4.7)	150.7 (±4.7)	148.9 (±4.5)	0.179

Table 2. Serum 25-hydroxyvitamin D concentrations at baseline and through 10 weeks of supplementation in non-pregnant and pregnant participants [1].

	Non-pregnant NH	Pregnant PH	Pregnant PL		
# Enrolled	16	14	14		
Vitamin D3 regimen					
Loading dose	70,000 IU	70,000 IU	0		
Weekly doses	35,000 IU	35,000 IU	14,000 IU		
Duration of supplementation	10 weeks	27–30 weeks gestation until delivery	27–30 weeks gestation until delivery		
Dates of enrollment	17 Aug–6 Sep 2009	3–16 Feb 2010	3–16 Feb 2010		
Participants with [25(OH)D] measured during 10th week (days 63 to 70), *n* (%)	14 (88%)	10 (71%)	9 (64%)	*p* value [2]	
Number of specimens per participant, Median	6	6	3	PH *vs.* NH	PH *vs.* PL
Baseline [25(OH)D]					
Mean [95% CI]	57 [47,69]	35 [30,42]	31 [26,38]	<0.001	0.341
Range (min, max)	27, 93	21, 55	20, 57		
Attained [25(OH)D] in 10th week					
Mean [95% CI]	139 [121,160]	98 [89,109]	76 [61,95]	<0.001	0.038
Range (min, max)	85, 238	71, 153	36, 119		
Δ[25(OH)D] in 10th week					
Mean [95% CI]	76 [61,96]	57 [44,73]	36 [22,61]	0.082	0.128
Range on days 63 to 70	28, 160	19, 130	7, 75		
Δ[25(OH)D] at days 63 to 70 per daily vitamin D3 dose (nmol/L/mcg)					
Mean [95% CI]	0.61 [0.48, 0.79]	0.46 [0.34,0.61]	0.73 [0.38,1.38]	0.220	0.081
Area under the Δ[25(OH)D]-time curve (nmol·d/L) to day 63/65 (AUC$_{63}$) [3]	3500 [2886,4245]	2925 [2331,3670]	1678 [923,3053]	0.383	0.020

Table 2. *Cont.*

Participants with mean [25(OH)D] ≥ 50 nmol/L in 10th week, #/n (%) [4]	14/14 (100%)	10/10 (100%)	8/9 (89%)	1.000	0.166
Participants with mean [25(OH)D] ≥ 80 nmol/L in 10th week, #/n (%) [4]	14/14 (100%)	9/10 (90%)	5/9 (56%)	0.152	0.127
PTH					
Baseline (n = 28), mean [95% CI]	-	2.10 [1.26,3.52]	1.53 [0.94,2.49]		
Final (n = 22), mean [95% CI]	-	1.63 [1.01,2.66]	2.49 [1.61,3.85]	-	0.011 [5]
Cord serum [25(OH)D] (n = 23)					
Mean [95% CI]	-	117 [99,137]	98 [84,115]	-	0.074
Range (min, max)	-	74, 168	53, 124		
Cord [25(OH)D] ≥ 50 nmol/L, #/n (%)	-	12/12 (100%)	11/11 (100%)	-	1.000
Cord [25(OH)D] ≥ 80 nmol/L, #/n (%)	-	11/12 (92%)	10/11 (91%)	-	0.949

[1] Summary measures are geometric means with 95% confidence intervals, unless otherwise indicated. [2] Linear regression models (GEE was implemented where there were repeated measures for the same individuals) unless otherwise indicated; all p values < 0.05 remained significant after correction for multiple pairwise comparisons using the Holm method. [3] AUC for each group was the geometric mean (and 95% confidence intervals) of individual participants' AUCs; the analyses included 33 participants who were followed-up to at least week 10 (day 63 or 65, depending on serum sampling schedule): NH, $n = 14$ participants; PH, $n =10$; PL, $n = 9$. Comparison of the AUC based on only 3 datapoints (baseline, day 21/28/35, and day 63/65) was undertaken as a sensitivity analysis because group PL participants only had [25(OH)D] measured at a maximum of three visits at which blood collection was scheduled; the latter analysis involved the same 33 participants as in the preceding analysis. [4] Proportion of participants in each group with average [25(OH)D] ≥ 50 nmol/L or ≥80 nmol/L in specimens collected on days 63 to 70; comparisons between groups were assessed by binomial regression. None of the pairwise comparisons were statistically significant after correction for multiplicity using the Holm method. [5] p value for the group-by-time interaction term in a GEE model (exchangeable correlation and robust standard errors), using log-transformed PTH as the outcome, indicating that the change from baseline over time significantly differed between the two groups.

3.2. Effect of Prenatal Vitamin D3 Supplementation on Vitamin D Status

Mean [25(OH)D] rose gradually above baseline in all groups during follow-up (Table 2; Figure 3). Final mean [25(OH)D] during the 10th week of supplementation was significantly higher in PH *versus* PL (98 *vs.* 76 nmol/L, respectively; $p = 0.038$) and significantly lower *versus* NH (98 *vs.* 139 nmol/L; $p < 0.001$) (Table 2). However, Δ[25(OH)D] in PH was not significantly lower in the 10th week compared to NH (Table 2). The [25(OH)D] threshold of 50 nmol/L was attained by nearly all participants, but only the higher-dose regimen reliably led to [25(OH)D] ≥ 80 nmol/L by the 10th week in pregnant women. During the 10th week, there were no notable inter-dose fluctuations in NH and PH (Figure 4); mean [25(OH)D] at days 65, 67, and 70 differed from day 63 by <6 nmol/L (all p values > 0.5). There was substantial inter-subject variability in the response to vitamin D supplementation, with one PL participant demonstrating only a 7 nmol/L final increase in [25(OH)D] above her baseline. Among participants who received the higher-dose regimen, there was as much as a 7-fold difference between the lowest and highest responders based on Δ[25(OH)D] at week 10 (Table 2). Three participants in NH had [25(OH)D] > 200 nmol/L, but the highest [25(OH)D] in any pregnant participant was 153 nmol/L. There was no significant association between baseline vitamin D status and Δ[25(OH)D] (data not shown).

Figure 3. Changes in serum 25-hydroxyvitamin D concentration from baseline resulting from weekly vitamin D3 administration to non-pregnant women who received an initial dose of 70,000 IU and then 35,000 IU/week thereafter (NH), pregnant women who received an initial dose of 70,000 IU and then 35,000 IU/week thereafter (PH), and pregnant women who received 14,000 IU/week (PL). Lines connect the group means at each follow-up visit.

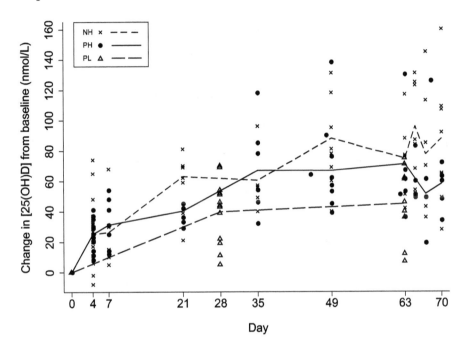

Figure 4. Lack of inter-dose fluctuations in mean serum 25-hydroxyvitamin D concentrations among non-pregnant (NH) and pregnant women (PH) during the 10th week of supplementation with 35,000 IU vitamin D3 per week, with the most recent dose administered on day 63. Lines connect the group means at each day; 95% confidence intervals are represented by vertical capped bars.

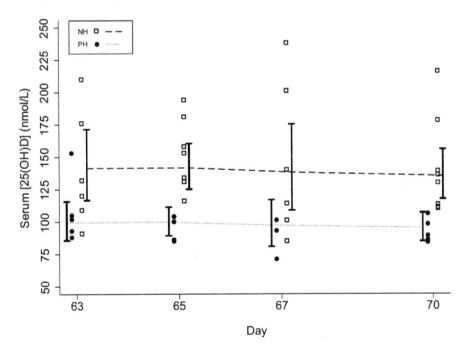

Non-linear parametric models representing the change in [25(OH)D] as a continuous function of time yielded inferences regarding baseline and modeled steady-state mean [25(OH)D] that were consistent with the empiric cross-sectional estimates (Table 3) and provided appropriate fits to the data (Figure 5). Extended models indicated that the Δ[25(OH)D] at modeled steady-state was 19 nmol/L greater in PH compared to PL ($p = 0.044$) (Table 3). Mean modeled steady-state Δ[25(OH)D] was lower in PH compared to NH but the difference was not statistically significant (Table 3).

Table 3. Estimates of the change in serum 25-hydroxyvitamin D concentration over time in response to weekly vitamin D3 supplementation in non-pregnant women who received an initial dose of 70,000 IU and then 35,000 IU/week (NH), pregnant women who received an initial dose of 70,000 IU and then 35,000 IU/week (PH), and pregnant women who received a weekly dose of 14,000 IU/week (PL). Results are based on negative exponential models, and shown as mean (lower 95% confidence bound, upper 95% confidence bound).

		Model 1	Model 2	Model 3	Model 4	Model 5
		Non-pregnant (NH)	Pregnant, higher-dose (PH)	Pregnant, lower-dose (PL)	Pregnant (PL & PH)	Higher dose (NH & PH)
Number of participants		16	14	14	28	29
Number of specimens		89	75	36	111	162
Baseline [25(OH)D]	nmol/L	58 [48,69]	36 [29,42]	31 [25,38]	31 [25,37]	57 [47,67]
Δ[25(OH)D] at steady-state (a)	nmol/L	79 [60,97]	62 [48,75]	45 [23,67]	43 [29,57]	77 [62,93]
Δ[25(OH)D] at steady-state per daily dose equivalent	nmol/L/mcg D3 per day	0.63 [0.48, 0.78]	0.49 [0.38, 0.60]	0.90 [0.47,1.34]	-	-
Steady-state [25(OH)D] ($[25(OH)D]_{t0} + a$)	nmol/L	137 [116,157]	97 [87,108]	76 [54,98]	74 [61,87]	134 [117,151]
Decay rate (k)	days^{-1}	0.08 [0.03,0.12]	0.11 [0.07,0.15]	0.07 [−0.01,0.16]	0.11 [0.07, 0.15]	0.09 [0.06, 0.12]
Group (g)	0 (Ref)	-	-	-	PW-C	NP-H
	1	-	-	-	PW-H	PW-H
Difference in [25(OH)D] between groups at baseline (β)	nmol/L	-	-	-	4 [−4,13]	−21 [−33,−9]
Difference in Δ[25(OH)D] between groups at steady-state (d)	nmol/L	-	-	-	19 [1,37] $p = 0.044$	−15 [−34,5] $p = 0.131$
Adjusted R^2		0.55	0.71	0.63	0.72	0.69

Figure 5. Negative exponential models predicting serum 25-hydroxyvitamin D concentrations in response to weekly vitamin D3 supplementation in non-pregnant women who received an initial dose of 70,000 IU and then 35,000 IU/week (NH), pregnant women who received an initial dose of 70,000 IU and then 35,000 IU/week (PH), and pregnant women who received a weekly dose of 14,000 IU/week (PL). Vertical bars represent the 95% confidence intervals of the empiric geometric means at each scheduled follow-up time.

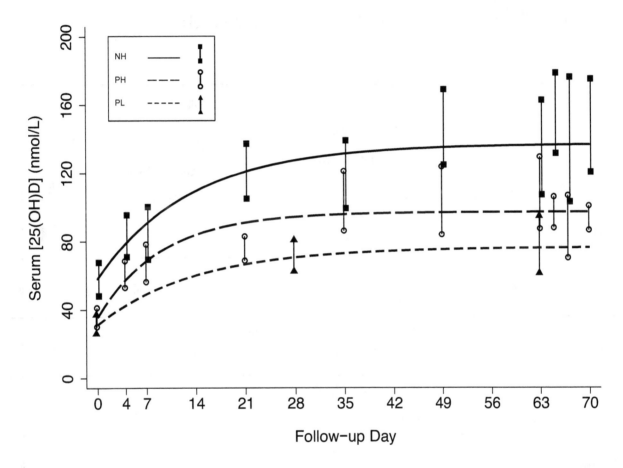

Mean cord serum [25(OH)D] was higher in PH (117 nmol/L) *versus* PL (98 nmol/L) but the difference was not significant (Table 2). The proportions of newborns with [25(OH)D] ≥ 80 nmol/L (PH: 92%; PL: 91%) and ≥50 nmol/L (PH: 100%; PL: 100%) were similar in the two groups. There was a moderate association between cord and maternal [25(OH)D] ($\rho = 0.67$, $p < 0.001$).

3.3. Ancillary Biochemical Parameters

Mean albumin-adjusted serum [Ca] increased significantly within the reference range during follow-up in PH but it did not change significantly in the comparison groups (Table 4; Figure 6). The increase in PH was significantly greater than in PL or NH (Table 4). There was a single episode of albumin-adjusted [Ca] > 2.60 mmol/L in a PH participant during an episode of acute gastroenteritis that occurred after two weeks of supplementation. Her albumin-adjusted [Ca] of 2.61 mmol/L declined to 2.39 mmol/L in a repeat specimen on the same day, the illness was self-limited, and there was no other biochemical or clinical evidence of vitamin D toxicity; furthermore, the participant continued to receive the supplement and had increasing [25(OH)D] (range, 52 to 98 nmol/L during follow-up) but did not develop any further episodes of hypercalcemia or elevations in urine ca:cr. There were no episodes of confirmed hypercalcemia according to *a priori* study definitions.

Table 4. Albumin-adjusted serum calcium concentration at baseline, the 1st to 5th week of follow-up, and the 6th to 10th week of follow-up in non-pregnant women who received an initial dose of 70,000 IU vitamin D3 and 35,000 IU/week (NH), pregnant women who received an initial dose of 70,000 IU vitamin D3 and 35,000 IU/week (PH), and pregnant women who received 14,000 IU/week (PL).

	n [1]			Albumin-adjusted serum calcium concentration (mmol/L) Mean ± SD Minimum, Maximum			*p* value, PH *vs.* NH [2]	*p* value, PH *vs.* PL [2]	# Episodes >2.60 mmol/L		
Follow-up period	NH	PH	PL	NH	PH	PL			NH	PH	PL
Baseline	16	14	14	2.39 ± 0.08 2.22, 2.5	2.39 ±0.04 2.3, 2.45	2.42 ±0.05 2.35, 2.52	-	-	0	0	0
1st to 5th week	31	27	14	2.40 ± 0.07 2.25, 2.6	2.45 ±0.07 [3] 2.32, 2.61	2.42 ±0.07 2.33, 2.55	0.020	0.012	0	1 [4]	0
6th to 10th week	43	33	12	2.38 ± 0.07 2.2, 2.52	2.44 ±0.07 [5] 2.27, 2.57	2.42 ±0.05 2.33, 2.52	0.009	0.055	0	0	0
Total	88	74	40	2.39 ± 0.07 2.2, 2.6	2.43 ±0.07 2.27, 2.61	2.42 ±0.06 2.33, 2.55	0.991	0.104	0	1	0
Cord Serum	-	12	11	-	2.69 ± 0.12 2.37, 2.82	2.73 ± 0.13 2.56, 2.94	-	0.414	0	0	0

[1] Number of specimens (there may have been multiple specimens from a single participant during a given follow-up period). [2] Group-by-time interactions using GEE with robust standard errors. [3] Significant increase from baseline *p* < 0.001; remained significant after adjustment for multiple testing. [4] Isolated value of 2.61 mmol/L derived from uncorrected total serum calcium concentration of 2.67 mmol/L and serum albumin of 42.9 g/L. Repeat albumin-adjusted serum calcium later on the same day was 2.39 mmol/L (unadjusted [Ca] = 2.37 mmol/L). [5] Significant increase from baseline, *p* = 0.008; remained significant after adjustment for multiple testing. Not significantly different from 1st to 5th weeks, *p* = 0.654.

Figure 6. Mean albumin-adjusted serum calcium concentrations in the three participant groups. (**A**) Mean albumin-adjusted serum calcium concentration in pregnant participants who received an initial dose of 70,000 IU and then 35,000 IU/week (PH) and pregnant participants who received a weekly dose of 14,000 IU/week (PL); (**B**) Mean albumin-adjusted serum calcium concentration in non-pregnant participants who received an initial dose of 70,000 IU and then 35,000 IU/week (NH). Vertical bars represent the 95% confidence intervals of the means at each scheduled follow-up time. Horizontal line indicates the upper limit of the reference range (2.60 mmol/L).

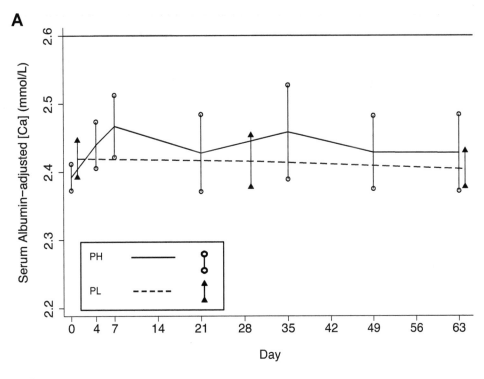

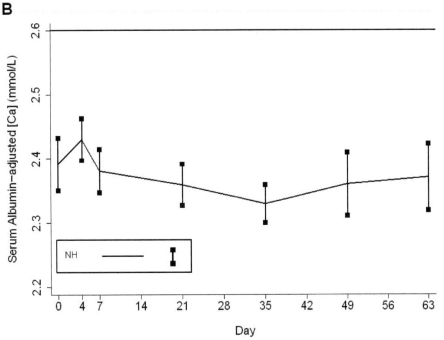

Urine ca:cr rose initially during follow-up in all groups but appeared to plateau in PL and decline in PH and NH during the latter half of the follow-up period (Table 5; Figure 7). There were five episodes of ca:cr > 1.0 mmol/mmol (Table 5). One participant in group PL had two consecutive episodes on days 42 and 44 and thus met the definition for persistent hypercalciuria by study criteria; however, [Ca] was normal and despite continued supplementation, the ca:cr was within the normal limits thereafter. The higher-dose intervention (PH) suppressed the average PTH concentration, which was significantly different from the increase observed in PL ($p = 0.011$) (Table 2).

Table 5. Urine calcium:creatinine ratio in random spot urine specimens collected at baseline, 1st to 5th weeks of follow-up, and 6th week to the end of the supplementation period in non-pregnant women who received an initial dose of 70,000 IU vitamin D3 and 35,000 IU/week (NH), pregnant women who received an initial dose of 70,000 IU vitamin D3 and 35,000 IU/week (PH), and pregnant women who received 14,000 IU/week (PL).

	n[1]			Urinary calcium-creatinine ratio (mmol/mmol) Mean[2] Minimum, Maximum			p value PH vs. NH[3]	p value PH vs. PL[3]	# Episodes >1.0 mmol/mmol (# Participants ever having >1.0 mmol/mmol)		
Follow-up period	NH	PH	PL	NH	PH	PL			NH	PH	PL
Baseline	16	14	14	0.23 0.04, 0.58	0.10 0.01, 0.44	0.21 0.06, 0.91	-	-	0 (0)	0 (0)	0 (0)
1st to 5th weeks	49	36	12	0.36[4] 0.04, 1.47	0.24[5] 0.02, 0.95	0.24 0.07, 0.64	0.164	0.105	3 (2)	0 (0)	0 (0)
6th week to end	62	53	33	0.26 0.03, 0.91	0.18[6] 0.01, 0.96	0.30 0.05, 1.05	0.164	0.500	0 (0)	0 (0)	2 (1)
Total	127	103	59	0.29 0.03, 1.47	0.19 0.01, 0.96	0.26 0.05, 1.05	0.014	0.047	3 (2)	0 (0)	2 (1)

[1] Number of specimens (there may have been multiple specimens from a single participant during a given follow-up period). [2] Geometric means. [3] Group by time interactions using GEE with robust standard errors. [4] The p value for the test of the difference from baseline was 0.018; however, this was not statistically significant after adjustment for multiple testing (adjusted critical p value of 0.017). [5] The increase from baseline was statistically significant ($p < 0.001$) and remained so after adjustment for multiple testing (adjusted critical p value of 0.025). [6] Not significantly different from baseline after adjustment for multiple testing ($p = 0.042$, adjusted critical p of 0.025); and, not significantly different from the period of 1st to 5th weeks ($p = 0.136$).

Figure 7. Mean urine calcium:creatinine ratio in the three participant groups.(**A**) Mean urine calcium:creatinine ratio in pregnant participants who received an initial dose of 70,000 IU and then 35,000 IU/week (PH) and pregnant participants who received a weekly dose of 14,000 IU/week (PL), and (**B**) Mean urine calcium:creatinine ratio in non-pregnant participants who received an initial dose of 70,000 IU and then 35,000 IU/week (NH). Vertical bars represent the 95% confidence intervals of the means at each scheduled follow-up time.

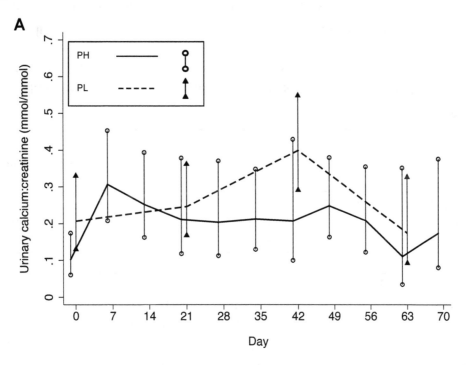

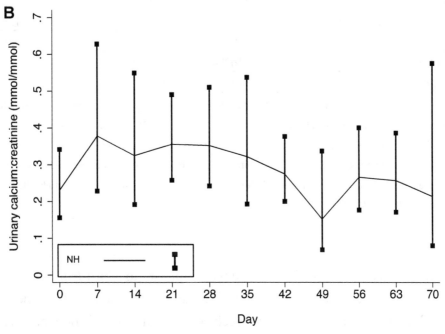

3.4. Clinical Outcomes

There were no known supplement-related clinical adverse events. One pregnant participant in the lower-dose group (PL) developed new-onset mild hypertension unassociated with any significant morbidity or biochemical abnormalities (highest serum [25(OH)D] was 86 nmol/L); her pregnancy ended in an uncomplicated term delivery. The frequency of possible hypercalcemia symptoms was similar during follow-up in PH when compared to PL (odds ratio, 0.82; 95% CI, 0.35 to 1.92; $p = 0.65$). Groups PH and PL were similar with respect to pregnancy and newborn outcomes (Table 6). Anthropometric measures at birth did not significantly differ between the two groups (data not shown).

Table 6. Pregnancy and newborn outcomes among women who received an initial dose of 70,000 IU vitamin D3 and 35,000 IU/week (PH) or 14,000 IU/week (PL) during the third trimester.

	PH	PL	*p* value (for between-group difference)
n	12	12	
Gestational age at birth, weeks (by LMP) [1]			
Mean (±SD)	39.2 (±2.3)	38.5 (±2.7)	0.512
Range	33.6–42.3	32.7–43.2	
Preterm, # (%)	1 (8%)	3 (25%)	0.590
Birth weight (g)			
Mean (±SD) [2]	2774 (±456)	2604 (±379)	0.332
Range	2210–4000	2020–3120	
# (%) SGA [3]	9 (75%)	8 (67%)	1.000
# (%) LBW	2 (17%)	4 (33%)	0.640
Delivery mode, # (%) Cesarean section [4]	6 (50%)	6 (50%)	1.000
Sex, # (%) female	6 (50%)	6 (50%)	1.000
Live births [5] **, # (%)**	12 (100%)	12 (100%)	-
Alive at 1 month of age, # (%)	12 (100%)	12 (100%)	-

[1] In a sample of 113 deliveries at the study site (October 2009 to January 2010) for which there was a recalled first day of last menstrual period, the mean gestational age at birth was 39.7 weeks (±2.2). [2] In a consecutive sample of 362 liveborn infants delivered at the study site (October 2009 to January 2010), the mean birth weight was 2780 g (±440). [3] Based on US newborn birthweight reference [19]. [4] In a consecutive sample of 369 deliveries at the study site (October 2009 to January 2010), there were 199 cesarean deliveries (54%). [5] In a sample of 369 deliveries at the study site (Oct 2009 to Jan 2010), there were 7 stillbirths (2%).

4. Discussion

This study demonstrated the biochemical dose response to third-trimester high-dose weekly antenatal vitamin D3 supplementation. Among Bangladeshi women with a mean [25(OH)D] of 33 nmol/L, 70,000 IU followed by 35,000 IU/week of vitamin D3 until delivery yielded an average [25(OH)D] that was about 20 nmol/L higher than an antenatal dose of 14,000 IU/week (the IOM vitamin D upper limit at the time the study was conducted). Similar to our conclusions from analyses of single-dose vitamin D3 pharmacokinetics in the same study setting (and involving an overlapping group of participants) [13], we found that the minor differences between pregnant *vs.* non-pregnant participants receiving the same dose were within the margins of error given the small sample size. However, based on the present analysis, we could not exclude the possibility of a slightly diminished 25(OH)D response to a weekly dose of vitamin D during the third trimester of pregnancy.

To our knowledge, the 35,000 IU/week regimen used in this study is the highest vitamin D3 maintenance dose studied in pregnancy under controlled conditions. Devlin *et al.* (1986) reported that a daily dose of 1000 IU vitamin D3 administered to 15 French women during the third trimester modestly raised mean maternal serum [25(OH)D] from 55 nmol/L to 65 nmol/L [20]. The largest published study of vitamin D3 supplementation in pregnancy was conducted by Bruce Hollis and colleagues in South Carolina, in which 502 pregnant women at 12 to 16 weeks gestation were randomized to 400 IU/day, 2000 IU/day, or 4000 IU/day vitamin D3 [21]. This population was more vitamin D-replete at baseline (mean [25(OH)D] = 60 nmol/L) compared to the present study. Based on data from the 350 participants (70%) followed until delivery, the 2000 IU/day and 4000 IU/day regimens raised [25(OH)D] to means of 105 nmol/L (rise of 47 nmol/L) and 119 nmol/L (rise of 60 nmol/L), respectively, at one month before delivery [21]. The Δ[25(OH)D] in the 2000 IU/day group in the Hollis study was similar to the response we observed in the 14,000 IU/day group (equivalent regimen) in the present study, substantiating the consistency of vitamin D3 dose-response modeling across diverse populations of pregnant women. In a separate trial in South Carolina, Wagner *et al.* reported comparatively less robust responses to 2000 IU/day and 4000 IU/day during pregnancy, which may have been attributable to non-adherence to the supplementation regimen [22].

The lower dose produced a more efficient 25(OH)D response per mcg of vitamin D3 when compared to the high-dose regimen: 0.73 *vs.* 0.46 nmol/L/mcg/day in the empiric estimates, and 0.90 *versus* 0.49 nmol/L/mcg/day based on the pharmacokinetic model. These estimates, as well as those from the non-pregnant cohort that received the higher-dose regimen (0.61 nmol/L/mcg/day based on 10th-week data, and 0.63 nmol/L/mcg/day based on the parametric model), were similar to the values conventionally cited for non-pregnant adults: ~0.70 nmol/L/mcg/day [23,24]. However, analyses by Barger-Lux *et al.* (1998) [25] and Aloia *et al.* (2008) [24], as well the recent IOM report (2010) [1], have demonstrated that the Δ[25(OH)D] per mcg is a curvilinear inverse function of vitamin D intake at doses <50 mcg/day, but nearly proportional to intake at >50 mcg/day [24], which may explain the greater observed efficiency of the lower dose.

A unique aspect of this study was the measurement of biochemical parameters *between* weekly doses at the end of the supplementation period. These data showed an absence of inter-dose perturbations in calcium homeostasis that might have otherwise been missed by sampling serum only at the time of the "trough" [25(OH)D] (*i.e.*, immediately preceding administration of a weekly dose). Although the study may have been too small to detect minor inter-dose fluctuations in [25(OH)D], the data supported the appropriateness of administering weekly doses of 35,000 IU instead of daily administration of 5000 IU.

In pregnant participants, the higher-dose vitamin D regimen had a significant suppressive effect on maternal PTH secretion, relative to the lower dose, as indicated by the change in average PTH concentrations from baseline to delivery, similar to previous observations by Wagner *et al.* in South Carolina [22]. However, since the role of PTH as a vitamin D status biomarker during pregnancy is unclear [26], the clinical significance of the apparent dose-response effect of vitamin D on PTH requires further study.

Both the higher and lower vitamin D3 regimens administered to pregnant women attained fetal [25(OH)D] ≥ 50 nmol/L. Therefore, in this small sample, we did not observe a clear benefit of the higher-dose over the lower-dose regimen with respect to neonatal vitamin D status. In a related study at the same study site, we observed a mean cord [25(OH)D] of 50 nmol/L (range of 29 to 80 nmol/L) in a group of neonates born to women who had received a single vitamin D3 dose of 70,000 IU at 30 weeks gestation [13], and previous studies in South Asia have found cord serum [25(OH)D] ranging from 17 to 59 nmol/L [27–30].

Appreciable increases in serum calcium in the higher-dose relative to the lower-dose group highlighted a dose-dependent effect of vitamin D3 supplementation on calcium homeostasis. We previously reported that mean serum calcium concentrations rose slightly but significantly during the first week after administration of a single 70,000 IU dose of vitamin D3 in both pregnant and non-pregnant participant groups [13]. However, in the present analyses of weekly-dose vitamin D3, a significant increase in serum [Ca] from baseline was only observed in pregnant women who received the higher dose. Pregnancy is associated with an elevation in the maternal serum concentration of the active vitamin D metabolite, 1,25-dihydroxyvitamin D (1,25(OH)2D) [31,32], which appears to be primarily attributable to classic renal 1α-hydroxylation of 25(OH)D [33]. However, placental trophoblasts and decidual cells [34] are capable of extra-renal 1α-hydroxylation which could theoretically predispose the pregnant woman to exaggerated physiological responses to increases in [25(OH)D] [9]. Similar to the participants who received only a single dose of 70,000 IU [13], maternal serum calcium values in the weekly-dose participants were all below the threshold for defining hypercalcemia used by the IOM in setting the 1997 dietary reference intakes (DRIs) for vitamin D (2.75 mmol/L) [35] and in the revised DRIs in 2010 (2.63 mmol/L) [1]. Cord blood calcium concentrations were also within reference limits, and [25(OH)D] were well below the range that has been associated with toxicity in adults [36] and older children [37]. Pregnancy and newborn clinical outcomes were within the expected range for the study population, but we were unable to draw conclusions from this study regarding clinical effects of vitamin D. Nonetheless, this study together with the recent findings of Hollis and Wagner and colleagues in South Carolina [21,22] demonstrate that vitamin D3 doses during pregnancy up to 25% above the current IOM UL of 4000 IU/day do not induce hypercalcemia, and have not led to any observed short-term clinical adverse effects.

There were several important limitations of this study. First, precision of estimates of pharmacokinetic parameters and between-group comparisons, as well as the generalizability of inferences regarding maternal-fetal safety of high-dose vitamin D supplementation, were limited by the small number of participants, stringent inclusion/exclusion criteria, and enrolment of pregnant and non-pregnant participants at one clinic site. Moreover, the lower-dose pregnancy group had less frequent blood sampling (a cost-savings measure given the relative lack of safety concerns for this group) and only 9 of 14 enrolled women contributed endpoint samples during the 10th week of supplementation. The supplementation period may not have been long enough to ensure that all participants reached a steady-state [25(OH)D]. Conclusions based on comparisons between pregnant and non-pregnant women were tempered by the differences in baseline characteristics, including season of enrolment and the relatively higher socioeconomic status of the non-pregnant participants. In addition, there were too few participants to consider modifiers of Δ[25(OH)D]. Most importantly, the present results do not yet provide sufficient evidence that the regimens studied are beneficial or safe for use in clinical or public health practice; rather, they serve to inform application of these dose regimens in future research studies.

5. Conclusions

This detailed analysis of the response to high-dose weekly vitamin D3 administered during the third-trimester of pregnancy demonstrated a dose-responsiveness to oral vitamin D3 in Bangladeshi women that echoed observations in other settings, and was generally in accordance with established pharmacokinetic characteristics of vitamin D3. Nonetheless, increases in the mean calcium concentration (within the normal range) and suppression of PTH secretion among pregnant women receiving the higher-dose regimen (70,000 IU initial dose followed by weekly doses of 35,000 IU) highlighted the physiological impact of the intervention and the need to cautiously address potential pregnancy-specific sensitivities to vitamin D supplementation.

Prior to undertaking large trials to test the effects of prenatal micronutrient interventions on pregnancy and birth outcomes, preliminary dose-finding and safety studies are essential, particularly when the intervention is a fat-soluble vitamin at a dose above the conventional upper limit of tolerability (*i.e.*, 4000 IU/day for vitamin D, as established by the Institute of Medicine [1]). The most direct application of the present observations is to guide the design of future trials of vitamin D3 (at doses up to 35,000 IU per week) aimed at confirming safety and establishing the health benefits of antenatal vitamin D supplementation in South Asia, where many potentially vitamin D-responsive outcomes (e.g., infant growth and infectious disease morbidity) are major public health priorities. Following from our preliminary pharmacokinetic studies, we have conducted a placebo-controlled trial of 35,000 IU/ week during the third trimester (*n* = 160), with follow-up of infants to monitor growth to one year of age (NCT01126528). Future trials in Dhaka will address the dose-dependency of the effects of prenatal vitamin D supplementation on infant growth and morbidity.

Acknowledgments

We appreciate the efforts of the following individuals: staff at icddr,b and Shimantik, including Taufiq Rahman, Sultana Mahabbat-e Khoda, Eliza Roy, Ashish Chowdhury, and Kazi Moksedur Rahman; Reinhold Vieth (Mount Sinai Hospital, Toronto) for performing the measurement of 25-hydroxyvitamin D concentrations and verifying the concentration of the vitamin D3 supplement; Brendon Pezzack for assistance with manuscript preparation. We also thank Diasorin Inc. (Stillwater, MN) for donating the kits used in the Liaison Total assay, and Popular Pharmaceuticals Inc. (Dhaka, Bangladesh) for supplying the Vigantol Oil. Daniel Roth was supported by The Alberta Heritage Foundation for Medical Research (Canada) and The Canadian Institutes of Health Research. The study was sponsored by the Center for Global Health, Johns Hopkins University and the Department of International Health at The Johns Hopkins Bloomberg School of Public Health.

Conflict of Interest

The authors declare no conflict of interest.

Appendix

Non-Linear Modeling of Change in 25[(OH)D] over Time

Mean changes in [25(OH)D] over time in each group were modeled as continuous non-linear parametric functions. Consistent with the first-order process that characterizes 25(OH)D metabolism in the physiological range of vitamin D inputs, Heaney's group has shown empirically that a negative exponential growth function is well suited to model the gradual rise in [25(OH)D] over time (*t*) to a steady-state plateau in response to daily (Heaney *et al.*, 2003 [23]) or weekly (Heaney *et al.*, 2011 [38]) oral vitamin D3 supplementation:

$$[25(OH)D]_t = [25(OH)D]_{t=0} + \alpha(1 - e^{-kt}) \tag{1}$$

A particular advantage of this model is that despite its non-linearity, the coefficients are easily interpreted: *a* is the Δ[25(OH)D] above baseline at steady-state and *k* is the slope that defines the rate of the rise (the higher is *k*, the more rapidly the steady-state is reached). The steady-steady is the [25(OH)D] at which the rate of 25(OH)D formation theoretically equals the rate of 25(OH)D utilization/catabolism. Furthermore, the model could be readily extended to permit comparisons between groups of participants (g), with the aim of estimating the average difference (d) between the groups' [25(OH)D] at steady-state (see below for derivation of the extended model):

$$[25(OH)D]_t = [25(OH)D]_{t=0} + \beta g + (gd + \alpha_0)(1 - e^{-kt}) \tag{2}$$

Regression coefficients were estimated by a non-linear least-squares approach, assuming a log-normal error distribution of [25(OH)D] and standard error estimation that accounted for the intra-subject correlation of repeated measures.

To derive an extended negative exponential growth function that enabled comparison of the steady-state concentrations between the two groups, we first considered a generic model for the negative exponential growth function, where [25(OH)D] at time *t* is a function of the baseline concentration [25(OH)D] at t=0, the slope of the exponential rise, *k*, and the asymptotic maximal rise above baseline, *a*, at steady-state (*t* = infinity):

$$[25(OH)D]_t = [25(OH)D]_{t=0} + \alpha(1 - e^{-kt})$$

We can consider Equation (1) with respect to two different groups, *g*, such that if:

$$[25(OH)D]_t = [25(OH)D]_{t=0} + \alpha_0(1 - e^{-kt}) \text{ if } g = 0$$

Then,

$$[25(OH)D]_t = [25(OH)D]_{t=0} + \alpha_0(1 - g)(1 - e^{-kt}) \tag{3}$$

Similarly for group *g* = 1, if:

$$[25(OH)D]_t = [25(OH)D]_{t=0} + \alpha_1(1 - e^{-kt}) \text{ if } g = 1$$

Then,

$$[25(OH)D]_t = [25(OH)D]_{t=0} + \alpha_1 g(1 - e^{-kt}) \tag{4}$$

Combining Equation (3) and Equation (4) into one model, and allowing the intercept to vary by group:

$$[25(OH)D]_t = [25(OH)D]_{t=0} + \beta g + \alpha_1 g(1 - e^{-kt}) + \alpha_0(1 - g)(1 - e^{-kt}) \qquad (5)$$

Solving further:

$$[25(OH)D]_t = [25(OH)D]_{t=0} + \beta g + [\alpha_1 g + \alpha_0(1 - g)](1 - e^{-kt})$$

$$[25(OH)D]_t = [25(OH)D]_{t=0} + \beta g + [\alpha_1 g + \alpha_0 - \alpha_0 g](1 - e^{-kt})$$

$$[25(OH)D]_t = [25(OH)D]_{t=0} + \beta g + [g(\alpha_1 - \alpha_0) + \alpha_0](1 - e^{-kt}) \qquad (6)$$

Since we are specifically interested in measuring the difference between a_1 and a_0, we can invoke a new coefficient d, whereby:

$$d = \alpha_1 - \alpha_0 \qquad (7)$$

Then, substituting Equation (7) into Equation (6) yields:

$$[25(OH)D]_t = [25(OH)D]_{t=0} + \beta g + (gd + \alpha_0)(1 - e^{-kt})$$

References

1. Ross, A.C.; Taylor, C.L.; Yaktine, A.L.; Del Valle, H.B. Committee to Review Dietary Reference Intakes for Vitamin D and Calcium, Institute of Medicine. Dietary Reference Intakes for Calcium and Vitamin D; The National Academies Press: Washington, DC, USA, 2010.
2. De-Regil, L.M.; Palacios, C.; Ansary, A.; Kulier, R.; Pena-Rosas, J.P. Vitamin D supplementation for women during pregnancy. *Cochrane Database Syst. Rev.* **2012**, *2*, doi: 10.1002/14651858. CD008873.pub2.
3. Finkelstein, J.L.; Mehta, S.; Duggan, C.; Manji, K.P.; Mugusi, F.M.; Aboud, S.; Spiegelman, D.; Msamanga, G.I.; Fawzi, W.W. Maternal vitamin D status and child morbidity, anemia, and growth in human immunodeficiency virus-exposed children in Tanzania. *Pediatr. Infect. Dis. J.* **2012**, *31*, 171–175.
4. Belderbos, M.E.; Houben, M.L.; Wilbrink, B.; Lentjes, E.; Bloemen, E.M.; Kimpen, J.L.; Rovers, M.; Bont, L. Cord blood vitamin D deficiency is associated with respiratory syncytial virus bronchiolitis. *Pediatrics* **2011**, *127*, e1513–e1520.
5. Morales, E.; Guxens, M.; Llop, S.; Rodriguez-Bernal, C.L.; Tardon, A.; Riano, I.; Ibarluzea, J.; Lertxundi, N.; Espada, M.; Rodriguez, A.; *et al.* Circulating 25-hydroxyvitamin D3 in pregnancy and infant neuropsychological development. *Pediatrics* **2012**, *130*, e913–e920.
6. Bischoff-Ferrari, H.; Shao, A.; Dawson-Hughes, B.; Hathcock, J.; Giovannucci, E.; Willett, W. Benefit–risk assessment of vitamin D supplementation. *Osteoporosis Int.* **2010**, *21*, 1121–1132.
7. Vieth, R. What is the optimal vitamin D status for health? *Prog. Biophys. Mol. Biol.* **2006**, *92*, 26–32.
8. Hollis, B.W. Circulating 25-hydroxyvitamin D levels indicative of vitamin D sufficiency: Implications for establishing a new effective dietary intake recommendation for vitamin D. *J. Nutr.* **2005**, *135*, 317–322.

9.   Roth, D.E. Vitamin D supplementation during pregnancy: Safety considerations in the design and interpretation of clinical trials. *J. Perinatol.* **2011**, *31*, 449–459.

10. Black, R.E.; Allen, L.H.; Bhutta, Z.A.; Caulfield, L.E.; de Onis, M.; Ezzati, M.; Mathers, C.; Rivera, J. Maternal and child undernutrition: Global and regional exposures and health consequences. *Lancet* **2008**, *371*, 243–260.

11. Islam, M.Z.; Lamberg-Allardt, C.; Karkkainen, M.; Outila, T.; Salamatullah, Q.; Shamim, A.A. Vitamin D deficiency: A concern in premenopausal Bangladeshi women of two socio-economic groups in rural and urban region. *Eur. J. Clin. Nutr.* **2002**, *56*, 51–56.

12. Roth, D.E.; Shah, M.R.; Black, R.E.; Baqui, A.H. Vitamin D status of infants in northeastern rural Bangladesh: Preliminary observations and a review of potential determinants. *J. Health Popul. Nutr.* **2010**, *28*, 458–469.

13. Roth, D.E.; Mahmud, A.; Raqib, R.; Black, R.E.; Baqui, A.H. Pharmacokinetics of a single oral dose of vitamin D3 (70,000 IU) in pregnant and non-pregnant women. *Nutr. J.* **2012**, *11*, doi:10.1186/1475-2891-11-114.

14. Wagner, D.; Hanwell, H.E.; Vieth, R. An evaluation of automated methods for measurement of serum 25-hydroxyvitamin D. *Clin. Biochem.* **2009**, *42*, 1549–1556.

15. Carter, G.D.; Berry, J.L.; Gunter, E.; Jones, G.; Jones, J.C.; Makin, H.L.; Sufi, S.; Wheeler, M.J. Proficiency testing of 25-hydroxyvitamin D (25-OHD) assays. *J. Steroid. Biochem. Mol. Biol.* **2010**, *121*, 176–179.

16. Perkins, S.L.; Livesey, J.F.; Belcher, J. Reference intervals for 21 clinical chemistry analytes in arterial and venous umbilical cord blood. *Clin. Chem.* **1993**, *39*, 1041–1044.

17. Vieth, R.; Chan, P.C.; MacFarlane, G.D. Efficacy and safety of vitamin D3 intake exceeding the lowest observed adverse effect level. *Am. J. Clin. Nutr.* **2001**, *73*, 288–294.

18. Gordon, A.Y.; Salzman, P. Optimality of the holm procedure among general step-down multiple testing procedures. *Stat. Probab. Lett.* **2008**, *78*, 1878–1884.

19. Oken, E.; Kleinman, K.P.; Rich-Edwards, J.; Gillman, M.W. A nearly continuous measure of birth weight for gestational age using a United States national reference. *BMC Pediatr.* **2003**, *3*, doi:10.1186/1471-2431-3-6.

20. Delvin, E.E.; Salle, B.L.; Glorieux, F.H.; Adeleine, P.; David, L.S. Vitamin D supplementation during pregnancy: Effect on neonatal calcium homeostasis. *J. Pediatr.* **1986**, *109*, 328–334.

21. Hollis, B.W.; Johnson, D.; Hulsey, T.C.; Ebeling, M.; Wagner, C.L. Vitamin D supplementation during pregnancy: Double blind, randomized clinical trial of safety and effectiveness. *J. Bone Miner Res.* **2011**, *26*, 2341–2357.

22. Wagner, C.L.; McNeil, R.; Hamilton, S.A.; Winkler, J.; Rodriguez Cook, C.; Warner, G.; Bivens, B.; Davis, D.J.; Smith, P.G.; Murphy, M.; *et al.* A randomized trial of vitamin D supplementation in 2 community health center networks in south carolina. *Am. J. Obstet. Gynecol.* **2013**, *208*, 137.e1–137.e13.

23. Heaney, R.P.; Davies, K.M.; Chen, T.C.; Holick, M.F.; Barger-Lux, M.J. Human serum 25-hydroxycholecalciferol response to extended oral dosing with cholecalciferol. *Am. J. Clin. Nutr.* **2003**, *77*, 204–210.

24. Aloia, J.F.; Patel, M.; Dimaano, R.; Li-Ng, M.; Talwar, S.A.; Mikhail, M.; Pollack, S.; Yeh, J.K. Vitamin D intake to attain a desired serum 25-hydroxyvitamin D concentration. *Am. J. Clin. Nutr.* **2008**, *87*, 1952–1958.

25. Barger-Lux, M.J.; Heaney, R.P.; Dowell, S.; Chen, T.C.; Holick, M.F. Vitamin D and its major metabolites: Serum levels after graded oral dosing in healthy men. *Osteoporos. Int.* **1998**, *8*, 222–230.

26. Wagner, C.L.; Hollis, B.W. Beyond PTH: Assessing vitamin D status during early pregnancy. *Clin. Endocrinol.* **2011**, *75*, 285–286.

27. Goswami, R.; Gupta, N.; Goswami, D.; Marwaha, R.K.; Tandon, N.; Kochupillai, N. Prevalence and significance of low 25-hydroxyvitamin D concentrations in healthy subjects in delhi. *Am. J. Clin. Nutr.* **2000**, *72*, 472–475.

28. Sachan, A.; Gupta, R.; Das, V.; Agarwal, A.; Awasthi, P.K.; Bhatia, V. High prevalence of vitamin D deficiency among pregnant women and their newborns in northern India. *Am. J. Clin. Nutr.* **2005**, *81*, 1060–1064.

29. Bhalala, U.; Desai, M.; Parekh, P.; Mokal, R.; Chheda, B. Subclinical hypovitaminosis D among exclusively breastfed young infants. *Indian Pediatr.* **2007**, *44*, 897–901.

30. Doi, M.; Sultana Rekha, R.; Ahmed, S.; Okada, M.; Kumar Roy, A.; El Arifeen, S.; Ekstrom, E.C.; Raqib, R.; Wagatsuma, Y. Association between calcium in cord blood and newborn size in Bangladesh. *Br. J. Nutr.* **2011**, *106*, 1398–1407.

31. Kovacs, C.S. Vitamin D in pregnancy and lactation: Maternal, fetal, and neonatal outcomes from human and animal studies. *Am. J. Clin. Nutr.* **2008**, *88*, 520S–528S.

32. Papapetrou, P.D. The interrelationship of serum 1,25-dihydroxyvitamin D, 25-hydroxyvitamin D and 24,25-dihydroxyvitamin D in pregnancy at term: A meta-analysis. *Hormones (Athens)* **2010**, *9*, 136–144.

33. Kovacs, C.S.; Kronenberg, H.M. Maternal-fetal calcium and bone metabolism during pregnancy, puerperium, and lactation. *Endocr. Rev.* **1997**, *18*, 832–872.

34. Zehnder, D.; Evans, K.N.; Kilby, M.D.; Bulmer, J.N.; Innes, B.A.; Stewart, P.M.; Hewison, M. The ontogeny of 25-hydroxyvitamin D(3) 1alpha-hydroxylase expression in human placenta and decidua. *Am. J. Pathol.* **2002**, *161*, 105–114.

35. Standing Committee on the Scientific Evaluation of Dietary Reference Intakes; Food and Nutrition Board; Institute of Medicine. *DRI: Dietary Reference Intakes for Calcium, Phosphorus, Magnesium, Vitamin D, and Fluoride*; National Academy Press: Washington, DC, USA, 1997.

36. Hathcock, J.N.; Shao, A.; Vieth, R.; Heaney, R. Risk assessment for vitamin D. *Am. J. Clin. Nutr.* **2007**, *85*, 6–18.

37. Joshi, R. Hypercalcemia due to hypervitaminosis D: Report of seven patients. *J. Trop. Pediatr.* **2009**, *55*, 396–398.

38. Heaney, R.P.; Recker, R.R.; Grote, J.; Horst, R.L.; Armas, L.A. Vitamin D(3) is more potent than vitamin D(2) in humans. *J. Clin. Endocrinol. Metab.* **2011**, *96*, E447–E452.

3

Vitamin D—Effects on Skeletal and Extraskeletal Health and the Need for Supplementation

Matthias Wacker and Michael F. Holick *

Vitamin D, Skin and Bone Research Laboratory, Section of Endocrinology, Nutrition, and Diabetes, Department of Medicine, Boston University Medical Center, 85 East Newton Street, M-1013, Boston, MA 02118, USA; E-Mail: mwacker@bu.edu

* Author to whom correspondence should be addressed; E-Mail: mfholick@bu.edu;

Abstract: Vitamin D, the sunshine vitamin, has received a lot of attention recently as a result of a meteoric rise in the number of publications showing that vitamin D plays a crucial role in a plethora of physiological functions and associating vitamin D deficiency with many acute and chronic illnesses including disorders of calcium metabolism, autoimmune diseases, some cancers, type 2 diabetes mellitus, cardiovascular disease and infectious diseases. Vitamin D deficiency is now recognized as a global pandemic. The major cause for vitamin D deficiency is the lack of appreciation that sun exposure has been and continues to be the major source of vitamin D for children and adults of all ages. Vitamin D plays a crucial role in the development and maintenance of a healthy skeleton throughout life. There remains some controversy regarding what blood level of 25-hydroxyvitamin D should be attained for both bone health and reducing risk for vitamin D deficiency associated acute and chronic diseases and how much vitamin D should be supplemented.

Keywords: vitamin D; 25-hydroxyvitamin D; vitamin D deficiency; osteoporosis; fractures; cancer; type 2 diabetes mellitus; cardiovascular diseases; autoimmune diseases; infectious diseases

1. Introduction

Vitamin D has been produced by phytoplankton for more than 500 million years [1] and is thought to be the oldest of all hormones whose function initially could have been the protection of ultraviolet-sensitive macromolecules including proteins, DNA and RNA, when these early forms of life were exposed to sunlight for photosynthesis. Later, after the evolution of ocean dwelling animals with vertebral skeletons ventured onto land, the maintenance of calcium homeostasis was a major physiological problem (as opposed to living in the calcium-rich ocean). It was vitamin D that ensured the efficient intestinal calcium absorption from dietary sources and ultimately was essential for the development and maintenance of a calcified mammalian skeleton [2]. Obtaining vitamin D from either sunlight or diet is still critical for most vertebrates for their skeletal health [1,3–5]. Over time, vitamin D has evolved into a hormone having numerous extraskeletal effects by regulating up to estimated 2000 genes [6,7].

Ethnical and gender differences in skin pigmentation indicate the evolutionary importance of a sufficient vitamin D supply. The varying degrees of depigmentation that evolved in order to permit UVB-induced synthesis of previtamin D_3 when hominids migrated outside the tropics can be considered as a compromise solution to the conflicting physiological requirements of vitamin D synthesis and photoprotection that differ depending on latitude and thus warrant different degrees of skin pigmentation. An evolutionary selection pressure towards a lighter skin coloration going along with a higher ability to produce vitamin D seems not only to be exerted by living in geographic regions with a lower UV intensity but also by being female. Gender differences in skin pigmentation with females being lighter skinned than males in all populations for which data about the skin reflectance was available could be explained by the higher needs of vitamin D during pregnancy and lactation [8].

2. Vitamin D—Sources

The main sources of vitamin D are sunlight, supplements and diet [7] (Table 1).

Table 1. Sources of vitamin D_2 and vitamin D_3 [7]. Note: This table is modified and reproduced with permission from [7], Copyright © 2007 Massachusetts Medical Society.

Source	Vitamin D Content IU = 25 ng
	Chemical structures of vitamin D_2 [9] and vitamin D_3 [10].

Vitamin D_2 (Ergocalciferol)   Vitamin D_3 (Cholecalciferol)

Table 1. *Cont.*

Natural sources	
Cod liver oil	~400–1000 IU/tsp vitamin D_3
Egg yolk	~20 IU/yolk vitamin D_3 or D_2
Mackerel, canned	~250 IU/3.5 oz vitamin D_3
Salmon, canned	~300–600 IU/3.5 oz vitamin D_3
Salmon, fresh farmed	~100–250 IU/3.5 oz vitamin D_3, vitamin D_2
Sardines, canned	~300 IU/3.5 oz vitamin D_3
Shiitake mushrooms, fresh	~100 IU/3.5 oz vitamin D_2
Shiitake mushrooms, sun dried	~1600 IU/3.5 oz vitamin D_2
Sunlight/UVB radiation	~20,000 IU equivalent to exposure to 1 minimal erythemal dose (MED) in a bathing suit. Thus, exposure of arms and legs to 0.5 MED is equivalent to ingesting ~3000 IU vitamin D_3
Tuna, canned	236 IU/3.5 oz vitamin D_3
Fortified foods	
Fortified breakfast cereals	~100 IU/serving usually vitamin D_3
Fortified butter	56 IU/3.5 oz usually vitamin D_3
Fortified cheeses	100 IU/3 oz usually vitamin D_3
Fortified margarine	429/3.5 oz usually vitamin D_3
Fortified milk	100 IU/8 oz usually vitamin D_3
Fortified orange juice	100 IU/8 oz vitamin D_3
Fortified yogurts	100 IU/8 oz usually vitamin D_3
Infant formulas	100 IU/8 oz vitamin D_3
Pharmaceutical Sources in the United States	
Drisdol (vitamin D_2) liquid	8000 IU/mL
Vitamin D_2 (Ergocalciferol)	50,000 IU/capsule
Supplemental Sources	
Multivitamin	400, 500, and 1000 IU vitamin D_3 or vitamin D_2
Vitamin D_3	400, 800, 1000, 2000, 5000, 10,000, 14,000, and 50,000 IU

Exposure of human skin to solar UVB radiation (wavelengths: 290–315 nm) leads to the conversion of 7-dehydrocholesterol to previtamin D_3 in the skin. Previtamin D_3 is then rapidly converted to vitamin D_3 (cholecalciferol) by temperature- and membrane-dependent processes [7,11,12] (Figure 1).

Figure 1. Schematic representation of the synthesis and metabolism of vitamin D for regulating calcium, phosphorus and bone metabolism [7]. During exposure to sunlight, 7-dehydrocholesterol in the skin is converted to previtamin D_3. Previtamin D_3 immediately converts by a heat dependent process to vitamin D_3 [7,11,12]. Excessive exposure to sunlight degrades previtamin D_3 and vitamin D_3 into inactive photoproducts [13]. Vitamin D_2 and vitamin D_3 from dietary sources is incorporated into chylomicrons, transported by the lymphatic system into the venous circulation [14]. Vitamin D (D represents D_2 or D_3) made in the skin or ingested in the diet can be stored in and then released from fat cells. Vitamin D in the circulation is bound to the vitamin D binding protein which transports it to the liver where vitamin D is converted by the vitamin D-25-hydroxylase to

25-hydroxyvitamin D [25(OH)D]. This is the major circulating form of vitamin D that is used by clinicians to measure vitamin D status [7,15] (although most reference laboratories report the normal range to be 20–100 ng/mL, the preferred healthful range is 30–60 ng/mL) [7]. It is biologically inactive and must be converted in the kidneys by the 25-hydroxyvitamin D-1α-hydroxylase (1-OHase) to its biologically active form 1,25-dihydroxyvitamin D [1,25(OH)$_2$D] [7,15–17]. Serum phosphorus, calcium, fibroblast growth factors (FGF-23) and other factors can either increase (+) or decrease (−) the renal production of 1,25(OH)$_2$D [7]. 1,25(OH)$_2$D feedback regulates its own synthesis and decreases the synthesis and secretion of parathyroid hormone (PTH) in the parathyroid glands [6,7]. 1,25(OH)$_2$D increases the expression of the 25-hydroxyvitamin D-24-hydroxylase (24-OHase) to catabolize 1,25(OH)$_2$D to the water soluble biologically inactive calcitroic acid which is excreted in the bile [7,18]. 1,25(OH)$_2$D enhances intestinal calcium absorption in the small intestine by stimulating the expression of the epithelial calcium channel (ECaC) and the calbindin 9K (calcium binding protein; CaBP) [7,19,20]. 1,25(OH)$_2$D is recognized by its receptor in osteoblasts causing an increase in the expression of receptor activator of NFκB ligand (RANKL). Its receptor RANK on the preosteoclast binds RANKL which induces the preosteoclast to become a mature osteoclast. The mature osteoclast removes calcium and phosphorus from the bone to maintain blood calcium and phosphorus levels [7,17]. Adequate calcium and phosphorus levels promote the mineralization of the skeleton [7]. Note: This figure is reproduced with permission from [21], Copyright © 2007 Michael F. Holick.

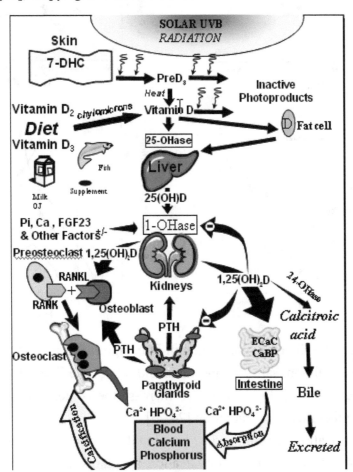

The amount of vitamin D production in the skin depends on the incident angle of the sun and thus on latitude, season and time of the day. It is highest when the sun is in the zenith and a flattening of the incident angle leads to a reduced vitamin D production [17]. Whole body exposure to sunlight with one minimal erythema dose (MED), *i.e.*, the minimal dose leading to pink coloration of the skin 24 h after exposure, leads to vitamin D levels comparable to oral intake of 10,000 to up to 25,000 IU vitamin D_2 [16,22]. However, sun exposure during most of the winter at latitudes above and below ~33 degrees North and South, respectively, doesn't lead to any production of vitamin D_3 in the skin [16,23] (Figure 2). Other factors influencing the cutaneous vitamin D production adversely are an increase in skin pigmentation, aging, especially age >65 years and the topical application of a sunscreen [17].

Figure 2. Influence of season, time of day, and latitude on the synthesis of previtamin D_3 in Northern (**A** and **C**) and Southern hemispheres (**B** and **D**). The hour indicated in **C** and **D** is the end of the 1-h exposure time. Note: This figure is reproduced with permission from [13], Copyright © 2010 Humana Press.

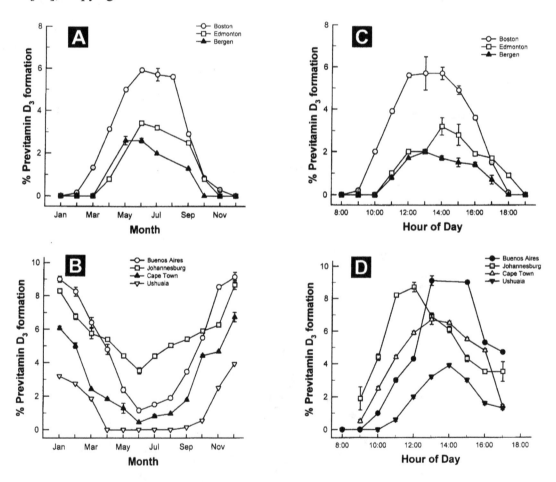

The number of foods naturally containing vitamin D in significant amounts is very limited. Among these are oily fish such as salmon, sardines and tuna, and oils of the liver of some fish such as cod as well as sun-exposed mushrooms [7] (Table 1). To increase the content of vitamin D_2 in mushrooms producers are irradiating them with UV radiation [24,25].

In the 1930s, the fortification of milk, sodas, bread and even beer became popular [26]; however, after several cases of presumed vitamin D intoxication in infants in the 1950s in Great Britain [27] strict regulations limiting vitamin D fortification to only margarine were introduced in Europe [14,28]. Due to a relatively high prevalence of lactose intolerance leading to an avoidance of milk by many adults, the fortification of orange juice in the US was introduced as a novel approach of enhancing the vitamin D status of the public in the 2003 and proved to be as effective as oral supplementation [26,29]. Other fortified foods include margarine, yogurt, infant formula, butter, cheese and breakfast cereals [7] (Table 1).

Vitamin D_2 and vitamin D_3 are available as oral over-the-counter supplements. In the US, only vitamin D_2 is available as prescription drug [7,17]. Although there has been debate as to whether vitamin D_2 is as effective as vitamin D_3 in maintaining vitamin D status [30–36], other studies in children and adults have demonstrated that they are equally effective [29,37–40].

3. Vitamin D—Metabolism

Vitamin D from cutaneous synthesis or dietary/supplemental intake, is transported to the fat where it can be stored or to the liver for the first step of activation, the hydroxylation to 25-hydroxyvitamin D [25(OH)D], which is the major circulating form of vitamin D [7,15] and measured to assess a patient's vitamin D status [7,16,41,42] (Figure 1).

25(OH)D is metabolized in the kidneys by the mitochondrial enzyme 25-hydroxyvitamin D-1α-hydroxylase (CYP27B1) to generate the systemically circulating active form, 1,25-dihydroxyvitamin D [1,25(OH)$_2$D] [7,15–17]. The renal synthesis of 1,25(OH)$_2$D is regulated by several factors including serum phosphorus, calcium, fibroblast growth factor 23 (FGF-23), parathormone (PTH) and itself [7]. CYP27B1 is also expressed extrarenally in a multitude of tissues [17,43], including bone, placenta, prostate, keratinocytes, macrophages, T-lymphocytes, dendritic cells, several cancer cells [44], and the parathyroid gland [45] and enables the production of 1,25(OH)$_2$D. This active form of vitamin D is locally active and exerts auto- or paracrine effects [15,17].

1,25(OH)$_2$D induces its own destruction by rapidly inducing the 25-hydroxyvitamin D-24-hydroxylase (CYP24A1), which leads to the multistep catabolism of both 25(OH)D and 1,25(OH)$_2$D into biologically inactive, water-soluble metabolites including calcitroic acid [7,18] (Figure 1).

4. Vitamin D Receptor (VDR)—Distribution and Function

1,25(OH)$_2$D, either produced in the kidneys [7] or extrarenally in the target tissues [15,17], is the ligand of the vitamin D receptor (VDR) whose widespread distribution across many tissues explains the myriad of physiological actions of vitamin D. By interacting with the VDR, a transcription factor [17,46], 1,25(OH)$_2$D regulates directly and indirectly the expression of up to 2000 genes [6,7], many of whose promoters contain specific vitamin D response elements (VDRE). The VDR partners with other transcription factors, most importantly the retinoid X receptor (RXR) [47], and coactivators and corepressors provide target gene specificity [48–50]. A membrane-bound VDR may also exist and mediate more immediate, non-genomic actions of 1,25(OH)$_2$D [44,51,52].

5. Prevalence of Vitamin D Deficiency and Insufficiency

25(OH)D is the vitamin D metabolite that is measured to assess a patient's vitamin D status [7,17]. Vitamin D deficiency is diagnosed when 25(OH)D <20 ng/mL [16,53], vitamin D insufficiency is defined as 25(OH)D of 21–29 ng/mL, and 25(OH)D >30 ng/mL is considered sufficient, with 40–60 ng/mL being the preferred range [16]. Vitamin D intoxication usually doesn't occur until 25(OH)D >150 ng/mL [7,16,23].

These reference values are in part based on the finding, that the decline of parathyroid hormone (PTH) concentrations with increasing 25(OH)D levels in adults reached its nadir asymptotically at a 25(OH)D of ~30–40 ng/mL in several studies [7,16,23,54–56]. However, a recent cross-sectional analysis of more than 300,000 paired serum PTH and 25(OH)D levels revealed no threshold, even at 25(OH)D levels >60 ng/mL, above which a further increase of the 25(OH)D level failed to further suppress PTH levels. The analysis also showed a strong age-dependency of the PTH-25(OH)D relationship [57].

According to studies in Canada, 30%–50% of children and adults are vitamin D deficient [58–60]. The National Health and Nutrition Examination Surveys 2001–2006 showed a prevalence of vitamin D deficiency of 33% [60,61]. Studies in Indian school children revealed a prevalence of severe vitamin D deficiency (<9 ng/mL) in more than 35% [62] and over 80% of pregnant women in India had 25(OH)D levels <22.5 ng/mL [63]. Also reports from Africa [64], Australia [65], Brazil [66], Middle East [67,68], Mongolia [69], and New Zealand [70] documented a high risk for vitamin D deficiency in both adults and children [60,71].

Based on these findings, it has been estimated that 1 billion people worldwide are vitamin D deficient or insufficient [7,60] (Figure 3A–C).

Figure 3. (**A**) Prevalence at risk of vitamin D deficiency defined as a 25-hydroxyvitamin D <12–20 ng/mL by age and sex: United States, 2001–2006. (**B**) Mean intake of vitamin D (IU) from food and food plus dietary supplements from Continuing Survey of Food Intakes by Individuals (CSFII) 1994–1996, 1998 and the Third National Health and Nutrition Examination Survey (NHANES III) 1988–1994. (**C**) Reported incidence of vitamin D deficiency defined as a 25-hydroxyvitamin D <20 ng/mL around the globe including Australia (AU), Canada (CA), China (CH), India (IN), Korea (KR), Malaysia (MA), Middle East (ME), Mongolia (MO), New Zealand (NZ), North Africa (NA), Northern Europe (NE), United States (USA) [60]. Note: This figure is reproduced with permission from [60], Copyright © 2012 The Endocrine Society.

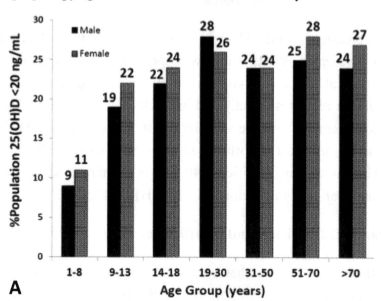

Figure 3. *Cont.*

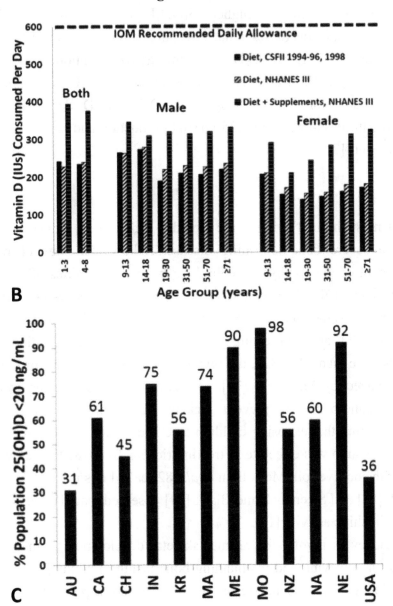

6. Vitamin D and Calcium and Phosphorus Metabolism

Vitamin D plays an important role in the calcium and phosphorus metabolism and helps ensure adequate levels of these minerals for metabolic functions and bone mineralization [7]. 1,25(OH)$_2$D increases the efficiency of intestinal calcium absorption from 10%–15% to 30%–40% by interacting with the VDR-RXR and thereby promoting the expression of an epithelial calcium channel and a calcium-binding protein [7,19,20]. Based on several experiments conducted in rodents [72,73] it has been estimated that 1,25(OH)$_2$D also increases the intestinal phosphorus absorption from 50%–60% to approximately 80% [7,14].

Vitamin D also mediates indirect effects on calcium and phosphorus by regulating the PTH levels. The parathyroid glands have CYP27B1 activity and the local production of 1,25(OH)$_2$D using 25(OH)D as substrate could inhibit the synthesis of PTH [74]. However, 25(OH)D could also directly suppress PTH synthesis by directly activating the VDR [75]. Vitamin D deficiency is associated with lower levels of serum-ionized calcium, a stimulus leading to increased PTH levels. Conversely, higher calcium levels that are associated with higher 25(OH)D levels, suppress the PTH secretion. PTH increases tubular calcium and decreases renal phosphorus reabsorption [14] (Figure 1). PTH also stimulates the production of 1,25(OH)$_2$D with the above mentioned effects on calcium and phosphorus homeostasis [7,14]. Moreover, both PTH and 1,25(OH)$_2$D stimulate osteoblasts to mobilize skeletal calcium stores [7,17] (Figure 1). Vitamin D deficiency leads to secondary hyperparathyroidism with PTH-enhanced 1,25(OH)$_2$D production and is often associated with normal to high 1,25(OH)$_2$D levels [7].

7. Bone Health

In the mid-1600s most children living in the crowded and polluted industrialized cities in Northern Europe developed a severe bone-deforming disease, rickets, that was characterized by growth retardation, enlargement of the epiphyses of the long bones, deformities of the legs, bending of the spine, knobby projections of the ribcage, and weak and toneless muscles [14,76] (Figure 4). Autopsy studies in children in the Netherlands and Boston in the early 1900s showed a rickets prevalence of 80%–90% [14]. In the 19th and 20th century, the major discoveries regarding the pathogenesis and prevention of rickets were made. In 1822, the importance of sun exposure for the prevention and cure of rickets was recognized by Sniadecki [77]. In 1890, these observations were extended and the recommendation of sun baths to prevent rickets was promoted by Palm [78]. In 1919, Huldschinski [79,80] found that exposing children to UV radiation from a sun quartz lamp (mercury arc lamp) or carbon arc lamp was effective in treating rickets. In 1918, Mellanby *et al.* [81] prevented rickets in puppies with cod liver oil. McCollum *et al.* [82] called this new nutritional factor vitamin D. Hess and Weinstock [83] and Steenbock and Black [84] observed that UV irradiation of various foods and oils imparted antirachitic activity [14].

Vitamin D sufficiency is pivotal for normal skeletal development both *in utero* [7,85] and in childhood [14], and for achieving and maintaining bone health in adults [23]. This is due to the fact that vitamin D sufficiency leads to an adequate calcium-phosphorus product ($Ca^{2+} \times HPO4^{2-}$) resulting in an effective bone mineralization [14]. Maternal vitamin D insufficiency during pregnancy was associated with a significant reduction in bone mineral acquisition in infants [85] that still persisted 9 years after birth [86]. In children whose epiphyseal plates haven't closed, vitamin D deficiency with 25(OH)D levels <15 ng/mL causes chondrocyte disorganization and hypertrophy at the mineralization front as well as skeletal mineralization defects. This results in bone deformities and short stature, the typical signs of vitamin D deficiency rickets [14,87].

In adults low 25(OH)D and high PTH also lead to a low serum calcium × phosphorus product, resulting in osteomalacia, *i.e.*, a defective mineralization of the collagen matrix causing a reduction of structural support and being associated with an increased risk of fracture [17,28]. Results from the National Health and Nutrition Examination Survey III (NHANES III) showed that bone density in the hip was directly related to the serum 25(OH)D level in both genders of all ethnicities [88,89]. A German study examined 25(OH)D serum levels and transiliac crest bone specimens of 675 individuals mainly in the 6th and 7th decade of life (401 males, mean age 58.7 ± 17 years, and 274 females, mean age: 68.3 ± 17.3 years) dying of unnatural death, such as a motor vehicle accident.

The bone biopsies were taken within 48 h after death as well as the blood samples. Various previous experiments had shown that the 25(OH)D serum levels were stable for at least 10 days postmortem. While there's no uniformly accepted osteoid volume cut-off for the histologic diagnosis of osteomalacia, the study showed a prevalence of osteomalacia of over 25% when using a threshold of >2% osteoid volume/bone volume (OV/BV) for the diagnosis of osteomalacia and a prevalence of >43% when using a threshold of 1.2% OV/BV as described by Delling in 1975 [90]. Osteomalacia was absent in all individuals with 25(OH)D >30 ng/mL, suggesting this as minimum serum level for maintenance of bone health. However, no minimum 25(OH)D level could be determined that was inevitably associated with mineralization defects [91].

One possible explanation is that obtaining a single blood level of 25(OH)D doesn't provide information about the long-term vitamin D status of the individual. It is possible that for example that the subject became ill during the winter and stopped ingesting foods containing vitamin D or decreased sun exposure during the summer that would acutely lower blood levels of 25(OH)D without causing osteomalacia.

Figure 4. Sister (right) and brother (left) ages 4 years and 6.5 years, respectively, demonstrating classic knock-knees and bow legs, growth retardation, and other skeletal deformities [14]. Note: This figure is reproduced with permission from [14], Copyright © 2006 American Society for Clinical Investigation.

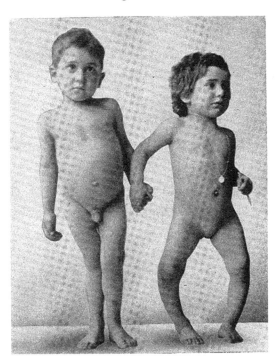

8. Osteoporosis and Fractures

As a decrease in 25(OH)D leads to secondary hyperparathyroidism associated with osteoclastogenesis and an increase in bone resorption exceeding osteoblast-mediated bone formation [88], this can precipitate and exacerbate osteopenia and osteoporosis in adults [17,92,93].

Osteoporosis has a prevalence of ~1/3 in women 60–70 years of age and of ~2/3 in women 80 years of age or older [7]. It's estimated that currently 10 million Americans have osteoporosis with

1.5 to 2 million osteoporosis-related fractures annually [94]. An osteoporosis-related fracture will be experienced by one in eight men over age 50 years in their lifetime [95].

Vitamin D promotes bone health by maintaining the PTH levels in a physiologically healthy level, stimulating osteoblastic activity, and promoting bone mineralization as well as reducing risk of falls thereby reducing risk of fracture [93,96].

According to data from the Women's Health Initiative [97], the odds ratio of risk for hip fracture was inversely related to the serum 25(OH)D level [88]. There's evidence that patients with 25(OH)D levels >30 ng/mL have a lower risk of fracture. Several studies have been conducted to evaluate the effect of vitamin D supplementation on the fracture risk, with some studies showing a significant reduction of the risk of fractures while others didn't [98]. One of these showed that the supplementation with calcium (1200 mg) and vitamin D_3 (800 IU/day) decreased the number of hip fractures by 43% (p = 0.043) and the total number of nonvertebral fractures by 32% [99]. The RECORD study however, did not show a reduction in fracture risk with supplementation with vitamin D (800 IU/day), or calcium (1000 mg/day), or both [100], but often compliance was poor and serum 25(OH)D levels were not measured at the end of the study in most participants [7,98,100]. A meta-analysis of more than 30,000 participants did show that supplementation with vitamin D (≥792 IU/day) led to a significant reduction in the risk of fracture; the risk of hip fracture was reduced by 30%, the risk of any non-vertebral fracture by 14% [98–106].

9. Muscular Health and Falls

Vitamin D exerts multiple effects on muscle health [107]. Its active form 1,25(OH)$_2$D could be produced locally in muscle cells as suggested by the recent identification of CYP27B1 bioactivity in regenerating mouse muscle and skeletal muscle cells [108], however other studies have failed to detect this enzyme in muscle cells [109]. 1,25(OH)$_2$D is thought to modulate muscle function via the VDR, which seems to be expressed in skeletal muscles [109–113], by regulating gene transcription and promoting *de-novo* protein synthesis [107]. Also, rapid non-genomic pathways involving a membrane-bound vitamin D receptor could exist and affect the calcium handling involving the sarcoplasmic reticulum and the calcium signaling in muscle cells [109]. Several studies indicate that the muscle function depends on the VDR genotype in the muscle cell [114,115]. The possibility of a direct interaction between 25(OH)D and the VDR has been proposed in CYP27B1$^{-/-}$ cells [109,116]. However, the existence of a VDR in muscle cells is discussed highly controversially, as a more recent study failed to detect the VDR in muscle cells and as the antibodies used for immunocytochemical staining to detect the VDR in previous studies have been shown to be not exclusively specific for the VDR and could explain potentially false-positive results in these previous studies [117].

Vitamin D deficiency is associated with diffuse muscle pain, muscle weakness [7,118], predominantly in the proximal muscle groups [115], and a reduction in performance speed [107,119]. This is caused by muscle atrophy of mainly type II muscle fibers [115]. Proximal muscle weakness in severe vitamin D deficiency could also be caused by secondary hyperparathyroidism and resultant hypophosphatemia [60,106,120].

There is a positive association between 25(OH)D, lower extremity function, proximal muscle strength and physical performance [107,121,122]. Muscle strength [123] and postural and dynamic balance [124] were increased by vitamin D supplementation [107]. The effect of vitamin D supplementation on the risk of falls was examined in a randomized, controlled multi-dose study, showing that the supplementation of 800 IU/day lowered the adjusted-incidence rate ratio of falls by 72% compared to those taking placebo over 5 months [125]. A meta-analysis of 8 randomized controlled trials (n = 2426) showed that supplemental vitamin D of 700–1000 IU/day or a serum 25(OH)D of ≥24 ng/mL reduced the risk of falls by 19% and 23% respectively. No benefit was observed with lower supplemental doses or lower serum 25(OH)D concentrations [126].

10. Cancer

Living at higher latitudes with lower UV exposure and thus lower vitamin D production is associated with an increased risk for the occurrence of a variety of cancers and with an increased likelihood of dying from them, as compared to living at lower latitudes [7,17,127,128]. A recent review of ecological studies associating solar UVB exposure-vitamin D and cancers found strong inverse correlations with solar UVB irradiance for 15 types of cancer: bladder, breast, cervical, colon, endometrial, esophageal, gastric, lung, ovarian, pancreatic, rectal, renal, and vulvar cancer; and Hodgkin's and non-Hodgkin's lymphoma [129].

An inverse association between 25(OH)D and the incidence of several cancers and mortality from these cancers has been shown in case-control studies, prospective and retrospective studies [130–140], especially for cancers of the colon, breast and prostate [7]. Regarding colon cancer, the Nurses' Health cohort study (n = 32,826) showed an inverse association of the odds ratios for colorectal cancer with the median 25(OH)D serum levels. At 16.2 ng/mL the odds ratio was 1 and 0.53 at 39.9 ng/mL ($p \leq 0.01$) [7,140].

These associational studies have certain limitations regarding the establishment of a causality between vitamin D status and a reduced risk of cancer, e.g., as low serum 25(OH)D levels are also linked with confounding factors related to higher cancer risk, including obesity (vitamin D is sequestered in adipose tissue), and lack of physical activity (correlated with less time outdoors and less solar exposure) [138]. However, a population-based, double-blind, randomized placebo-controlled trial of 4 years duration with more than thousand postmenopausal women, whose principal secondary outcome was cancer incidence, showed that the supplementation with calcium (1400–1500 mg/day) and vitamin D_3 (1100 IU/day) reduced the relative risk (RR) of cancer by ~60% (p < 0.01). The repetition of a cancer free survival analysis after the first 12 months revealed, that the relative risk for the calcium + vitamin D group was reduced by ~77% (confidence interval [CI]: 0.09–0.60; p < 0.005). Multiple regression models also showed that both treatment and serum 25(OH)D concentrations were significant, independent predictors of cancer risk [137].

Mounting evidence suggests a biological plausibility for anti-carcinogenic effects of vitamin D, which could explain these results. 1,25(OH)$_2$D, which has been shown to be produced locally by various cancer cells metabolizing the substrate 25(OH)D [38], inhibits carcinogenesis by several mechanisms [141]. 1,25(OH)$_2$D exerts anti-proliferative effects on cancer cells by promoting cyclin-dependent kinase (CDK) inhibitor synthesis, and by influencing several growth factors and their signaling pathways including insulin-like growth factor 1 (IGF-1), transforming growth factor β (TGFβ), Wnt/β-catenin, MAP kinase 5 (MAPK5) and nuclear factor κB (NF-kB) [142] (Figure 5).

Figure 5. Metabolism of 25-hydroxyvitamin D [25(OH)D] to 1,25 dihydroxyvitamin D 1,25(OH)$_2$D for non-skeletal functions. When a monocyte/macrophage is stimulated through its toll-like receptor 2/1 (TLR2/1) by an infective agent such as Mycobacterium tuberculosis (TB), or its lipopolysaccharide (LPS) the signal upregulates the expression of vitamin D receptor (VDR) and the 25-hydroxyvitamin D-1-hydroxylase (1-OHase). 25(OH)D levels >30 ng/mL provides adequate substrate for the 1-OHase to convert it to 1,25(OH)$_2$D. 1,25(OH)$_2$D returns to the nucleus where it increases the expression of cathelicidin which is a peptide capable of promoting innate immunity and inducing the destruction of infective agents such as TB. It is also likely that the 1,25(OH)$_2$D produced in the monocytes/macrophage is released to act locally on activated T (AT) and activated B (AB) lymphocytes which regulate cytokine and immunoglobulin synthesis respectively [143–147]. When 25(OH)D levels are ~30 ng/mL, it reduces risk of many common cancers [130–140]. It is believed that the local production of 1,25(OH)$_2$D in the breast, colon, prostate, and other cells regulates a variety of genes that control proliferation. Once 1,25(OH)$_2$D completes the task of maintaining normal cellular proliferation and differentiation, it induces the 25-hydroxyvitamin D-24-hydroxylase (24-OHase). The 24-OHase enhances the metabolism of 1,25(OH)$_2$D to calcitroic acid which is biologically inert [7,18]. Thus, the local production of 1,25(OH)$_2$D does not enter the circulation and has no influence on calcium metabolism. The parathyroid glands have 1-OHase activity [45] and the local production of 1,25(OH)$_2$D inhibits the expression and synthesis of PTH [74]. The production of 1,25(OH)$_2$D in the kidney enters the circulation and is able to downregulate renin production in the kidney [148,149] and to stimulate insulin secretion in the β-islet cells of the pancreas [148,150]. Note: This figure is reproduced with permission from [21], Copyright © 2007 Michael F. Holick.

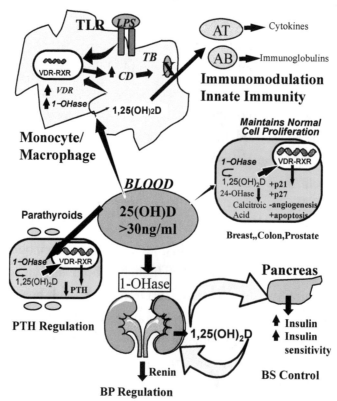

Apoptosis is characterized as programmed cell death permitting the removal of damaged cells including cancer cells in multicellular organisms without impairing the cellular microenvironment. Defective apoptosis plays a major role in the development and progression of cancer [151]. It has been shown, that both immunobiological mechanisms of cancer immunosurveillance and cancer immunoediting [152], as well as chemotherapeutic agents and radiation, utilize the apoptotic pathway to induce cancer cell death [151,153]. $1,25(OH)_2D_3$ might exert anti-carcinogenic effects by promoting various pro-apoptotic mechanisms including the downregulation of the anti-apoptotic gene Bcl-2 [154] and by upregulating of the pro-apoptotic gene Bax [155], $1,25(OH)_2D_3$ induces differentiation, partly by reducing the expression of the *c-myc* oncogene [141,156]. It regulates the prostaglandin (PG) metabolism and signaling, thus decreasing PG-mediated promotion of carcinogenesis [141,157]. It suppresses tumor angiogenesis, e.g., mediated by $1,25(OH)_2D$'s effects on the PG synthesis and by regulating the expression of crucial factors controlling the angiogenesis. $1,25(OH)_2D_3$ suppresses tumor invasion and metastasis by various mechanisms [141], e.g., by decreasing the expression and activity of cell invasion-associated serine proteases and metalloproteinases and inducing their inhibitors [158], and by inducing *E*-cadherin expression, contributing to adhesive properties of cells [141,159]. Other effects mediated by $1,25(OH)_2D$ are thought to be the induction of autophagy as process to trigger the death of cancer cells and to block tumor growth and by inducing enzymes involved in antioxidant defense mechanisms and DNA-repair [142]. $1,25(OH)_2D$ also regulates androgen and estrogen receptor signaling, thereby inhibiting tumor growth of some sex hormone-dependent tumors such as prostate and breast cancer. It has also been shown to reduce the expression of aromatase, thereby inhibiting breast cancer growth [141].

11. Vitamin D and Cardiovascular Risk

Most epidemiological and prospective studies as well as meta-analyses [148,160–163] suggest a significant inverse association between 25(OH)D serum levels and cardiovascular risk. The prospective Intermountain Heart Collaborative Study with more than 40,000 participants revealed that 25(OH)D <15 ng/mL compared to 25(OH)D >30 ng/mL was associated with highly significant increases in the prevalence of type 2 diabetes mellitus, hypertension, hyperlipidemia, and peripheral vascular disease, coronary artery disease, myocardial infarction, heart failure, and stroke ($p < 0.0001$), as well as with incident death (all-cause mortality was used as primary survival measure), heart failure, coronary artery disease/myocardial infarction ($p < 0.0001$), stroke ($p = 0.003$), and their composite ($p < 0.0001$) [164].

A meta-analysis examining the association between vitamin D status and the risk of cerebrovascular events including >1200 stroke cases found that the pooled relative risk for stroke was 52% higher when comparing 25(OH)D levels ≤12.4 ng/mL with 25(OH)D levels >18.8 ng/mL [165].

Many of these associations are well established, causation however is yet to be proven [166]. Individuals spending less time exercising outdoors in the sun, e.g., have a higher risk of developing cardiovascular diseases, and those individuals also will likely have lower 25(OH)D levels coincidentally [166,167]. Also, obesity, a condition associated with cardiovascular disease [168], is associated with a lower vitamin D status due to a sequestration and volumetric dilution of the lipophilic vitamin D in the fat tissue [23,166,169,170], potentially explaining the described correlations [166]. Despite these limitations many studies suggest a biological plausibility for the beneficial effects of vitamin D on cardiovascular risk factors and cardiovascular health.

The vitamin D receptor is present in endothelium, vascular smooth muscle, and cardiomyocytes [162,166] and may protect against atherosclerosis through the inhibition of macrophage cholesterol uptake and foam cell formation, reduced vascular smooth muscle cell proliferation, and reduced expression of adhesion molecules in endothelial cells [166] and through inhibition of cytokine release from lymphocytes [162]. Several meta-analyses indicate an inverse association between vitamin D status and hypertension [171]. Studies showed, that antihypertensive effects were associated with raising 25(OH)D levels with vitamin D supplementation [172–174] or UVB exposure [175].

Mechanistically, this effect could be partly mediated by vitamin D's capability to suppress the levels of PTH, which can cause arrhythmias and lead to myocardial hypertrophy and increased blood pressure [148,176]. $1,25(OH)_2D_3$ has also been shown to suppress the levels of renin and could contribute to vitamin D's potential antihypertensive properties [148,149].

A meta-analysis examining the association between vitamin D status or vitamin D supplementation, and incident type 2 diabetes showed that individuals with 25(OH)D levels >25 ng/mL compared to those with 25(OH)D <14 ng/mL had a 43% lower risk of developing type 2 diabetes and that a vitamin D supplementation with >500 IU/day compared to <200 IU/day reduced the risk by 13% [177]. In the Nurses' Health Study >83,000 women were followed-up prospectively and it was shown, that a combined daily intake of >1200 mg calcium and >800 IU vitamin D was associated with a 33% lower risk of type 2 diabetes with RR of 0.67 (CI: 0.49–0.90) compared with an intake of <600 mg calcium and 400 IU vitamin D [178]. A prospective study following-up more than 2000 participants showed, that the risk of progression from prediabetes to diabetes was reduced by 62% when comparing the highest quartile of 25(OH)D levels with the lowest quartile [179,180].

This could be explained by experimental findings indicating that vitamin D exerts various antidiabetic effects. The VDR is expressed in pancreatic beta cells and $1,25(OH)_2D$ stimulates insulin secretion [148,150]. Improvement in vitamin D status also leads to a improvement of insulin sensitivity, mediated for example by upregulation of insulin receptors [148], and modulates inflammation, which is also thought to play a role in type 2 diabetes [150,179] (Figure 5).

12. Vitamin D's Role in Autoimmune Disease

Ecological studies have shown that the prevalence of certain autoimmune diseases was associated with latitude, suggesting a potential role of sunlight exposure, and thus vitamin D production, on the pathogenesis of type 1 diabetes mellitus, multiple sclerosis and Crohn's disease [181]. The increased prevalence at higher latitudes has been shown for multiple sclerosis (MS) [181,182], inflammatory bowel disease [183], rheumatoid arthritis [184] and type 1 diabetes [181,182,185].

A few case-control studies relate the vitamin D status to the risk of developing these autoimmune diseases [181]. One of them, a prospective, nested case-control study analyzed serum samples and the data of disability databases of more than seven million US military personnel, and showed, that among whites (148 cases, 296 controls), the risk of multiple sclerosis significantly decreased with increasing levels of 25(OH)D (odds ratio for a 20 ng/mL increase in 25(OH)D was 0.59 (95% CI: 0.36–0.97). When comparing the highest quintile of 25(OH)D with the lowest, the odds ratio for developing MS was 0.38 (95% CI: 0.19–0.75; $p = 0.006$), with an particularly strong inverse association for 25(OH)D levels measured before age 20 years [186].

A study addressing vitamin D's effect on multiple sclerosis showed the safety of high-dose vitamin D (~14,000 IU/day). It appeared to have immunomodulatory effects including a persistent reduction in T-cell proliferation and resulted in a trend for fewer relapse events [187]. When examining the association between 25(OH)D serum levels and the relapse rate in MS patients before and after supplementation with ~3000 IU vitamin D per day, a significant strong inverse relationship between the relapse incidence rate and the 25(OH)D level ($p < 0.0001$) was found [188].

An inverse association between maternal 25(OH)D levels and the risk for type 1 diabetes in the offspring has been shown in a population-based, nested cohort study of ~30,000 pregnant women. Compared to the upper quartile of 25(OH)D levels, the odds of type 1 diabetes in the women with the lowest quartile was more than twofold higher [189]. A birth-cohort study with >10,000 children showed, that regular supplementation with 2000 IU vitamin D per day in the first year of life was associated with a 88% reduction of the risk for type 1 diabetes later in life when compared to those without supplementation [190]. However, another study did not show a statistically significant association between taking cod liver oil or other vitamin D supplements in the first year of life and the risk of type 1 diabetes mellitus [191].

Merlino *et al.* [192] showed in a prospective cohort study of 29,368 women of ages 55–69 years without a history of rheumatoid arthritis at study baseline, that greater intake (highest versus lowest tertile) of vitamin D was inversely associated with risk of rheumatoid arthritis (RR 0.67; 95% CI: 0.44–1.00; p for trend =0.05).

These associations indicate a contributory role of vitamin D in the pathophysiology of autoimmune diseases. This is further supported by various experimental findings showing vitamin D's capability to regulate chemokine production, counteracting autoimmune inflammation and to induce differentiation of immune cells in a way that promotes self-tolerance. This involves the enhancement of the innate and the inhibition of the adaptive immune system by regulating the interactions between lymphocytes and antigen presenting cells. By increasing the quantity of Th2 lymphocytes and by inducing proliferation of dendritic cells with tolerance properties, vitamin D exerts anti-inflammatory and immunoregulatory effects [181].

Immune cells possess both the enzymatic machinery to produce 1,25(OH)$_2$D and a VDR. This could explain, why certain polymorphisms in the VDR gene seem to affect the risk for multiple autoimmune diseases, the time of onset of disease and disease activity [181,193–197].

13. Vitamin D and Infectious Diseases

The plethora of effects of vitamin D on regulating the immune system plays a role in fighting infectious diseases [198]. Vitamin D enhances the innate immunity against various infections [143], especially tuberculosis, influenza and viral upper respiratory tract infections [198].

Historically, cod liver oil (one of only a few natural sources of vitamin D) was given to tuberculosis patients in 19th and 20th century [199–201]. Later in the nineteenth century, tuberculosis patients were treated in sanatoriums with heliotherapy, *i.e.*, sun exposure. In 1903, Niels Ryberg Finsen was awarded the Nobel prize for medicine "in recognition of his contribution to the treatment of diseases, especially lupus vulgaris (tuberculosis of the skin), with concentrated light radiation, whereby he has opened a new avenue for medical science" [199,202]. After vitamin D had been identified as the active ingredient in cod-liver oil [199,203], vitamin D_2 was used successfully in the treatment of lupus vulgaris in several studies. In 1946 a report in *Proc. R. Soc. Med.* [204] stated that there was no room for doubt that calciferol (vitamin D) in adequate dosage will cure a substantial proportion of cases of lupus vulgaris [199,204]. In 1947 the first reference to successful treatment of pulmonary tuberculosis with vitamin D was published [199,205]. In the wake of the antibiotic era both heliotherapy and vitamin D therapy for treating tuberculosis patients were quickly forgotten [199,206]. However recent studies have suggested that vitamin D may have an important role to play in reducing risk for acquiring one of the most common and deadly infectious diseases that plague third world countries [206].

One case-control study examining the association between vitamin D status and tuberculosis showed, that the mean 25(OH)D levels were statistically significant different ($p < 0.005$) between patients with pulmonary and extrapulmonary tuberculosis (10.7 ng/mL) and controls (19.5 ng/mL) [207]. In another study, 25(OH)D levels <10 ng/mL were significantly associated with active tuberculosis (OR 2.9; 95% CI: 1.3–6.5; $p = 0.008$) [208]. A meta-analysis showed, that low serum 25(OH)D levels were associated with higher risk of active tuberculosis, and that the pooled effect size in random effects meta-analysis was 0.68 (95% CI: 0.43–0.93), representing a medium to large effect [209]. A double-blind, placebo-controlled study in Mongolian school children ($n = 120$) examining the effect of vitamin D supplementation (800 IU/day) on tuberculin skin test conversion to positive showed a trend towards fewer conversions in the vitamin D group ($p = 0.06$), suggesting a potential role of vitamin D in reducing the rate of acquisition of latent tuberculosis infection [210].

Several interventional studies examining the effect of vitamin D supplementation in patients with active tuberculosis have been conducted. Some of them showed an improved immunity against mycobacteria [211], a significantly improved sputum conversion rate and a higher rate of radiological improvement [212], and a significantly hastened sputum culture conversion in participants with the tt genotype of the TaqI vitamin D receptor polymorphism [213]. There was also a higher rate of tuberculosis symptom improvement and a significantly higher weight gain ($p < 0.005$) in children [214]. A prospective, randomized placebo-controlled trial examining the effect of adjunctive vitamin D supplementation in patients receiving antimicrobial therapy showed that vitamin D supplementation led to an accelerated sputum smear conversion and an accelerated resolution of inflammation [215]. Another study however in which three doses of 100,000 IU vitamin D_3 each were given during 8 months did not lead to a reduction in the clinical severity score or mortality [216].

Some studies examined the effect of vitamin D supplementation on the risk of influenza [217,218].

In 1981, R. Edgar Hope-Simpson proposed that a "seasonal stimulus" was intimately associated with solar radiation and explained the remarkable seasonality of epidemic influenza [219,220]. As the vitamin D status changes during the seasons, it has been suggested, that vitamin D could be this "seasonal stimulus" [219]. A randomized trial of vitamin D_3 supplementation (1200 IU/day) in school children ($n = 334$) showed a significantly reduced risk for influence A as determined by both antibody and sputum testing compared to the placebo group (RR 0.58; 95% CI: 0.34–0.99; $p = 0.04$) [218].

One study using questionnaires to retrospectively determine the occurrence of influenza-like disease in participants of 10 different clinical trials ($n = 569$), receiving 1111–6800 IU/day, however did not show a significant difference in the incidence and severity of influenza-like disease [217].

The NHANES III study ($n > 18$) revealed an inverse association between serum 25(OH)D levels and recent upper respiratory tract infections (URTI). Lower 25(OH)D levels were independently associated with recent URTI compared with 25(OH)D levels of $\geq$30 ng/mL (OR 1.36; 95% CI: 1.01–1.84 for <10 ng/mL and OR 1.24; 95% CI: 1.07–1.43 for 10 to <30 ng/mL). In individuals with asthma or chronic obstructive airway disease this association was stronger (OR of 5.67 in asthma respectively OR of 2.26 in chronic obstructive airway disease) [221]. A study in Finish men ($n = 800$) found a significant association between 25(OH)D serum levels <16 ng/mL and significantly more days of absence from duty due to respiratory infections ($p = 0.004$) [222]. In Indian children ($n = 150$) vitamin D deficiency has been associated with a significantly higher risk of acute lower respiratory infections [223].

A study with >200 participants whose primary endpoint was the effect of vitamin D supplementation on bone loss also revealed, that the vitamin D_3 supplementation for 2 years with 800 IU/day and for 1 year with 2000 IU/day was associated with a significantly reduced risk of cold and influenza symptoms, an effect that was magnified with the supplementation of 2000 IU/day [198,224]. Other studies however did not show a statistically significant difference, possibly due to poor compliance [225,226]. Certain VDR polymorphisms were also associated with a significantly increased risk of acute lower respiratory tract infections [227].

Several mechanisms could explain vitamin D's potentially beneficial effects on infectious diseases. Monocytes and macrophages can sense pathogen-associated molecular patterns (PAMPs) of, e.g., tuberculosis by utilizing their toll-like receptors (TLRs). This induces both VDR and CYP27B1, which increases the local production of 1,25(OH)$_2$D that is dependent on the serum 25(OH)D concentration [145,228]. 1,25(OH)$_2$D enhances the innate immune system by inducing the production of antimicrobial peptides like cathelicidin, reactive oxygen species by the (reduced) nicotinamide adenine dinucleotide phosphate (NADPH) oxidase and potentially reactive nitrogen species by inducible nitric oxide synthase (iNOS), and by inducing autophagy [143–147] (Figure 4).

14. Vitamin D and Respiratory Diseases

Although some studies did not find a consistent association between 25(OH)D levels in cord blood, maternal vitamin D intake or status during pregnancy and the risk for asthma in childhood [229–236], in children with asthma, 25(OH)D levels seem to correlate positively with asthma control [237] and lung function [238], and inversely with corticosteroid use [239]. A few interventional studies examining vitamin D's effect on asthma exist [229]. One of them showed as secondary outcome that vitamin D_3 supplementation (1200 IU/day) in school children was associated with a significant 83% reduced risk for asthma exacerbations [218]. Presumably vitamin D's immunmodulatory and pulmonary effects could play a role [229].

15. Prevention and Treatment of Vitamin D Deficiency

According to the Endocrine Society Practice Guidelines a screening for vitamin D deficiency by measuring the 25(OH)D serum level is only recommended for individuals at risk (the most important risk factors are listed in Figure 6), and not for the general population [16]. To prevent vitamin D deficiency, the Institute of Medicine (IOM) recommends, that infants should immediately receive a daily supplementation of vitamin D of 400 IUs during the first year of life. Individuals between 1 and 70 years should receive 600 IU of vitamin D daily and adults >70 years should receive a daily dose of 800 IU vitamin D [53] (Table 2). The serum 25(OH)D level increases for every 100 IU/day by

~0.6–1.0 ng/mL [29,37,240,241]. The doses recommended by IOM will likely increase the 25(OH)D level to 20 ng/mL, which they considered to be adequate for bone health, but not to levels >30 ng/mL, as recommended by the Endocrine Society.

That's why the Endocrine Society recommended in its Practice Guidelines that infants during their first year of life receive a daily supplementation of 400–1000 IU (up to 2000 IU is safe), children and adolescents between 1 and 18 years a daily supplementation of 600–1000 IU (up to 4000 IU is safe), and adults >18 years a daily supplementation of 1500–2000 IU (up to 10,000 IU is safe) for the prevention of vitamin D deficiency [16,53] (Table 2).

Figure 6. A Schematic representation of the major causes for vitamin D deficiency and potential health consequences. Note: This figure is reproduced with permission from [21], Copyright © 2007 Michael F. Holick.

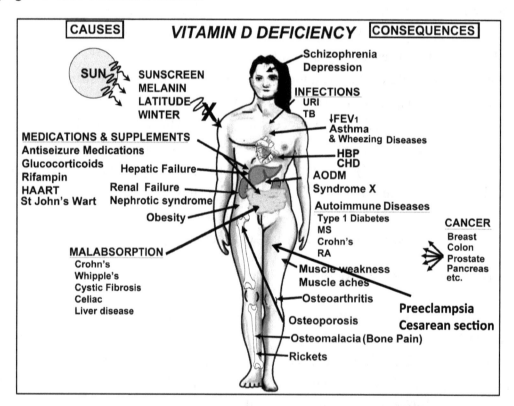

Table 2. Recommendations of the Institute of Medicine and the Endocrine Society Practice Guidelines for daily vitamin D supplementation to prevent vitamin D deficiency. This table is reproduced with permission from [16], Copyright © 2011 The Endocrine Society.

| Life Stage Group | IOM Recommendations | | | | Endocrine Society's Recommendations | |
	AI	EAR	RDA	UL	Daily Allowance (IU/day)	UL (IU)
Infants						
0 to 6 months	400 IU (10 μg)			1000 IU (25 μg)	400–1000	2000
6 to 12 months	400 IU (10 μg)			1500 IU (38 μg)	400–1000	2000
Children						
1–3 years		400 IU (10 μg)	600 IU (15 μg)	2500 IU (63 μg)	600–1000	4000
4–8 years		400 IU (10 μg)	600 IU (15 μg)	3000 IU (75 μg)	600–1000	4000

Table 2. *Cont.*

Males					
9–13 years	400 IU (10 µg)	600 IU (15 µg)	4000 IU (100 µg)	600–1000	4000
14–18 years	400 IU (10 µg)	600 IU (15 µg)	4000 IU (100 µg)	600–1000	4000
19–30 years	400 IU (10 µg)	600 IU (15 µg)	4000 IU (100 µg)	1500–2000	10,000
31–50 years	400 IU (10 µg)	600 IU (15 µg)	4000 IU (100 µg)	1500–2000	10,000
51–70 years	400 IU (10 µg)	600 IU (15 µg)	4000 IU (100 µg)	1500–2000	10,000
>70 years	400 IU (10 µg)	800 IU (20 µg)	4000 IU (100 µg)	1500–2000	10,000
Females					
9–13 years	400 IU (10 µg)	600 IU (15 µg)	4000 IU (100 µg)	600–1000	4000
14–18 years	400 IU (10 µg)	600 IU (15 µg)	4000 IU (100 µg)	600–1000	4000
19–30 years	400 IU (10 µg)	600 IU (15 µg)	4000 IU (100 µg)	1500–2000	10,000
31–50 years	400 IU (10 µg)	600 IU (15 µg)	4000 IU (100 µg)	1500–2000	10,000
51–70 years	400 IU (10 µg)	600 IU (15 µg)	4000 IU (100 µg)	1500–2000	10,000
>70 years	400 IU (10 µg)	800 IU (20 µg)	4000 IU (100 µg)	1500–2000	10,000
Pregnancy					
14–18 years	400 IU (10 µg)	600 IU (15 µg)	4000 IU (100 µg)	600–1000	4000
19–30 years	400 IU (10 µg)	600 IU (15 µg)	4000 IU (100 µg)	1500–2000	10,000
31–50 years	400 IU (10 µg)	600 IU (15 µg)	4000 IU (100 µg)	1500–2000	10,000
Lactation *					
14–18 years	400 IU (10 µg)	600 IU (15 µg)	4000 IU (100 µg)	600–1000	4000
19–30 years	400 IU (10 µg)	600 IU (15 µg)	4000 IU (100 µg)	1500–2000	10,000
31–50 years	400 IU (10 µg)	600 IU (15 µg)	4000 IU (100 µg)	1500–2000	10,000

* Mother's requirement 4000–6000 (mother's intake for infant's requirement if infant is not receiving 400 IU/day); AI = Adequate Intake; EAR = Estimated Average Requirement; IU = International Units; RDA = Recommended Dietary Allowance; UL = Tolerable Upper Intake Level.

However, obese individuals, patients with malabsorption syndromes, and patients on glucocorticoids, anti-seizure and AIDS medications may require higher doses of vitamin D than individuals without these conditions [16]. The Endocrine Society's Clinical Practice Guidelines also recommended sensible sun exposure, which for most individuals is the main physiological source of vitamin D, and provided a list of the foods rich in vitamin D, and encouraged taking a daily vitamin D supplement to ensure adequate 25(OH)D levels.

The Endocrine Society's Practice Guidelines also recommended treatment strategies for patients with vitamin D deficiency depending on age and underlying medical conditions. For vitamin D deficient infants 0–1 years old, a treatment with 2000 IU/day of vitamin D_2 or vitamin D_3 or with 50,000 IU of vitamin D_2 or vitamin D_3 once weekly for 6 weeks was suggested, followed by maintenance therapy of 400–1000 IU/day. For vitamin D deficient children aged 1–18 years who are vitamin D deficient, treatment with 2000 IU/day of vitamin D_2 or vitamin D_3 or with 50,000 IU of vitamin D_2 once a week, both for at least 6 weeks, was suggested, followed by maintenance therapy of 600–1000 IU/day. Vitamin D deficient adults should be treated with 50,000 IU of vitamin D_2 or vitamin D_3 once a week for 8 weeks or with ~6000 IU/day of vitamin D_2 or vitamin D_3, followed by maintenance therapy of 1500–2000 IU/day. In obese patients, patients with malabsorption syndromes, and patients on medications affecting vitamin D metabolism, two to three times higher doses are (at least 6000–10,000 IU/day) of vitamin D to treat vitamin D deficiency are recommended, followed by maintenance therapy of at least 3000–6000 IU/day [16]. This strategy of giving 50,000 IU of vitamin D twice monthly to treat or prevent recurrence of vitamin D deficiency or insufficiency was without any toxicity for up to six years [242] (Figure 7).

Figure 7. (**A**) Mean serum 25-hydroxyvitamin D [25(OH)D] levels in all patients: includes patients treated with 50,000 IU vitamin D_2 every 2 weeks (maintenance therapy, $n = 81$), including those patients with vitamin D insufficiency who were initially treated with 8 weeks of 50,000 IU vitamin D_2 weekly prior to maintenance therapy ($n = 39$). Error bars represent standard error of the mean, mean result over 5 years shown. Time 0 is initiation of treatment, results shown as mean values averaged for 6 month intervals. When mean 25(OH)D in each 6 month group was compared to mean initial 25(OH)D, a significant difference was shown with $p < 0.001$ up until month 43 and $p < 0.001$ when all remaining values after month 43 were compared to mean initial 25(OH)D. (**B**) Mean serum 25(OH)D levels in patients receiving maintenance therapy only: Levels for 37 patients who were vitamin D insufficient (25(OH)D levels <30 ng/mL) and 5 patients who were vitamin D sufficient (25(OH)D levels ≥30 ng/mL) who were treated with maintenance therapy of 50,000 IU vitamin D_2 every two weeks. Error bars represent standard error of the mean, mean result over 5 years shown. Time 0 is initiation of treatment, results shown as mean values averaged for 6 month intervals. When mean 25(OH)D in each 6 month group were compared to mean initial 25(OH)D, a significant difference was shown with $p < 0.001$ up until month 37 and $p < 0.001$ when all remaining values after month 43 were compared to mean initial 25(OH)D. (**C**) Serum calcium levels: Results for all 81 patients who were treated with 50,000 IU of vitamin D_2. Error bars represent standard error of the mean. Time 0 is initiation of treatment, results shown as mean values averaged for 6 month intervals. Normal serum calcium: 8.5–10.2 mg/dL. Note: This figure is reproduced with permission from [242], Copyright © 2009 American Medical Association.

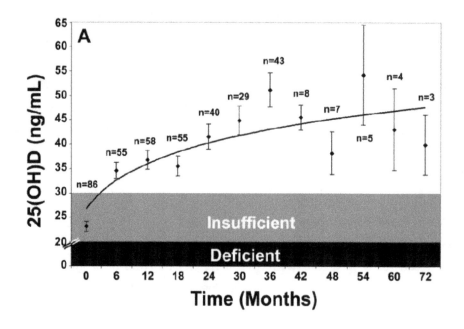

Figure 7. *Cont.*

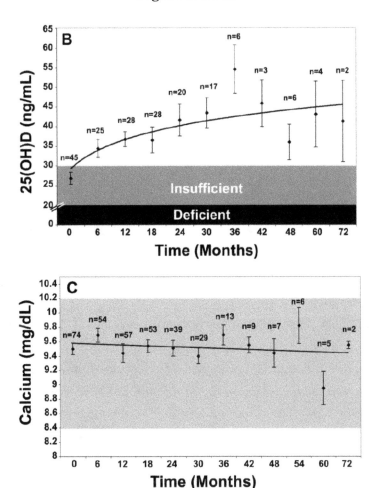

However, certain conditions like granulomatous conditions [243], genetic disorders [244] or rare polymorphisms of enzymes involved in vitamin D metabolism [245] are associated with an increased risk for vitamin D toxicity.

16. Conclusion

What continues to be needed are randomized controlled interventional studies with high power and using sufficiently high doses of vitamin D examining vitamin D's effects on various health outcomes.

However, the present body of evidence of experimental findings, ecological, case-control, retro- and prospective observational and interventional studies is substantial and suggests a pivotal role of vitamin D for a plethora of physiological functions and health outcomes including neuropsychiatric disorders [246], justifying the recommendation to enhance children's and adults' vitamin D status by following recommendations for sensible sun exposure, ingesting foods that contain vitamin D and vitamin D supplementation. Increasing the vitamin D status worldwide in the general adult and children population without rare conditions associated with an increased risk for vitamin D toxicity will help improve their overall health and well-being (Figure 6).

Acknowledgements

This work was supported in part by the UV Foundation (2880 Zanker Road, Suite 203, San Jose, CA 95134, USA) and the Mushroom Council (6620 Fletcher Lane, McLean, VA, USA).

Conflict of Interest

The authors declare no conflict of interest.

References

1. Holick, M. Phylogenetic and Evolutionary Aspects of Vitamin D from Phytoplankton to Humans. In *Verebrate Endocrinology: Fundamentals and Biomedical Implications*; Pang, P.K.T., Schreibman, M.P., Eds.; Academic Press, Inc.: Orlando, FL, USA, 1989.

2. Holick, M.F. Vitamin D: Evolutionary, physiological and health perspectives. *Curr. Drug Targets* **2011**, *12*, 4–18.

3. Yoshida, T.; Stern, P.H. How vitamin D works on bone. *Endocrinol. Metab. Clin. North Am.* **2012**, *41*, 557–569.

4. Sai, A.J.; Walters, R.W.; Fang, X.; Gallagher, J.C. Relationship between vitamin D, parathyroid hormone, and bone health. *J. Clin. Endocrinol. Metab.* **2011**, *96*, E436–E446.

5. Lips, P.; van Schoor, N.M. The effect of vitamin D on bone and osteoporosis. *Best Pract. Res. Clin. Endocrinol. Metab.* **2011**, *25*, 585–591.

6. Nagpal, S.; Na, S.; Rathnachalam, R. Noncalcemic actions of vitamin D receptor ligands. *Endocr. Rev.* **2005**, *26*, 662–687.

7. Holick, M.F. Vitamin D deficiency. *N. Engl. J. Med.* **2007**, *357*, 266–281.

8. Jablonski, N.G.; Chaplin, G. The evolution of human skin coloration. *J. Hum. Evol.* **2000**, *39*, 57–106.

9. Ergocalciferol. Available online: http://www.chemspider.com/Chemical-Structure.4444351.html (accessed on 21 December 2012).

10. Cholecalciferol. Available online: http://www.chemspider.com/Chemical-Structure.9058792.html (accessed on 21 December 2012).

11. Holick, M.F.; Tian, X.Q.; Allen, M. Evolutionary importance for the membrane enhancement of the production of vitamin D_3 in the skin of poikilothermic animals. *Proc. Natl. Acad. Sci. USA* **1995**, *92*, 3124–3126.

12. Tian, X.Q.; Chen, T.C.; Matsuoka, L.Y.; Wortsman, J.; Holick, M.F. Kinetic and thermodynamic studies of the conversion of previtamin D_3 to vitamin D_3 in human skin. *J. Biol. Chem.* **1993**, *268*, 14888–14892.

13. Chen, T.; Lu, Z.; Holick, M. Photobiology of Vitamin D. In *Vitamin D: Physiology, Molecular Biology, and Clinical Applications*, 2nd ed.; Holick, M.F., Ed.; Humana Press: New York, NY, USA, 2010; pp. 35–60.

14. Holick, M.F. Resurrection of vitamin D deficiency and rickets. *J. Clin. Invest.* **2006**, *116*, 2062–2072.

15. Jones, G. Phosphorus metabolism and management in chronic kidney disease: Expanding role for vitamin D in chronic kidney disease: Importance of blood 25-OH-D levels and extra-renal 1α-hydroxylase in the classical and nonclassical actions of 1α,25-dihydroxyvitamin D$_3$. *Semin. Dial.* **2007**, *20*, 316–324.

16. Holick, M.F.; Binkley, N.C.; Bischoff-Ferrari, H.A.; Gordon, C.M.; Hanley, D.A.; Heaney, R.P.; Murad, M.H.; Weaver, C.M. Evaluation, treatment, and prevention of vitamin D deficiency: An endocrine society clinical practice guideline. *J. Clin. Endocrinol. Metab.* **2011**, *96*, 1911–1930.

17. Holick, M.F. Vitamin D and health: Evolution, biologic functions, and recommended dietary intakes for vitamin D. *Clin. Rev. Bone Miner. Metab.* **2009**, *7*, 2–19.

18. Bosworth, C.R.; Levin, G.; Robinson-Cohen, C.; Hoofnagle, A.N.; Ruzinski, J.; Young, B.; Schwartz, S.M.; Himmelfarb, J.; Kestenbaum, B.; de Boer, I.H. The serum 24,25-dihydroxyvitamin D concentration, a marker of vitamin D catabolism, is reduced in chronic kidney disease. *Kidney Int.* **2012**, *92*, 693–700.

19. Christakos, S.; Dhawan, P.; Porta, A.; Mady, L.J.; Seth, T. Vitamin D and intestinal calcium absorption. *Mol. Cell. Endocrinol.* **2011**, *347*, 25–29.

20. Christakos, S. Recent advances in our understanding of 1,25-dihydroxyvitamin D$_3$ regulation of intestinal calcium absorption. *Arch. Biochem. Biophys.* **2012**, *523*, 73–76.

21. Holick, M.F. The vitamin D deficiency pandemic: A forgotten hormone important for health. *Public Health Rev.* **2010**, *32*, 267–283.

22. Holick, M.F. Environmental factors that influence the cutaneous production of vitamin D. *Am. J. Clin. Nutr.* **1995**, *61*, 638S–645S.

23. Holick, M.F.; Chen, T.C. Vitamin D deficiency: A worldwide problem with health consequences. *Am. J. Clin. Nutr.* **2008**, *87*, 1080S–1086S.

24. Urbain, P.; Singler, F.; Ihorst, G.; Biesalski, H.K.; Bertz, H. Bioavailability of vitamin D$_2$ from UV-B-irradiated button mushrooms in healthy adults deficient in serum 25-hydroxyvitamin D: A randomized controlled trial. *Eur. J. Clin. Nutr.* **2011**, *65*, 965–971.

25. Mau, J.-L.; Chen, P.-R.; Yang, J.-H. Ultraviolet irradiation increased vitamin D$_2$ content in edible mushrooms. *J. Agric. Food Chem.* **1998**, *46*, 5269–5272.

26. Tangpricha, V.; Koutkia, P.; Rieke, S.M.; Chen, T.C.; Perez, A.A.; Holick, M.F. Fortification of orange juice with vitamin D: A novel approach for enhancing vitamin D nutritional health. *Am. J. Clin. Nutr.* **2003**, *77*, 1478–1483.

27. Hypercalcaemia in infants and vitamin D. *Br. Med. J.* **1956**, *2*, 149.

28. Holick, M.F. Sunlight and vitamin D for bone health and prevention of autoimmune diseases, cancers, and cardiovascular disease. *Am. J. Clin. Nutr.* **2004**, *80*, 1678S–1688S.

29. Biancuzzo, R.M.; Young, A.; Bibuld, D.; Cai, M.H.; Winter, M.R.; Klein, E.K.; Ameri, A.; Reitz, R.; Salameh, W.; Chen, T.C.; Holick, M.F. Fortification of orange juice with vitamin D$_2$ or vitamin D$_3$ is as effective as an oral supplement in maintaining vitamin D status in adults. *Am. J. Clin. Nutr.* **2010**, *91*, 1621–1626.

30. Armas, L.A.G.; Hollis, B.W.; Heaney, R.P. Vitamin D$_2$ is much less effective than vitamin D$_3$ in humans. *J. Clin. Endocrinol. Metab.* **2004**, *89*, 5387–5391.

31. Trang, H.M.; Cole, D.E.; Rubin, L.A.; Pierratos, A.; Siu, S.; Vieth, R. Evidence that vitamin D_3 increases serum 25-hydroxyvitamin D more efficiently than does vitamin D_2. *Am. J. Clin. Nutr.* **1998**, *68*, 854–858.

32. Houghton, L.A.; Vieth, R. The case against ergocalciferol (vitamin D_2) as a vitamin supplement. *Am. J. Clin. Nutr.* **2006**, *84*, 694–697.

33. Romagnoli, E.; Mascia, M.L.; Cipriani, C.; Fassino, V.; Mazzei, F.; D'Erasmo, E.; Carnevale, V.; Scillitani, A.; Minisola, S. Short and long-term variations in serum calciotropic hormones after a single very large dose of ergocalciferol (vitamin D_2) or cholecalciferol (vitamin D_3) in the elderly. *J. Clin. Endocrinol. Metab.* **2008**, *93*, 3015–3020.

34. Heaney, R.P.; Recker, R.R.; Grote, J.; Horst, R.L.; Armas, L.A.G. Vitamin D_3 is more potent than vitamin D_2 in humans. *J. Clin. Endocrinol. Metab.* **2011**, *96*, E447–E452.

35. Leventis, P.; Kiely, P.D. The tolerability and biochemical effects of high-dose bolus vitamin D_2 and D_3 supplementation in patients with vitamin D insufficiency. *Scand. J. Rheumatol.* **2009**, *38*, 149–153.

36. Tripkovic, L.; Lambert, H.; Hart, K.; Smith, C.P.; Bucca, G.; Penson, S.; Chope, G.; Hyppönen, E.; Berry, J.; Vieth, R.; Lanham-New, S. Comparison of vitamin D_2 and vitamin D_3 supplementation in raising serum 25-hydroxyvitamin D status: A systematic review and meta-analysis. *Am. J. Clin. Nutr.* **2012**, *95*, 1357–1364.

37. Holick, M.F.; Biancuzzo, R.M.; Chen, T.C.; Klein, E.K.; Young, A.; Bibuld, D.; Reitz, R.; Salameh, W.; Ameri, A.; Tannenbaum, A.D. Vitamin D_2 is as effective as vitamin D_3 in maintaining circulating concentrations of 25-hydroxyvitamin D. *J. Clin. Endocrinol. Metab.* **2008**, *93*, 677–681.

38. Thacher, T.D.; Obadofin, M.O.; O'Brien, K.O.; Abrams, S.A. The Effect of vitamin D_2 and vitamin D_3 on intestinal calcium absorption in Nigerian children with rickets. *J. Clin. Endocrinol. Metab.* **2009**, *94*, 3314–3321.

39. Gordon, C.M.; Williams, A.L.; Feldman, H.A.; May, J.; Sinclair, L.; Vasquez, A.; Cox, J.E. Treatment of hypovitaminosis D in infants and toddlers. *J. Clin. Endocrinol. Metab.* **2008**, *93*, 2716–2721.

40. Rapuri, P.B.; Gallagher, J.C.; Haynatzki, G. Effect of vitamins D_2 and D_3 supplement use on serum 25OHD concentration in elderly women in summer and winter. *Calcif. Tissue Int.* **2004**, *74*, 150–156.

41. Hollis, B. Assessment of vitamin D nutritional and hormonal status: What to measure and how to do it. *Calcif. Tissue Int.* **1996**, *58*, 4–5.

42. DeLuca, H.F. Overview of general physiologic features and functions of vitamin D. *Am. J. Clin. Nutr.* **2004**, *80*, 1689S–1696S.

43. Zehnder, D.; Bland, R.; Williams, M.C.; McNinch, R.W.; Howie, A.J.; Stewart, P.M.; Hewison, M. Extrarenal expression of 25-hydroxyvitamin D(3)1 alpha-hydroxylase. *J. Clin. Endocrinol. Metab.* **2001**, *86*, 888–894.

44. Lehmann, B.; Meurer, M. Vitamin D metabolism. *Dermatol. Ther.* **2010**, *23*, 2–12.

45. Ritter, C.S.; Haughey, B.H.; Armbrecht, H.J.; Brown, A.J. Distribution and regulation of the 25-hydroxyvitamin D3 1α-hydroxylase in human parathyroid glands. *J. Steroid Biochem. Mol. Biol.* **2012**, *130*, 73–80.

46. Rosen, C.J.; Adams, J.S.; Bikle, D.D.; Black, D.M.; Demay, M.B.; Manson, J.E.; Murad, M.H.; Kovacs, C.S. The nonskeletal effects of vitamin D: An endocrine society scientific statement. *Endocr. Rev.* **2012**, *33*, 456–492.

47. Carlberg, C.; Bendik, I.; Wyss, A.; Meier, E.; Sturzenbecker, L.J.; Grippo, J.F.; Hunziker, W. Two nuclear signalling pathways for vitamin D. *Nature* **1993**, *361*, 657–660.

48. McKenna, N.J.; Lanz, R.B.; O'Malley, B.W. Nuclear receptor coregulators: Cellular and molecular biology. *Endocr. Rev.* **1999**, *20*, 321–344.

49. Smith, C.L.; O'Malley, B.W. Coregulator function: A key to understanding tissue specificity of selective receptor modulators. *Endocr. Rev.* **2004**, *25*, 45–71.

50. Dunlop, T.W.; Vaisanen, S.; Frank, C.; Carlberg, C. The genes of the coactivator TIF2 and the corepressor SMRT are primary 1alpha,25(OH)2D3 targets. *J. Steroid Biochem. Mol. Biol.* **2004**, *89–90*, 257–260.

51. Fleet, J.C. Vitamin D receptors: Not just in the nucleus anymore. *Nutr. Rev.* **1999**, *57*, 60–62.

52. Norman, A.W. Minireview: Vitamin D receptor: New assignments for an already busy receptor. *Endocrinology* **2006**, *147*, 5542–5548.

53. Institute of Medicine of the National Academies. *Dietary Reference Intakes for Calcium and Vitamin D*; Catharine Ross, A., Taylor, C.L., Yaktine, A.L., Eds.; The National Academy of Sciences: Washington, DC, USA, 2011.

54. Chapuy, M.C.; Schott, A.M.; Garnero, P.; Hans, D.; Delmas, P.D.; Meunier, P.J. Healthy elderly French women living at home have secondary hyperparathyroidism and high bone turnover in winter. EPIDOS Study Group. *J. Clin. Endocrinol. Metab.* **1996**, *81*, 1129–1133.

55. Holick, M.F.; Siris, E.S.; Binkley, N.; Beard, M.K.; Khan, A.; Katzer, J.T.; Petruschke, R.A.; Chen, E.; de Papp, A.E. Prevalence of vitamin D inadequacy among postmenopausal north American women receiving osteoporosis therapy. *J. Clin. Endocrinol. Metab.* **2005**, *90*, 3215–3224.

56. Thomas, M.K.; Lloyd-Jones, D.M.; Thadhani, R.I.; Shaw, A.C.; Deraska, D.J.; Kitch, B.T.; Vamvakas, E.C.; Dick, I.M.; Prince, R.L.; Finkelstein, J.S. Hypovitaminosis D in medical inpatients. *N. Engl. J. Med.* **1998**, *338*, 777–783.

57. Valcour, A.; Blocki, F.; Hawkins, D.M.; Rao, S.D. Effects of age and serum 25-OH-vitamin D on serum parathyroid hormone levels. *J. Clin. Endocrinol. Metab.* **2012**, *97*, 3989–3995.

58. Whiting, S.J.; Langlois, K.A.; Vatanparast, H.; Greene-Finestone, L.S. The vitamin D status of Canadians relative to the 2011 Dietary Reference Intakes: An examination in children and adults with and without supplement use. *Am. J. Clin. Nutr.* **2011**, *94*, 128–135.

59. Hanley, D.A.; Cranney, A.; Jones, G.; Whiting, S.J.; Leslie, W.D.; Cole, D.E.; Atkinson, S.A.; Josse, R.G.; Feldman, S.; Kline, G.A.; Rosen, C. Vitamin D in adult health and disease: A review and guideline statement from Osteoporosis Canada. *CMAJ* **2010**, *182*, E610–E618.

60. Holick, M.F.; Binkley, N.C.; Bischoff-Ferrari, H.A.; Gordon, C.M.; Hanley, D.A.; Heaney, R.P.; Murad, M.H.; Weaver, C.M. Guidelines for preventing and treating vitamin D deficiency and insufficiency revisited. *J. Clin. Endocrinol. Metab.* **2012**, *97*, 1153–1158.

61. Looker, A.C.; Johnson, C.L.; Lacher, D.A.; Pfeiffer, C.M.; Schleicher, R.L.; Sempos, C.T. Vitamin D status: United States, 2001–2006. *NCHS Data Brief* **2011**, *59*, 1–8.

62. Marwaha, R.K.; Tandon, N.; Reddy, D.R.H.; Aggarwal, R.; Singh, R.; Sawhney, R.C.; Saluja, B.; Ganie, M.A.; Singh, S. Vitamin D and bone mineral density status of healthy schoolchildren in northern India. *Am. J. Clin. Nutr.* **2005**, *82*, 477–482.

63. Sachan, A.; Gupta, R.; Das, V.; Agarwal, A.; Awasthi, P.K.; Bhatia, V. High prevalence of vitamin D deficiency among pregnant women and their newborns in northern India. *Am. J. Clin. Nutr.* **2005**, *81*, 1060–1064.

64. Prentice, A.; Schoenmakers, I.; Jones, K.; Jarjou, L.; Goldberg, G. Vitamin D deficiency and its health consequences in Africa. *Clin. Rev. Bone Miner. Metab.* **2009**, *7*, 94–106.

65. Van der Mei, I.A.; Ponsonby, A.L.; Engelsen, O.; Pasco, J.A.; McGrath, J.J.; Eyles, D.W.; Blizzard, L.; Dwyer, T.; Lucas, R.; Jones, G. The high prevalence of vitamin D insufficiency across Australian populations is only partly explained by season and latitude. *Environ. Health Perspect.* **2007**, *115*, 1132–1139.

66. Maeda, S.S.; Kunii, I.S.; Hayashi, L.; Lazaretti-Castro, M. The effect of sun exposure on 25-hydroxyvitamin D concentrations in young healthy subjects living in the city of Sao Paulo, Brazil. *Braz. J. Med. Biol. Res.* **2007**, *40*, 1653–1659.

67. Sedrani, S.H. Low 25-hydroxyvitamin D and normal serum calcium concentrations in Saudi Arabia: Riyadh region. *Ann. Nutr. Metab.* **1984**, *28*, 181–185.

68. El-Hajj Fuleihan, G. Vitamin D Deficiency in the Middle East and Its Health Consequences. In *Vitamin D: Physiology, Molecular Biology, and Clinical Applications*; Holick, M.F., Ed.; Humana Press: New York, NY, USA, 2010; pp. 469–494.

69. Rich-Edwards, J.W.; Ganmaa, D.; Kleinman, K.; Sumberzul, N.; Holick, M.F.; Lkhagvasuren, T.; Dulguun, B.; Burke, A.; Frazier, A.L. Randomized trial of fortified milk and supplements to raise 25-hydroxyvitamin D concentrations in schoolchildren in Mongolia. *Am. J. Clin. Nutr.* **2011**, *94*, 578–584.

70. Rockell, J.; Skeaff, C.; Williams, S.; Green, T. Serum 25-hydroxyvitamin D concentrations of New Zealanders aged 15 years and older. *Osteoporos. Int.* **2006**, *17*, 1382–1389.

71. Prentice, A. Vitamin D deficiency: A global perspective. *Nutr. Rev.* **2008**, *66*, S153–S164.

72. Marks, J.; Srai, S.K.; Biber, J.; Murer, H.; Unwin, R.J.; Debnam, E.S. Intestinal phosphate absorption and the effect of vitamin D: A comparison of rats with mice. *Exp. Physiol.* **2006**, *91*, 531–537.

73. Chen, T.C.; Castillo, L.; Korycka-Dahl, M.; DeLuca, H.F. Role of vitamin D metabolites in phosphate transport of rat intestine. *J. Nutr.* **1974**, *104*, 1056–1060.

74. Segersten, U.; Correa, P.; Hewison, M.; Hellman, P.; Dralle, H.; Carling, T.; Åkerström, G.; Westin, G. 25-Hydroxyvitamin D(3)-1α-hydroxylase expression in normal and pathological parathyroid glands. *J. Clin. Endocrinol. Metab.* **2002**, *87*, 2967–2972.

75. Ritter, C.S.; Armbrecht, H.J.; Slatopolsky, E.; Brown, A.J. 25-Hydroxyvitamin D3 suppresses PTH synthesis and secretion by bovine parathyroid cells. *Kidney Int.* **2006**, *70*, 654–659.

76. Rajakumar, K. Vitamin D, cod-liver oil, sunlight, and rickets: A historical perspective. *Pediatrics* **2003**, *112*, e132–e135.

77. Mozołowski, W. Jędrzej Sniadecki (1768–1838) on the cure of rickets. *Nature* **1939**, *143*, 121.

78. Palm, T.A. The geographical distribution and etiology of rickets. *Practitioner* **1890**, *45*, 270–342.

79. Huldschinsky, K. Heilung von Rachitis durch künstliche Höhensonne. *Dtsch. Med. Wochenschr.* **1919**, *45*, 712–713.

80. Huldschinsky, K. *The Ultra-Violet Light Treatment of Rickets*; Alpine Press: Newark, NJ, USA, 1928; pp. 3–19.

81. Mellanby, T. The part played by an "accessory factor" in the production of experimental rickets. *J. Physiol.* **1918**, *52*, 11–14.

82. McCollum, E.F.; Simmonds, N.; Becker, J.E.; Shipley, P.G. Studies on experimental rickets; and experimental demonstration of the existence of a vitamin which promotes calcium deposition. *J. Biol. Chem.* **1922**, *53*, 293–312.

83. Hess, A.F.; Weinstock, M. Antirachitic properties imparted to inert fluids and to green vegetables by ultraviolet irradiation. *J. Biol. Chem.* **1924**, *62*, 301–313.

84. Steenbock, H.; Black, A. The reduction of growth-promoting and calcifying properties in a ration by exposure to ultraviolet light. *J. Biol. Chem.* **1924**, *61*, 408–422.

85. Cooper, C.; Javaid, K.; Westlake, S.; Harvey, N.; Dennison, E. Developmental origins of osteoporotic fracture: The role of maternal vitamin D insufficiency. *J. Nutr.* **2005**, *135*, 2728S–2734S.

86. Javaid, M.K.; Crozier, S.R.; Harvey, N.C.; Gale, C.R.; Dennison, E.M.; Boucher, B.J.; Arden, N.K.; Godfrey, K.M.; Cooper, C. Maternal vitamin D status during pregnancy and childhood bone mass at age 9 years: A longitudinal study. *Lancet* **2006**, *367*, 36–43.

87. Holick, M.F. Vitamin D and bone health. *J. Nutr.* **1996**, *126*, 1159S–1164S.

88. Adams, J.S.; Hewison, M. Update in vitamin D. *J. Clin. Endocrinol. Metab.* **2010**, *95*, 471–478.

89. Bischoff-Ferrari, H.A.; Kiel, D.P.; Dawson-Hughes, B.; Orav, J.E.; Li, R.; Spiegelman, D.; Dietrich, T.; Willett, W.C. Dietary calcium and serum 25-hydroxyvitamin D status in relation to BMD among U.S. adults. *J. Bone Miner. Res.* **2009**, *24*, 935–942.

90. Delling, G. *Endokrine Osteopathien; Morphologie, Histomorphometrie und Differentialdiagnose. Endocrine Bone Diseases; Morphology, Histomorphometry and Differential Diagnosis*; Fischer: Stuttgart, Germany, 1975.

91. Priemel, M.; von Domarus, C.; Klatte, T.O.; Kessler, S.; Schlie, J.; Meier, S.; Proksch, N.; Pastor, F.; Netter, C.; Streichert, T.; *et al.* Bone mineralization defects and vitamin D deficiency: Histomorphometric analysis of iliac crest bone biopsies and circulating 25-hydroxyvitamin D in 675 patients. *J. Bone Miner. Res.* **2010**, *25*, 305–312.

92. Holick, M.F. Vitamin D: Importance in the prevention of cancers, type 1 diabetes, heart disease, and osteoporosis. *Am. J. Clin. Nutr.* **2004**, *79*, 362–371.

93. Holick, M.F. Optimal vitamin D status for the prevention and treatment of osteoporosis. *Drugs Aging* **2007**, *24*, 1017–1029.

94. Becker, D.; Kilgore, M.; Morrisey, M. The societal burden of osteoporosis. *Curr. Rheumatol. Rep.* **2010**, *12*, 186–191.

95. Khosla, S.; Amin, S.; Orwoll, E. Osteoporosis in Men. *Endocr. Rev.* **2008**, *29*, 441–464.

96. Dawson-Hughes, B.; Heaney, R.P.; Holick, M.F.; Lips, P.; Meunier, P.J.; Vieth, R. Estimates of optimal vitamin D status. *Osteoporos. Int.* **2005**, *16*, 713–716.

97. Cauley, J.A.; LaCroix, A.Z.; Wu, L.; Horwitz, M.; Danielson, M.E.; Bauer, D.C.; Lee, J.S.; Jackson, R.D.; Robbins, J.A.; Wu, C.; *et al.* Serum 25-hydroxyvitamin D concentrations and risk for hip fractures. *Ann. Int. Med.* **2008**, *149*, 242–250.

98. Bischoff-Ferrari, H.A.; Willett, W.C.; Orav, E.J.; Lips, P.; Meunier, P.J.; Lyons, R.A.; Flicker, L.; Wark, J.; Jackson, R.D.; Cauley, J.A.; *et al.* A pooled analysis of vitamin D dose requirements for fracture prevention. *N. Engl. J. Med.* **2012**, *367*, 40–49.

99. Chapuy, M.C.; Arlot, M.E.; Duboeuf, F.; Brun, J.; Crouzet, B.; Arnaud, S.; Delmas, P.D.; Meunier, P.J. Vitamin D_3 and calcium to prevent hip fractures in elderly women. *N. Engl. J. Med.* **1992**, *327*, 1637–1642.

100. Grant, A.M.; Avenell, A.; Campbell, M.K.; McDonald, A.M.; MacLennan, G.S.; McPherson, G.C.; Anderson, F.H.; Cooper, C.; Francis, R.M.; Donaldson, C.; *et al.* Null Oral vitamin D_3 and calcium for secondary prevention of low-trauma fractures in elderly people (Randomised Evaluation of Calcium Or vitamin D, RECORD): A randomised placebo-controlled trial. *Lancet* **2005**, *365*, 1621–1628.

101. Dawson-Hughes, B.; Harris, S.S.; Krall, E.A.; Dallal, G.E. Effect of calcium and vitamin D supplementation on bone density in men and women 65 years of age or older. *N. Engl. J. Med.* **1997**, *337*, 670–676.

102. Lips, P.; Graafmans, W.C.; Ooms, M.E.; Bezemer, P.D.; Bouter, L.M. Vitamin D supplementation and fracture incidence in elderly persons. A randomized, placebo-controlled clinical trial. *Ann. Int. Med.* **1996**, *124*, 400–406.

103. Meyer, H.E.; Smedshaug, G.B.; Kvaavik, E.; Falch, J.A.; Tverdal, A.; Pedersen, J.I. Can vitamin D supplementation reduce the risk of fracture in the elderly? A randomized controlled trial. *J. Bone Miner. Res.* **2002**, *17*, 709–715.

104. Jackson, R.D.; LaCroix, A.Z.; Gass, M.; Wallace, R.B.; Robbins, J.; Lewis, C.E.; Bassford, T.; Beresford, S.A.A.; Black, H.R.; Blanchette, P.; *et al.* Calcium plus vitamin D supplementation and the risk of fractures. *N. Engl. J. Med.* **2006**, *354*, 669–683.

105. Pfeifer, M.; Begerow, B.; Minne, H.W.; Abrams, C.; Nachtigall, D.; Hansen, C. Effects of a short-term vitamin D and calcium supplementation on body sway and secondary hyperparathyroidism in elderly women. *J. Bone Miner. Res.* **2000**, *15*, 1113–1118.

106. Pfeifer, M.; Begerow, B.; Minne, H.W.; Suppan, K.; Fahrleitner-Pammer, A.; Dobnig, H. Effects of a long-term vitamin D and calcium supplementation on falls and parameters of muscle function in community-dwelling older individuals. *Osteoporos. Int.* **2009**, *20*, 315–322.

107. Bischoff-Ferrari, H. Relevance of vitamin D in muscle health. *Rev. Endocr. Metab. Disord.* **2012**, *13*, 71–77.

108. Srikuea, R.; Zhang, X.; Park-Sarge, O.-K.; Esser, K.A. VDR and CYP27B1 are expressed in C2C12 cells and regenerating skeletal muscle: Potential role in suppression of myoblast proliferation. *Am. J. Physiol. Cell Physiol.* **2012**, *303*, C396–C405.

109. Ceglia, L.; Harris, S.S. Vitamin D and its role in skeletal muscle. *Calcif. Tissue Int.* **2012**, doi:10.1007/s00223-012-9645-y.

110. Simpson, R.U.; Thomas, G.A.; Arnold, A.J. Identification of 1,25-dihydroxyvitamin D3 receptors and activities in muscle. *J. Biol. Chem.* **1985**, *260*, 8882–8891.

111. Bischoff, H.A.; Borchers, M.; Gudat, F.; Duermueller, U.; Theiler, R.; Stähelin, H.B.; Dick, W. *In situ* detection of 1,25-dihydroxyvitamin D3 receptor in human skeletal muscle tissue. *Histochem. J.* **2001**, *33*, 19–24.

112. Costa, E.M.; Blau, H.M.; Feldman, D. 1,25-Dihydroxyvitamin D3 receptors and hormonal responses in cloned human skeletal muscle cells. *Endocrinology* **1986**, *119*, 2214–2220.

113. Boland, R.; Norman, A.; Ritz, E.; Hasselbach, W. Presence of a 1,25-dihydroxy-vitamin D3 receptor in chick skeletal muscle myoblasts. *Biochem. Biophys. Res. Commun.* **1985**, *128*, 305–311.

114. Pfeifer, M.; Begerow, B.; Minne, H.W. Vitamin D and muscle function. *Osteoporos. Int.* **2002**, *13*, 187–194.

115. Janssen, H.C.; Samson, M.M.; Verhaar, H.J. Vitamin D deficiency, muscle function, and falls in elderly people. *Am. J. Clin. Nutr.* **2002**, *75*, 611–615.

116. Lou, Y.-R.; Molnár, F.; Peräkylä, M.; Qiao, S.; Kalueff, A.V.; St-Arnaud, R.; Carlberg, C.; Tuohimaa, P. 25-Hydroxyvitamin D(3) is an agonistic vitamin D receptor ligand. *J. Steroid Biochem. Mol. Biol.* **2010**, *118*, 162–170.

117. Wang, Y.; DeLuca, H.F. Is the vitamin D receptor found in muscle? *Endocrinology* **2011**, *152*, 354–363.

118. Schott, G.D.; Wills, M.R. Muscle weakness in osteomalacia. *Lancet* **1976**, *307*, 626–629.

119. Bischoff-Ferrari, H.A.; Giovannucci, E.; Willett, W.C.; Dietrich, T.; Dawson-Hughes, B. Estimation of optimal serum concentrations of 25-hydroxyvitamin D for multiple health outcomes. *Am. J. Clin. Nutr.* **2006**, *84*, 18–28.

120. Glerup, H.; Mikkelsen, K.; Poulsen, L.; Hass, E.; Overbeck, S.; Andersen, H.; Charles, P.; Eriksen, E.F. Hypovitaminosis D myopathy without biochemical signs of osteomalacic bone involvement. *Calcif. Tissue Int.* **2000**, *66*, 419–424.

121. Wicherts, I.S.; van Schoor, N.M.; Boeke, A.J.P.; Visser, M.; Deeg, D.J.H.; Smit, J.; Knol, D.L.; Lips, P. Vitamin D status predicts physical performance and its decline in older persons. *J. Clin. Endocrinol. Metab.* **2007**, *92*, 2058–2065.

122. Bischoff-Ferrari, H.A.; Dietrich, T.; Orav, E.J.; Hu, F.B.; Zhang, Y.; Karlson, E.W.; Dawson-Hughes, B. Higher 25-hydroxyvitamin D concentrations are associated with better lower-extremity function in both active and inactive persons aged ≥60 y. *Am. J. Clin. Nutr.* **2004**, *80*, 752–758.

123. Bischoff, H.A.; Stähelin, H.B.; Dick, W.; Akos, R.; Knecht, M.; Salis, C.; Nebiker, M.; Theiler, R.; Pfeifer, M.; Begerow, B.; *et al.* Effects of vitamin D and calcium supplementation on falls: A randomized controlled trial. *J. Bone Miner. Res.* **2003**, *18*, 343–351.

124. Bischoff-Ferrari, H.; Conzelmann, M.; Stähelin, H.; Dick, W.; Carpenter, M.; Adkin, A.; Theiler, R.; Pfeifer, M.; Allum, J. Is fall prevention by vitamin D mediated by a change in postural or dynamic balance? *Osteoporos. Int.* **2006**, *17*, 656–663.

125. Broe, K.E.; Chen, T.C.; Weinberg, J.; Bischoff-Ferrari, H.A.; Holick, M.F.; Kiel, D.P. A higher dose of vitamin D reduces the risk of falls in nursing home residents: A randomized, multiple-dose study. *J. Am. Geriatr. Soc.* **2007**, *55*, 234–239.

126. Bischoff-Ferrari, H.A.; Dawson-Hughes, B.; Staehelin, H.B.; Orav, J.E.; Stuck, A.E.; Theiler, R.; Wong, J.B.; Egli, A.; Kiel, D.P.; Henschkowski, J. Fall prevention with supplemental and active

forms of vitamin D: A meta-analysis of randomised controlled trials. *BMJ* **2009**, *339*, doi:10.1136/bmj.b3692.

127. Apperly, F.L. The relation of solar radiation to cancer mortality in north America. *Cancer Res.* **1941**, *1*, 191–195.

128. Garland, C.F.; Garland, F.F. Do sunlight and vitamin D reduce the likelihood of colon cancer? *Int. J. Epidemiol.* **1980**, *9*, 227–231.

129. Grant, W.B. Ecological studies of the UVB-vitamin D-cancer hypothesis. *Anticancer Res.* **2012**, *32*, 223–236.

130. Drake, M.T.; Maurer, M.J.; Link, B.K.; Habermann, T.M.; Ansell, S.M.; Micallef, I.N.; Kelly, J.L.; Macon, W.R.; Nowakowski, G.S.; Inwards, D.J.; *et al.* Vitamin D insufficiency and prognosis in non-Hodgkin's lymphoma. *J. Clin. Oncol.* **2010**, *28*, 4191–4198.

131. Freedman, D.M.; Looker, A.C.; Chang, S.-C.; Graubard, B.I. Prospective study of serum vitamin D and cancer mortality in the United States. *J. Natl. Cancer Inst.* **2007**, *99*, 1594–1602.

132. Garland, C.F.; Garland, F.C.; Shaw, E.K.; Comstock, G.W.; Helsing, K.J.; Gorham, E.D. Serum 25-hydroxyvitamin D and colon cancer: Eight-year prospective study. *Lancet* **1989**, *334*, 1176–1178.

133. Garland, C.; Shekelle, R.B.; Barrett-Connor, E.; Criqui, M.H.; Rossof, A.H.; Paul, O. Dietary vitamin D and calcium and risk of colorectal cancer: A 19-year prospective study in men. *Lancet* **1985**, *1*, 307–309.

134. Garland, C.F.; Garland, F.C.; Gorham, E.D.; Lipkin, M.; Newmark, H.; Mohr, S.B.; Holick, M.F. The role of itamin D in cancer prevention. *Am. J. Public Health* **2006**, *96*, 252–261.

135. Giovannucci, E.; Liu, Y.; Rimm, E.B.; Hollis, B.W.; Fuchs, C.S.; Stampfer, M.J.; Willett, W.C. Prospective study of predictors of vitamin D status and cancer incidence and mortality in men. *J. Natl. Cancer Inst.* **2006**, *98*, 451–459.

136. John, E.M.; Schwartz, G.G.; Dreon, D.M.; Koo, J. Vitamin D and breast cancer risk: The NHANES I Epidemiologic Follow-up Study, 1971–1975 to 1992. National Health and Nutrition Examination Survey. *Cancer Epidemiol. Biomarkers Prev.* **1999**, *8*, 399–406.

137. Lappe, J.M.; Travers-Gustafson, D.; Davies, K.M.; Recker, R.R.; Heaney, R.P. Vitamin D and calcium supplementation reduces cancer risk: Results of a randomized trial. *Am. J. Clin. Nutr.* **2007**, *85*, 1586–1591.

138. Manson, J.E.; Mayne, S.T.; Clinton, S.K. Vitamin D and prevention of cancer—Ready for prime time? *N. Engl. J. Med.* **2011**, *364*, 1385–1387.

139. Shin, M.-H.; Holmes, M.D.; Hankinson, S.E.; Wu, K.; Colditz, G.A.; Willett, W.C. Intake of dairy products, calcium, and vitamin D and risk of breast cancer. *J. Natl. Cancer Inst.* **2002**, *94*, 1301–1310.

140. Feskanich, D.; Ma, J.; Fuchs, C.S.; Kirkner, G.J.; Hankinson, S.E.; Hollis, B.W.; Giovannucci, E.L. Plasma vitamin D metabolites and risk of colorectal cancer in women. *Cancer Epidemiol. Biomarkers Prev.* **2004**, *13*, 1502–1508.

141. Krishnan, A.V.; Feldman, D. Mechanisms of the anti-cancer and anti-inflammatory actions of vitamin D. *Annu. Rev. Pharmacol. Toxicol.* **2011**, *51*, 311–336.

142. Fleet, J.C.; Desmet, M.; Johnson, R.; Li, Y. Vitamin D and cancer: A review of molecular mechanisms. *Biochem. J.* **2012**, *441*, 61–76.

143. Vazirnia, A.; Liu, P.T. Vitamin D and the Innate Immune Response. In *Vitamin D and the Lung*; Litonjua, A.A., Ed.; Humana Press: New York, NY, USA, 2012; pp. 59–84.

144. Campbell, G.R.; Spector, S.A. Autophagy induction by vitamin D inhibits both *Mycobacterium tuberculosis* and human immunodeficiency virus type 1. *Autophagy* **2012**, *8*, 1523–1525.

145. Liu, P.T.; Stenger, S.; Li, H.; Wenzel, L.; Tan, B.H.; Krutzik, S.R.; Ochoa, M.T.; Schauber, J.; Wu, K.; Meinken, C.; *et al.* Toll-like receptor triggering of a vitamin D-mediated human antimicrobial response. *Science* **2006**, *311*, 1770–1773.

146. Sly, L.M.; Lopez, M.; Nauseef, W.M.; Reiner, N.E. 1α,25-Dihydroxyvitamin D$_3$-induced monocyte antimycobacterial activity is regulated by phosphatidylinositol 3-kinase and mediated by the NADPH-dependent phagocyte oxidase. *J. Biol. Chem.* **2001**, *276*, 35482–35493.

147. Baeke, F.; Takiishi, T.; Korf, H.; Gysemans, C.; Mathieu, C. Vitamin D: Modulator of the immune system. *Curr. Opin. Pharmacol.* **2010**, *10*, 482–496.

148. Pilz, S.; Tomaschitz, A.; März, W.; Drechsler, C.; Ritz, E.; Zittermann, A.; Cavalier, E.; Pieber, T.R.; Lappe, J.M.; Grant, W.B.; *et al.* Vitamin D, cardiovascular disease and mortality. *Clin. Endocrinol.* **2011**, *75*, 575–584.

149. Li, Y.C.; Qiao, G.; Uskokovic, M.; Xiang, W.; Zheng, W.; Kong, J. Vitamin D: A negative endocrine regulator of the renin-angiotensin system and blood pressure. *J. Steroid Biochem. Mol. Biol.* **2004**, *89–90*, 387–392.

150. Wolden-Kirk, H.; Overbergh, L.; Christesen, H.T.; Brusgaard, K.; Mathieu, C. Vitamin D and diabetes: Its importance for beta cell and immune function. *Mol. Cell. Endocrinol.* **2011**, *347*, 106–120.

151. Russo, A.; Terrasi, M.; Agnese, V.; Santini, D.; Bazan, V. Apoptosis: A relevant tool for anticancer therapy. *Ann. Oncol.* **2006**, *17*, vii115–vii123.

152. Dunn, G.P.; Old, L.J.; Schreiber, R.D. The Immunobiology of cancer immunosurveillance and immunoediting. *Immunity* **2004**, *21*, 137–148.

153. Kerr, J.F.R.; Winterford, C.M.; Harmon, B.V. Apoptosis. Its significance in cancer and cancer therapy. *Cancer* **1994**, *73*, 2013–2026.

154. Blutt, S.E.; McDonnell, T.J.; Polek, T.C.; Weigel, N.L. Calcitriol-induced apoptosis in LNCaP cells is blocked by overexpression of Bcl-2. *Endocrinology* **2000**, *141*, 10–17.

155. Deeb, K.K.; Trump, D.L.; Johnson, C.S. Vitamin D signalling pathways in cancer: Potential for anticancer therapeutics. *Nat. Rev. Cancer* **2007**, *7*, 684–700.

156. Rohan, J.N.P.; Weigel, N.L. 1Alpha,25-dihydroxyvitamin D$_3$ reduces c-Myc expression, inhibiting proliferation and causing G1 accumulation in C4-2 prostate cancer cells. *Endocrinology* **2009**, *150*, 2046–2054.

157. Hawk, E.T.; Viner, J.L.; Dannenberg, A.; DuBois, R.N. COX-2 in cancer—A player that's defining the rules. *J. Natl. Cancer Inst.* **2002**, *94*, 545–546.

158. Koli, K.; Keski-Oja, J. 1Alpha,25-dihydroxyvitamin D$_3$ and its analogues down-regulate cell invasion-associated proteases in cultured malignant cells. *Cell Growth Differ.* **2000**, *11*, 221–229.

159. Peña, C.; García, J.M.; Silva, J.; García, V.; Rodríguez, R.; Alonso, I.; Millán, I.; Salas, C.; de Herreros, A.G.; Muñoz, A.; Bonilla, F. E-cadherin and vitamin D receptor regulation by SNAIL and ZEB1 in colon cancer: Clinicopathological correlations. *Hum. Mol. Genet.* **2005**, *14*, 3361–3370.

160. Grandi, N.C.; Breitling, L.P.; Brenner, H. Vitamin D and cardiovascular disease: Systematic review and meta-analysis of prospective studies. *Prev. Med.* **2010**, *51*, 228–233.

161. Vacek, J.L.; Vanga, S.R.; Good, M.; Lai, S.M.; Lakkireddy, D.; Howard, P.A. Vitamin D deficiency and supplementation and relation to cardiovascular health. *Am. J. Cardiol.* **2012**, *109*, 359–363.

162. Wang, T.J.; Pencina, M.J.; Booth, S.L.; Jacques, P.F.; Ingelsson, E.; Lanier, K.; Benjamin, E.J.; D'Agostino, R.B.; Wolf, M.; Vasan, R.S. Vitamin D deficiency and risk of cardiovascular disease. *Circulation* **2008**, *117*, 503–511.

163. Eaton, C.B.; Young, A.; Allison, M.A.; Robinson, J.; Martin, L.W.; Kuller, L.H.; Johnson, K.C.; Curb, J.D.; van Horn, L.; McTiernan, A.; *et al.* Prospective association of vitamin D concentrations with mortality in postmenopausal women: Results from the Women's Health Initiative (WHI). *Am. J. Clin. Nutr.* **2011**, *94*, 1471–1478.

164. Anderson, J.L.; May, H.T.; Horne, B.D.; Bair, T.L.; Hall, N.L.; Carlquist, J.F.; Lappé, D.L.; Muhlestein, J.B. Relation of vitamin D deficiency to cardiovascular risk factors, disease status, and incident events in a general healthcare population. *Am. J. Cardiol.* **2010**, *106*, 963–968.

165. Sun, Q.; Pan, A.; Hu, F.B.; Manson, J.E.; Rexrode, K.M. 25-Hydroxyvitamin D levels and the risk of stroke. *Stroke* **2012**, *43*, 1470–1477.

166. Reid, I.R.; Bolland, M.J. Role of vitamin D deficiency in cardiovascular disease. *Heart* **2012**, *98*, 609–614.

167. Tall, A.R. Exercise to reduce cardiovascular risk—How much is enough? *N. Engl. J. Med.* **2002**, *347*, 1522–1524.

168. Wilson, P.W.; D'Agostino, R.B.; Sullivan, L.; Parise, H.; Kannel, W.B. Overweight and obesity as determinants of cardiovascular risk: The Framingham experience. *Arch. Intern. Med.* **2002**, *162*, 1867–1872.

169. Wortsman, J.; Matsuoka, L.Y.; Chen, T.C.; Lu, Z.; Holick, M.F. Decreased bioavailability of vitamin D in obesity. *Am. J. Clin. Nutr.* **2000**, *72*, 690–693.

170. Drincic, A.T.; Armas, L.A.G.; van Diest, E.E.; Heaney, R.P. Volumetric dilution, rather than sequestration best explains the low vitamin D status of obesity. *Obesity* **2012**, *20*, 1444–1448.

171. Burgaz, A.; Orsini, N.; Larsson, S.C.; Wolk, A. Blood 25-hydroxyvitamin D concentration and hypertension: A meta-analysis. *J. Hypertens.* **2011**, *29*, 636–645.

172. Witham, M.D.; Nadir, M.A.; Struthers, A.D. Effect of vitamin D on blood pressure: A systematic review and meta-analysis. *J. Hypertens.* **2009**, *27*, 1948–1954.

173. Wu, S.H.; Ho, S.C.; Zhong, L. Effects of vitamin D supplementation on blood pressure. *South Med. J.* **2010**, *103*, 729–737.

174. Elamin, M.B.; Abu Elnour, N.O.; Elamin, K.B.; Fatourechi, M.M.; Alkatib, A.A.; Almandoz, J.P.; Liu, H.; Lane, M.A.; Mullan, R.J.; Hazem, A.; *et al.* Vitamin D and cardiovascular outcomes: A systematic review and meta-analysis. *J. Clin. Endocrinol. Metab.* **2011**, *96*, 1931–1942.

175. Krause, R.; Bühring, M.; Hopfenmüller, W.; Holick, M.F.; Sharma, A.M. Ultraviolet B and blood pressure. *Lancet* **1998**, *352*, 709–710.

176. Fitzpatrick, L.; Bilezikian, J.; Silverberg, S. Parathyroid hormone and the cardiovascular system. *Curr. Osteoporos. Rep.* **2008**, *6*, 77–83.

177. Mitri, J.; Muraru, M.D.; Pittas, A.G. Vitamin D and type 2 diabetes: A systematic review. *Eur. J. Clin. Nutr.* **2011**, *65*, 1005–1015.

178. Pittas, A.G.; Dawson-Hughes, B.; Li, T.; van Dam, R.M.; Willett, W.C.; Manson, J.E.; Hu, F.B. Vitamin D and calcium intake in relation to type 2 diabetes in women. *Diabetes Care* **2006**, *29*, 650–656.

179. Holick, M.F. Nutrition: D-iabetes and D-eath D-efying vitamin D. *Nat. Rev. Endocrinol.* **2012**, *8*, 388–390.

180. Deleskog, A.; Hilding, A.; Brismar, K.; Hamsten, A.; Efendic, S.; Östenson, C.G. Low serum 25-hydroxyvitamin D level predicts progression to type 2 diabetes in individuals with prediabetes but not with normal glucose tolerance. *Diabetologia* **2012**, *55*, 1668–1678.

181. Antico, A.; Tampoia, M.; Tozzoli, R.; Bizzaro, N. Can supplementation with vitamin D reduce the risk or modify the course of autoimmune diseases? A systematic review of the literature. *Autoimmun. Rev.* **2012**, *12*, 127–136.

182. Ponsonby, A.-L.; McMichael, A.; van der Mei, I. Ultraviolet radiation and autoimmune disease: Insights from epidemiological research. *Toxicology* **2002**, *181–182*, 71–78.

183. Peyrin-Biroulet, L.; Oussalah, A.; Bigard, M.-A. Crohn's disease: The hot hypothesis. *Med. Hypotheses* **2009**, *73*, 94–96.

184. Vieira, V.M.; Hart, J.E.; Webster, T.F.; Weinberg, J.; Puett, R.; Laden, F.; Costenbader, K.H.; Karlson, E.W. Association between residences in U.S. northern latitudes and rheumatoid arthritis: A spatial analysis of the Nurses' Health Study. *Environ. Health Perspect.* **2010**, *118*, 957–961.

185. Mohr, S.; Garland, C.; Gorham, E.; Garland, F. The association between ultraviolet B irradiance, vitamin D status and incidence rates of type 1 diabetes in 51 regions worldwide. *Diabetologia* **2008**, *51*, 1391–1398.

186. Munger, K.L.; Levin, L.I.; Hollis, B.W.; Howard, N.S.; Ascherio, A. Serum 25-hydroxyvitamin D levels and risk of multiple sclerosis. *JAMA* **2006**, *296*, 2832–2838.

187. Burton, J.M.; Kimball, S.; Vieth, R.; Bar-Or, A.; Dosch, H.-M.; Cheung, R.; Gagne, D.; D'Souza, C.; Ursell, M.; O'Connor, P. A phase I/II dose-escalation trial of vitamin D3 and calcium in multiple sclerosis. *Neurology* **2010**, *74*, 1852–1859.

188. Pierrot-Deseilligny, C.; Rivaud-Pechoux, S.; Clerson, P.; de Paz, R.; Souberbielle, J.C. Relationship between 25-OH-D serum level and relapse rate in multiple sclerosis patients before and after vitamin D supplementation. *Ther. Adv. Neurol. Disord.* **2012**, *5*, 187–198.

189. Sørensen, I.M.; Joner, G.; Jenum, P.A.; Eskild, A.; Torjesen, P.A.; Stene, L.C. Maternal serum levels of 25-hydroxy-vitamin D during pregnancy and risk of type 1 diabetes in the offspring. *Diabetes* **2012**, *61*, 175–178.

190. Hyppönen, E.; Läärä, E.; Reunanen, A.; Järvelin, M.-R.; Virtanen, S.M. Intake of vitamin D and risk of type 1 diabetes: A birth-cohort study. *Lancet* **2001**, *358*, 1500–1503.

191. Stene, L.C.; Ulriksen, J.; Magnus, P.; Joner, G. Use of cod liver oil during pregnancy associated with lower risk of Type I diabetes in the offspring. *Diabetologia* **2000**, *43*, 1093–1098.

192. Merlino, L.A.; Curtis, J.; Mikuls, T.R.; Cerhan, J.R.; Criswell, L.A.; Saag, K.G. Vitamin D intake is inversely associated with rheumatoid arthritis: Results from the Iowa Women's Health Study. *Arthritis Rheum.* **2004**, *50*, 72–77.

193. Vogel, A.; Strassburg, C.P.; Manns, M.P. Genetic association of vitamin D receptor polymorphisms with primary biliary cirrhosis and autoimmune hepatitis. *Hepatology* **2002**, *35*, 126–131.

194. Ban, Y.; Taniyama, M.; Ban, Y. Vitamin D receptor gene polymorphism is associated with Graves' disease in the Japanese population. *J. Clin. Endocrinol. Metab.* **2000**, *85*, 4639–4643.

195. Škrabić, V.; Zemunik, T.; Šitum, M.; Terzić, J. Vitamin D receptor polymorphism and susceptibility to type 1 diabetes in the Dalmatian population. *Diabetes Res. Clin. Pract.* **2003**, *59*, 31–35.

196. Garcia-Lozano, J.R.; Gonzalez-Escribano, M.F.; Valenzuela, A.; Garcia, A.; Núñez-Roldán, A. Association of vitamin D receptor genotypes with early onset rheumatoid arthritis. *Eur. J. Immunogenet.* **2001**, *28*, 89–93.

197. Gómez-Vaquero, C.; Fiter, J.; Enjuanes, A.; Nogués, X.; Díez-Pérez, A.; Nolla, J.M. Influence of the BsmI polymorphism of the vitamin D receptor gene on rheumatoid arthritis clinical activity. *J. Rheumatol.* **2007**, *34*, 1823–1826.

198. Yamshchikov, A.V.; Desai, N.S.; Blumberg, H.M.; Ziegler, T.R.; Tangpricha, V. Vitamin D for treatment and prevention of infectious diseases: A systematic review of randomized controlled trials. *Endocr. Pract.* **2009**, *15*, 438–449.

199. Battersby, A.J.; Kampmann, B.; Burl, S. Vitamin D in early childhood and the effect on immunity to mycobacterium tuberculosis. *Clin. Dev. Immunol.* **2012**, *2012*, 430972.

200. Hart, P.D. Chemotherapy of tuberculosis; research during the past 100 years. *Br. Med. J.* **1946**, *2*, 805–849.

201. Everett, D. On the use of cod-liver oil in tubercular disease. *Prov. Med. Surg. J.* **1846**, *10*, 538–539.

202. The Nobel Prize in Physiology or Medicine 1903. Niels Ryberg Finsen. Available online: http://www.nobelprize.org/nobel_prizes/medicine/laureates/1903/ (accessed on 8 September 2012).

203. Rider, A.A. Elmer Verner McCollum—A biographical sketch (1879–1967). *J. Nutr.* **1970**, *100*, 1–10.

204. Dowling, G.B.; Thomas, E.W.; Wallace, H.J. Lupus Vulgaris treated with Calciferol. *Proc. R. Soc. Med.* **1946**, *39*, 225–227.

205. Phelan, J.J. Calciferol in pulmonary tuberculosis. *Lancet* **1947**, *1*, 764.

206. Martineau, A.R. Old wine in new bottles: Vitamin D in the treatment and prevention of tuberculosis. *Proc. Nutr. Soc.* **2012**, *71*, 84–89.

207. Sasidharan, P.K.; Rajeev, E.; Vijayakumari, V. Tuberculosis and vitamin D deficiency. *J. Assoc. Physicians India* **2002**, *50*, 554–558.

208. Wilkinson, R.J.; Llewelyn, M.; Toossi, Z.; Patel, P.; Pasvol, G.; Lalvani, A.; Wright, D.; Latif, M.; Davidson, R.N. Influence of vitamin D deficiency and vitamin D receptor polymorphisms on tuberculosis among Gujarati Asians in west London: A case-control study. *Lancet* **2000**, *355*, 618–621.

209. Nnoaham, K.E.; Clarke, A. Low serum vitamin D levels and tuberculosis: A systematic review and meta-analysis. *Int. J. Epidemiol.* **2008**, *37*, 113–119.

210. Ganmaa, D.; Giovannucci, E.; Bloom, B.R.; Fawzi, W.; Burr, W.; Batbaatar, D.; Sumberzul, N.; Holick, M.F.; Willett, W.C. Vitamin D, tuberculin skin test conversion, and latent tuberculosis in

Mongolian school-age children: A randomized, double-blind, placebo-controlled feasibility trial. *Am. J. Clin. Nutr.* **2012**, *96*, 391–396.

211. Martineau, A.R.; Wilkinson, R.J.; Wilkinson, K.A.; Newton, S.M.; Kampmann, B.; Hall, B.M.; Packe, G.E.; Davidson, R.N.; Eldridge, S.M.; Maunsell, Z.J.; *et al.* A single dose of vitamin D enhances immunity to mycobacteria. *Am. J. Respir. Crit. Care Med.* **2007**, *176*, 208–213.

212. Nursyam, E.W.; Amin, Z.; Rumende, C.M. The effect of vitamin D as supplementary treatment in patients with moderately advanced pulmonary tuberculous lesion. *Acta Med. Indones.* **2006**, *38*, 3–5.

213. Martineau, A.R.; Timms, P.M.; Bothamley, G.H.; Hanifa, Y.; Islam, K.; Claxton, A.P.; Packe, G.E.; Moore-Gillon, J.C.; Darmalingam, M.; Davidson, R.N.; *et al.* High-dose vitamin D_3 during intensive-phase antimicrobial treatment of pulmonary tuberculosis: A double-blind randomised controlled trial. *Lancet* **2011**, *377*, 242–250.

214. Morcos, M.M.; Gabr, A.A.; Samuel, S.; Kamel, M.; el Baz, M.; el Beshry, M.; Michail, R.R. Vitamin D administration to tuberculous children and its value. *Boll. Chim. Farm.* **1998**, *137*, 157–164.

215. Coussens, A.K.; Wilkinson, R.J.; Hanifa, Y.; Nikolayevskyy, V.; Elkington, P.T.; Islam, K.; Timms, P.M.; Venton, T.R.; Bothamley, G.H.; Packe, G.E.; *et al.* Vitamin D accelerates resolution of inflammatory responses during tuberculosis treatment. *Proc. Natl. Acad. Sci. USA* **2012**, *109*, doi:10.1073/pnas.1216789109.

216. Wejse, C.; Gomes, V.F.; Rabna, P.; Gustafson, P.; Aaby, P.; Lisse, I.M.; Andersen, P.L.; Glerup, H.; Sodemann, M. Vitamin D as supplementary treatment for tuberculosis. *Am. J. Respir. Crit. Care Med.* **2009**, *179*, 843–850.

217. Jorde, R.; Witham, M.; Janssens, W.; Rolighed, L.; Borchhardt, K.; de Boer, I.H.; Grimnes, G.; Hutchinson, M.S. Vitamin D supplementation did not prevent influenza-like illness as diagnosed retrospectively by questionnaires in subjects participating in randomized clinical trials. *Scand. J. Infect. Dis.* **2012**, *44*, 126–132.

218. Urashima, M.; Segawa, T.; Okazaki, M.; Kurihara, M.; Wada, Y.; Ida, H. Randomized trial of vitamin D supplementation to prevent seasonal influenza A in schoolchildren. *Am. J. Clin. Nutr.* **2010**, *91*, 1255–1260.

219. Cannell, J.J.; Vieth, R.; Umhau, J.C.; Holick, M.F.; Grant, W.B.; Madronich, S.; Garland, C.F.; Giovannucci, E. Epidemic influenza and vitamin D. *Epidemiol. Infect.* **2006**, *134*, 1129–1140.

220. Hope-Simpson, R.E. The role of season in the epidemiology of influenza. *J. Hyg. (Lond.)* **1981**, *86*, 35–47.

221. Ginde, A.; Mansbach, J.M.; Camargo, C.A. Association between serum 25-hydroxyvitamin D level and upper respiratory tract infection in the third national health and nutrition examination survey. *Arch. Intern. Med.* **2009**, *169*, 384–390.

222. Laaksi, I.; Ruohola, J.-P.; Tuohimaa, P.; Auvinen, A.; Haataja, R.; Pihlajamäki, H.; Ylikomi, T. An association of serum vitamin D concentrations <40 nmol/L with acute respiratory tract infection in young Finnish men. *Am. J. Clin. Nutr.* **2007**, *86*, 714–717.

223. Wayse, V.; Yousafzai, A.; Mogale, K.; Filteau, S. Association of subclinical vitamin D deficiency with severe acute lower respiratory infection in Indian children under 5 y. *Eur. J. Clin. Nutr.* **2004**, *58*, 563–567.

224. Aloia, J.F.; Li-Ng, M. Re: Epidemic influenza and vitamin D. *Epidemiol. Infect.* **2007**, *135*, 1095–1096.

225. Avenell, A.; Cook, J.A.; MacLennan, G.S.; MacPherson, G.C. Vitamin D supplementation to prevent infections: A sub-study of a randomised placebo-controlled trial in older people (RECORD trial, ISRCTN 51647438). *Age Ageing* **2007**, *36*, 574–577.

226. Li-Ng, M.; Aloia, J.F.; Pollack, S.; Cunha, B.A.; Mikhail, M.; Yeh, J.; Berbari, N. A randomized controlled trial of vitamin D3 supplementation for the prevention of symptomatic upper respiratory tract infections. *Epidemiol. Infect.* **2009**, *137*, 1396–1404.

227. Roth, D.E.; Jones, A.B.; Prosser, C.; Robinson, J.L.; Vohra, S. Vitamin D receptor polymorphisms and the risk of acute lower respiratory tract infection in early childhood. *J. Infect. Dis.* **2008**, *197*, 676–680.

228. Hewison, M. An update on vitamin D and human immunity. *Clin. Endocrinol.* **2012**, *76*, 315–325.

229. Brown, S.D.; Calvert, H.H.; Fitzpatrick, A.M. Vitamin D and asthma. *Dermato-Endocrinol.* **2012**, *4*, 137–145.

230. Camargo, C.A., Jr.; Rifas-Shiman, S.L.; Litonjua, A.A.; Rich-Edwards, J.W.; Weiss, S.T.; Gold, D.R.; Kleinman, K.; Gillman, M.W. Maternal intake of vitamin D during pregnancy and risk of recurrent wheeze in children at 3 y of age. *Am. J. Clin. Nutr.* **2007**, *85*, 788–795.

231. Camargo, C.A., Jr.; Ingham, T.; Wickens, K.; Thadhani, R.; Silvers, K.M.; Epton, M.J.; Town, G.I.; Pattemore, P.K.; Espinola, J.A.; Crane, J. Cord-blood 25-hydroxyvitamin D levels and risk of respiratory infection, wheezing, and asthma. *Pediatrics* **2011**, *127*, e180–e187.

232. Carroll, K.N.; Gebretsadik, T.; Larkin, E.K.; Dupont, W.D.; Liu, Z.; van Driest, S.; Hartert, T.V. Relationship of maternal vitamin D level with maternal and infant respiratory disease. *Am. J. Obstet. Gynecol.* **2011**, *205*, e211–e217.

233. Devereux, G.; Litonjua, A.A.; Turner, S.W.; Craig, L.C.; McNeill, G.; Martindale, S.; Helms, P.J.; Seaton, A.; Weiss, S.T. Maternal vitamin D intake during pregnancy and early childhood wheezing. *Am. J. Clin. Nutr.* **2007**, *85*, 853–859.

234. Erkkola, M.; Kaila, M.; Nwaru, B.I.; Kronberg-Kippila, C.; Ahonen, S.; Nevalainen, J.; Veijola, R.; Pekkanen, J.; Ilonen, J.; Simell, O.; *et al.* Maternal vitamin D intake during pregnancy is inversely associated with asthma and allergic rhinitis in 5-year-old children. *Clin. Exp. Allergy* **2009**, *39*, 875–882.

235. Gale, C.R.; Robinson, S.M.; Harvey, N.C.; Javaid, M.K.; Jiang, B.; Martyn, C.N.; Godfrey, K.M.; Cooper, C. Maternal vitamin D status during pregnancy and child outcomes. *Eur. J. Clin. Nutr.* **2008**, *62*, 68–77.

236. Rothers, J.; Wright, A.L.; Stern, D.A.; Halonen, M.; Camargo, C.A., Jr. Cord blood 25-hydroxyvitamin D levels are associated with aeroallergen sensitization in children from Tucson, Arizona. *J. Allergy Clin. Immunol.* **2011**, *128*, 1093–1099.

237. Chinellato, I.; Piazza, M.; Sandri, M.; Peroni, D.; Piacentini, G.; Boner, A.L. Vitamin D serum levels and markers of asthma control in Italian children. *J. Pediatr.* **2011**, *158*, 437–441.

238. Chinellato, I.; Piazza, M.; Sandri, M.; Peroni, D.G.; Cardinale, F.; Piacentini, G.L.; Boner, A.L. Serum vitamin D levels and exercise-induced bronchoconstriction in children with asthma. *Eur. Respir. J.* **2011**, *37*, 1366–1370.

239. Searing, D.A.; Zhang, Y.; Murphy, J.R.; Hauk, P.J.; Goleva, E.; Leung, D.Y. Decreased serum vitamin D levels in children with asthma are associated with increased corticosteroid use. *J. Allergy Clin. Immunol.* **2010**, *125*, 995–1000.

240. Heaney, R.P.; Davies, K.M.; Chen, T.C.; Holick, M.F.; Barger-Lux, M.J. Human serum 25-hydroxycholecalciferol response to extended oral dosing with cholecalciferol. *Am. J. Clin. Nutr.* **2003**, *77*, 204–210.

241. Godar, D.E.; Pope, S.J.; Grant, W.B.; Holick, M.F. Solar UV doses of adult Americans and vitamin D(3) production. *Dermato-Endocrinol.* **2011**, *3*, 243–250.

242. Pietras, S.M.; Obayan, B.K.; Cai, M.H.; Holick, M.F. Vitamin D2 treatment for vitamin D deficiency and insufficiency for up to 6 years. *Arch. Intern. Med.* **2009**, *169*, 1806–1808.

243. Jones, G. Pharmacokinetics of vitamin D toxicity. *Am. J. Clin. Nutr.* **2008**, *88*, 582S–586S.

244. Taylor, A.B.; Stern, P.H.; Bell, N.H. Abnormal regulation of circulating 25-hydroxyvitamin D in the Williams syndrome. *N. Engl. J. Med.* **1982**, *306*, 972–975.

245. Schlingmann, K.P.; Kaufmann, M.; Weber, S.; Irwin, A.; Goos, C.; John, U.; Misselwitz, J.; Klaus, G.; Kuwertz-Bröking, E.; Fehrenbach, H.; *et al.* Mutations in CYP24A1 and Idiopathic Infantile Hypercalcemia. *N. Engl. J. Med.* **2011**, *365*, 410–421.

246. Eyles, D.W.; Burne, T.H.J.; McGrath, J.J. Vitamin D, effects on brain development, adult brain function and the links between low levels of vitamin D and neuropsychiatric disease. *Front. Neuroendocrinol.* **2012**, in press.

4

Vitamin D Level and Risk of Community-Acquired Pneumonia and Sepsis

Anna J. Jovanovich [1], Adit A. Ginde [2], John Holmen [3], Kristen Jablonski [1], Rebecca L. Allyn [4], Jessica Kendrick [1,4] and Michel Chonchol [1,*]

[1] Division of Renal Diseases and Hypertension, University of Colorado Denver, Denver, CO 80045 USA; E-Mails: Anna.Jovanovich@ucdenver.edu (A.J.J.); Kristen.Nowak@ucdenver.edu (K.J.); Jessica.Kendrick@ucdenver.edu (J.K.)

[2] Department of Emergency Medicine, University of Colorado Denver, Denver, CO 80045 USA; E-Mail: Adit.Ginde@ucdenver.edu

[3] Intermountain Healthcare, Salt Lake City, UT 84157, USA; E-Mail: John.Holmen@imail.org

[4] Denver Health Medical Center, Denver, CO 80204, USA; E-Mail: Rebecca.Allyn@ucdenver.edu

* Author to whom correspondence should be addressed; E-Mail: Michel.Chonchol@ucdenver.edu;

Abstract: Previous research has reported reduced serum 25-hydroxyvitamin D (25(OH)D) levels is associated with acute infectious illness. The relationship between vitamin D status, measured prior to acute infectious illness, with risk of community-acquired pneumonia (CAP) and sepsis has not been examined. Community-living individuals hospitalized with CAP or sepsis were age-, sex-, race-, and season-matched with controls. ICD-9 codes identified CAP and sepsis; chest radiograph confirmed CAP. Serum 25(OH)D levels were measured up to 15 months prior to hospitalization. Regression models adjusted for diabetes, renal disease, and peripheral vascular disease evaluated the association of 25(OH)D levels with CAP or sepsis risk. A total of 132 CAP patients and controls were 60 ± 17 years, 71% female, and 86% Caucasian. The 25(OH)D levels <37 nmol/L (adjusted odds ratio (OR) 2.57, 95% CI 1.08–6.08) were strongly associated with increased odds of CAP hospitalization. A total of 422 sepsis patients and controls were 65 ± 14 years, 59% female, and 91% Caucasian. The 25(OH)D levels <37 nmol/L (adjusted OR 1.75, 95% CI 1.11–2.77) were associated with increased odds of sepsis hospitalization. Vitamin D status was inversely associated with risk of CAP and sepsis hospitalization in a community-living adult population. Further clinical trials are needed to evaluate whether vitamin D supplementation can reduce risk of infections, including CAP and sepsis.

Keywords: vitamin D deficiency; sepsis; community-acquired pneumonia; infection; epidemiology

---

1. Introduction

Relatively little progress has been made in improving mortality associated with community-acquired pneumonia (CAP) [1] which is a leading cause of death in the United States [2]. Likewise, the incidence of sepsis continues to rise, the population-adjusted incidence of sepsis increased 8.7% per year between 1979 and 2000 [3]. While mortality associated with sepsis has improved [3], it remains a substantial cause of death in the United States [2].

The major circulating form of vitamin D, 25-hydroxyvitamin D (25(OH)D), and its active form, 1,25-dihydroxyvitamin D (1,25(OH)$_2$D), were originally recognized as important endocrine hormones in calcium homeostasis and bone health. However, studies over the past twenty years suggest a broader role of 25(OH)D in endothelial function, cell proliferation, and immunity. The vitamin D receptor (VDR) is essentially ubiquitous, including immune cells. It responds to 1,25(OH)$_2$D [4,5] and regulates antimicrobial peptides cathelicidin and beta-defensing [5]. Furthermore, 25(OH)D deficiency is common; 32% of the U.S. population have 25(OH)D levels <50 nmol/L and 77% have levels <75 nmol/L [6]. Large epidemiological studies have shown an association between 25(OH)D deficiency and chronic diseases [7] including diabetes [8], renal disease [9], and peripheral vascular disease [10].

Lower serum 25(OH)D levels are associated with increased risk of upper respiratory tract infection [11–13]. When measured during hospital admission for acute illness, 25(OH)D deficiency is associated with increased risk of mortality in patients with CAP [14], more severe sepsis [15], and mortality in septic patients [16]. Most studies linking infection risk with 25(OH)D levels measure 25(OH)D during acute illness, which may not reflect pre-illness 25(OH)D status. There are no data assessing existing 25(OH)D deficiency with risk of hospital admission for CAP or sepsis. In this case-control study of community-living adults, serum 25(OH)D levels and the risk of hospital admission for CAP and sepsis was evaluated.

2. Experimental Section

2.1. Data Source

A retrospective matched cohort study was performed using the Intermountain Healthcare Enterprise Data Warehouse, which incorporates comprehensive electronic health and administrative data for over 10 years [17]. Intermountain Healthcare is a non-profit organization with 22 hospitals and over 150 outpatient clinics that serves the states of Utah and southeastern Idaho. The latitude of the hospitals and outpatient clinics is approximately 40° N. Facilities range from major adult tertiary-level care centers to small clinics and hospitals that are the only source of care in rural communities.

There were 160,979 admissions from 2008 to 2010 [17]. The institutional review board at Intermountain Healthcare System and University of Colorado Denver approved the project.

2.2. Cohort Definition

Case and control selection occurred between 1 January 2008 and 31 December 2010. CAP cases were identified through ICD-9 codes (480–488) and confirmed with chest radiograph. There were 187,132 CAP admissions of which 43,460 had discharge ICD-9 codes indicating pneumonia. Of these, 11,455 had chest radiography confirming pneumonia. 4352 Sepsis cases were identified through ICD-9 codes (995.91, 995.92). Controls were randomly selected from a pool of 62,757 adult patients without a CAP or sepsis diagnosis admitted within the same time period and matched 1:1 with cases by age, sex, race, and season of 25(OH)D measurement. Cases and control had to have a serum 25(OH) level in the electronic medical record 3–15 months prior to admission; therefore, only 132 and 422 patients were included in the final CAP and sepsis analyses, respectively. These time points were chosen arbitrarily to assess the relationship between pre-infection serum 25(OH)D levels and infectious episodes.

2.3. 25(OH) D Measurements

Serum 25(OH)D level were measured in all participants using an INCSTAR 25(OH)D two step assay procedure with a coefficient of variation of less than 10%. The first step in the procedure involves the rapid extraction of 25(OH)D from the serum using acetonitrile. Following extraction, the treated sample is assayed by using an equilibrium radioimmunoassay procedure. This method is based on an antibody with specificity to 25(OH)D. The sample, antibody, and tracer are incubated at 20–25 °C for ninety minutes. A second antibody-precipitating complex is used to achieve phase separation. The radioimmunoassay method tends to overestimate the level of 25(OH)D because the antibody recognizes all forms of dihydroxy-vitamin D and D steroids.

2.4. Statistical Analysis

The associations of serum 25(OH)D levels with CAP or sepsis admission were evaluated separately. The χ^2 Test of Independence tested the distribution of categorical variables and the Wilcoxon Rank Sum tested for differences in 25(OH)D levels among cases and controls. Cox logistic regression was performed using log-transformed 25(OH)D as a continuous variable and non-transformed 25(OH)D as a categorical variable (<75 nmol/L *vs.* ≥75 nmol/L, <50 nmol/L *vs.* ≥50 nmol/L, and <37 nmol/L *vs.* ≥37 nmol/L). These thresholds were chosen using established definitions of 25(OH)D deficiency/insufficiency [18,19]. Models adjusted for diabetes, renal disease, and peripheral vascular disease, which were chosen as confounding variables on the basis of previous studies [20,21] and obtained from the Charlson Comorbidity Index score. Two-tailed values of $p < 0.05$ were considered statistically significant.

3. Results

3.1. Community-Acquired Pneumonia

The demographic and clinical characteristics of the 66 cases and 66 controls for the CAP cohort are described in Table 1. The mean (SD) age of the participants was 60 ± 17 years, 71% were female, and 86% were Caucasian. There was no statistically significant difference in median [IQR] 25(OH)D levels in controls *vs.* cases (79.3 [71.1–88.1] *vs.* 70.1 [62.2–79.6] nmol/L, $p = 0.33$). Renal disease was more prevalent in cases than controls (31.8% *vs.* 10.6%, $p = 0.003$). Serum 25(OH)D levels were recorded in 28 cases 3–5 months prior, in 18 cases 6–11 months prior, in 10 cases each 9–11 and 12–15 months prior to admission.

Table 1. Baseline characteristics for community-acquired pneumonia and sepsis cases and matched controls.

	Case	Control
Number		
CAP	66	66
Sepsis	211	211
Age in years		
CAP	60 ± 17	60 ± 17
Sepsis	65 ± 14	65 ± 14
Females		
CAP	47	47
Sepsis	125	125
Race—White		
CAP	57	57
Sepsis	189	189
Race—Hispanic		
CAP	6	6
Sepsis	13	13
Race—Other		
CAP	3	3
Sepsis	5	5
Diabetes		
CAP	24 (36.4%)	19 (28.8%)
Sepsis *	97 (46.0%)	64 (30.3%)
Renal Disease		
CAP *	21 (31.8%)	7 (10.6%)
Sepsis *	76 (36.0%)	46 (21.8%)
Peripheral Vascular		
CAP	13 (19.7%)	9 (13.6%)
Sepsis	61 (28.9%)	45 (21.3%)
25(OH)D (nmol/L) **		
CAP	70.1 [62.2–79.6]	79.3 [71.1–88.1]
Sepsis	61.2 [55.9–66.4]	69.1 [64.2–74.1]

Table 1. *Cont.*

25(OH)D >75 nmol/L		
CAP	34 (52.3%)	35 (53.0%)
Sepsis	84 (39.8%)	99 (46.9%)
25(OH)D 51–75 nmol/L		
CAP	19 (28.8%)	19 (28.8%)
Sepsis	56 (26.5%)	60 (28.4%)
25(OH)D 37–50 nmol/L		
CAP	7 (10.6%)	10 (15.2%)
Sepsis	31 (14.7%)	29 (13.7%)
25(OH)D <37 nmol/L		
CAP	9 (9.1%)	2 (3.0%)
Sepsis *	40 (19.0%)	23 (10.9%)

* $p < 0.05$; ** median [IQR]; CAP, community-acquired pneumonia; 25(OH)D, 25 hydroxyvitamin D.

In unadjusted logistic regression, log-transformed 25(OH)D as a continuous variable was not associated with CAP (0.99 [0.90–1.09], $p = 0.84$). A lack of association remained after adjustment for diabetes, renal disease, and peripheral vascular disease (OR 0.94 [0.59–1.48], $p = 0.78$). Likewise, 25(OH)D <75 nmol/L *vs.* ≥75 nmol/L and <50 nmol/L *vs.* ≥50 nmol/L were not associated with CAP in adjusted analyses (Table 2). However, when 25(OH)D was categorized as <37 nmol/L *vs.* ≥37 nmol/L, there was an association with increased odds of CAP (OR 2.57 [1.08–6.08], $p = 0.03$; Table 2) in the adjusted model.

Table 2. Adjusted odds ratios for Community-Acquired Pneumonia (CAP) and Sepsis Cases relative to controls by serum 25(OH)D levels.

Model [§]	OR (95% CI)	*p*-Value
25(OH)D <75 nmol/L *vs.* ≥75 nmol/L		
CAP	1.03 (0.51–2.09)	0.93
Sepsis	1.24 (0.84–1.83)	0.28
25(OH)D <50 nmol/L *vs.* ≥50 nmol/L		
CAP	0.96 (0.35–2.61)	0.94
Sepsis	1.75 (1.11–2.77)	0.02
25(OH)D <37 nmol/L *vs.* ≥37 nmol/L		
CAP	2.57 (1.08–6.08)	0.03
Sepsis	1.89 (1.09–3.31)	0.02

[§] Adjustments made for diabetes, renal disease, peripheral vascular disease; CAP, community-acquired pneumonia; 25(OH)D, 25 hydroxyvitamin D.

3.2. Sepsis

The demographic and clinical characteristics of the 211 cases and 211 controls for the sepsis cohort are described in Table 1. The mean (SD) age of the participants was 65 ± 14 years, 59% were female and 91% were Caucasian. There was no statistically significant difference in median [IQR] 25(OH)D levels in controls *vs.* cases (69.1 [64.2–74.1] nmol/L *vs.* 61.2 [55.9–66.4] nmol/L, $p = 0.05$).

Comorbid conditions were more prevalent in sepsis cases than in controls: diabetes (46.0% *vs.* 30.3%, *p* = 0.0009) and renal disease (36.0% *vs.* 21.2%, *p* = 0.001). Serum 25(OH)D levels were recorded in 93 cases 3–5 months prior, in 50 cases 6–11 months prior, in 47 cases 9–11 months prior, and 21 cases 12–15 months prior to admission.

In unadjusted logistic regression, log-transformed 25(OH)D as a continuous variable was not associated with sepsis (OR 0.99 [0.93–1.05], *p* = 0.70). A lack of association remained after adjustment for diabetes, renal disease, and peripheral vascular disease (OR 0.82 [0.64–1.05], *p* = 0.12). 25(OH)D <75 nmol/L *vs.* ≥75 nmol/L was not associated with sepsis in adjusted analyses (Table 2). However, when 25(OH)D was categorized as <50 nmol/L *vs.* ≥50 nmol/L and <37 nmol/L *vs.* ≥37 nmol/L, there was an association with increased odds of sepsis (Table 2, OR 1.75 [1.11–2.77], *p* = 0.02 and 1.89 [1.09–3.31], *p* = 0.02, respectively) in adjusted analyses.

4. Discussion

In a cohort of community-living adults, increased risk of hospitalization for CAP was associated with serum 25(OH)D levels <37 nmol/L and for sepsis with serum 25(OH)D levels <50 nmol/L. This association was not observed for 25(OH)D <75 nmol/L, suggesting that 25(OH)D <37 nmol/L confers a greater risk of infection than vitamin D insufficiency.

These findings are consistent with other epidemiologic studies linking vitamin D deficiency with increased risk of infection and infection-associated complications. A large observational study using National Health and Nutrition Examination Survey data showed that in a diverse cohort of 18,883 individuals greater than 12 years of age, those with a serum 25(OH)D level <25 nmol/L and a serum 25(OH)D 25–75 nmol/L had a 36% and 24% increased risk of upper respiratory tract infection, respectively, compared to those with a serum 25(OH)D ≥75 nmol/L [11]. Likewise, in a prospective observational study evaluating 25(OH)D levels in Finnish military recruits, 25(OH)D levels <40 nmol/L were associated with a higher likelihood of physician diagnosed respiratory tract infections and lost days of work in the subsequent six months [13]. Ginde and colleagues reported that upon presentation to an urban emergency department, 81 patients with sepsis and 25(OH)D levels <75 nmol/L were more likely to have severe sepsis compared to those with 25(OH)D levels ≥75 nmol/L (61% *vs.* 24%, *p* = 0.006) at initial evaluation and at 24 h (67% *vs.* 29%, *p* = 0.005) [15]. While other studies have measured 25(OH)D levels at acute illness onset, our study evaluates 25(OH)D levels at least 3 months prior to hospital admission, thus suggesting that there is an increased risk of CAP with a 25(OH)D level <37 nmol/L and sepsis with a 25(OH)D level <50 nmol/L. It also eliminates the potential for confounding by acute illness altering serum 25(OH)D levels.

Both the VDR and CYP27B1, the gene encoding 1-α-hydroxylase, which converts 25(OH)D to its active form 1,25(OH)$_2$D, are expressed in immune cells, suggesting that 25(OH)D has paracrine or autocrine function. Furthermore, 1-α-hydroxylase in macrophages is not regulated by parathyroid hormone (PTH) [22] but depends on circulating 25(OH)D concentrations or may be induced by cytokines [23]. When toll-like receptors on macrophages bind bacterial wall lipopolysaccharides (LPS), 1-α-hydroxylase and VDR expression is increased[4] resulting in local conversion of 25(OH)D to 1,25(OH)$_2$D, which in turn increases the expression of cathelicidin and beta-defensing, bactericidal proteins. There is evidence that cathelicidin transcription is particularly dependent on sufficient levels of 25(OH)D [4]. Indeed, in a study of critically ill patients with and without sepsis, Jeng and colleagues report a positive relationship between 25(OH)D levels and LL-37 (cathelicidin) levels [24].

In sepsis, 25(OH)D and 1,25(OH)$_2$D may have other effects beyond those associated with immunity such as endothelial function, coagulation, and hemodynamic stability. In rats with induced sepsis, pretreatment with 1,25(OH)$_2$D resulted in a more normal coagulation profile compared to placebo [25]. The VDR is also found in arterioles and the myocardium [26] and 1,25(OH)$_2$D has been shown to enhance the effect of inotropes [27] suggesting a possible positive hemodynamic effect of 1,25(OH)$_2$D in sepsis [25]. Taken together, sufficient circulating 25(OH)D levels, independent of the classic vitamin D-PTH axis, play a pivotal role in immunity. Moreover, 25(OH)D may also be protective against the adverse physiologic changes that occur in sepsis.

The findings of this study are consistent with other epidemiologic reports linking serum 25(OH)D <75 nmol/L with increased risk of infection and associated complications [11–16]. While other studies measured 25(OH)D levels during acute illness, this is the first to evaluate 25(OH)D levels ≥3 months prior to hospital admission for CAP or sepsis, eliminating potential confounding by acute illness altering serum 25(OH)D levels. This study has important strengths. Chest radiograph confirmed CAP ICD-9 codes. Serum 25(OH)D level was measured prior to the onset of illness, which is different from other studies that measured 25(OH)D at the time of presentation. This is important because vitamin D binding protein may be decreased resulting in potential urinary wasting of 25(OH)D in sepsis [24]. Finally, this study used a community-living cohort that included a relatively large number of patients with sepsis.

This study has several limitations. First, it is retrospective and observational so causation cannot be assumed. Second, the use of ICD-9 codes to identify admissions for sepsis limits details of cause and severity. Third, while cases and controls were well-matched and regression models adjusted for comorbidities, there may be other unmeasured confounders that could potentially affect the results. Fourth, ascertainment bias may exist because only cases and controls with a serum 25(OH)D level available prior to admission were considered. Additionally, no information is available on outcomes during the hospitalization.

5. Conclusions

In conclusion, serum 25(OH)D level <37 nmol/L in a community-living cohort was associated with increased risk of hospital admission for CAP and sepsis. Large randomized controlled trials are needed to establish whether or not 25(OH)D repletion will decrease CAP and sepsis incidence in community-living adult populations.

Acknowledgments

This work was supported by the National Institute of Health and the American Geriatrics Society Beeson Career Development Award [grant number K23AG040708] and the American Geriatrics Society Jahnigen Career Development Scholars Award to AG; the National Institute of Diabetes and Digestive and Kidney Diseases [grant numbers 1R01DK081473-01A, 1R01DK078112-01A2] to MC; the National Institute of Diabetes and Digestive and Kidney Diseases [grant number K23DK087859-01A1] to JK.

Author Contributions

Anna Jovanovich, John Holmen, Jessica Kendrick and Michel Chonchol had full access to all of the data in the study and take responsibility for the integrity of the data and the accuracy of the data analysis. Study concept and design: Jovanovich, Ginde, Holmen, Jablonski, ALlyn, Kendrick and Chonchol. Collection, management, analysis and interpretation of data: Jovanovich, Ginde, Holmen, Jablonski, Allyn, Kendrick and Chonchol. Preparation, review, or approval of manuscript: Jovanovich, Ginde, Holmen, Jablonski, Allyn, Kendrick and Chonchol.

Conflicts of Interest

The authors declare no conflict of interest.

References

1. Mandell, L.A.; Wunderink, R.G.; Anzueto, A.; Bartlett, J.G.; Campbell, G.D.; Dean, N.C.; Dowell, S.F.; File, T.M., Jr.; Musher, D.M.; Niederman, M.S.; *et al.* Infectious Diseases Society of America/American Thoracic Society consensus guidelines on the management of community-acquired pneumonia in adults. *Clin. Infect. Dis.* **2007**, *44*, S27–S72.
2. Deaths: Preliminary Data for 2009. National Vital Statistics Reports. CDC. 2011. Available online: http://www.cdc.gov/nchs/data/nvsr/nvsr59/nvsr59_04.pdf (accessed on 16 March 2011).
3. Martin, G.S.; Mannino, D.M.; Eaton, S.; Moss, M. The epidemiology of sepsis in the United States from 1979 through 2000. *N. Engl. J. Med.* **2003**, *348*, 1546–1554.
4. Liu, P.T.; Stenger, S.; Li, H.; Wenzel, L.; Tan, B.H.; Krutzik, S.R.; Ochoa, M.T.; Schauber, J.; Wu, K.; Meinken, C.; *et al.* Toll-like receptor triggering of a vitamin D-mediated human antimicrobial response. *Science* **2006**, *311*, 1770–1773.
5. White, J.H. Vitamin D metabolism and signaling in the human immune system. *Rev. Endocr. Metab. Disord.* **2012**, *13*, 21–29.
6. Ginde, A.A.; Liu, M.C.; Camargo, C.A., Jr. Demographic differences and trends of vitamin D insufficiency in the US population, 1988–2004. *Arch. Intern. Med.* **2009**, *169*, 626–632.
7. Holick, M.F. Vitamin D for health and in chronic kidney disease. *Semin. Dial.* **2005**, *18*, 266–275.
8. Scragg, R.; Sowers, M.; Bell, C.; Third National Health and Nutrition Examination Survey. Serum 25-hydroxyvitamin D, diabetes, and ethnicity in the Third National Health and Nutrition Examination Survey. *Diabetes Care* **2004**, *27*, 2813–2818.
9. Chonchol, M.; Scragg, R. 25-Hydroxyvitamin D, insulin resistance, and kidney function in the Third National Health and Nutrition Examination Survey. *Kidney Int.* **2007**, *71*, 134–139.
10. Melamed, M.L.; Muntner, P.; Michos, E.D.; Uribarri, J.; Weber, C.; Sharma, J.; Raggi, P. Serum 25-hydroxyvitamin D levels and the prevalence of peripheral arterial disease: Results from NHANES 2001 to 2004. *Arterioscler. Thromb. Vasc. Biol.* **2008**, *28*, 1179–1185.
11. Ginde, A.A.; Mansbach, H.M.; Camargo, C.A., Jr. Association between serum 25-hydroxyvitamin D level and upper respiratory tract infection in the Third National Health and Nutrition Examination Survey. *Arch. Intern. Med.* **2009**, *169*, 384–390.

12. Sabetta, J.R.; DePetrillo, P.; Cipriani, R.J.; Smardin, J.; Burns, L.A.; Landry, M.L. Serum 25-hydroxyvitamin D and the incidence of acute viral respiratory tract infection in healthy adults. *PLoS One* **2010**, *5*, e11088.

13. Laaksi, I.; Ruohola, J.P.; Tuohimaa, P.; Auvinen, A.; Haataja, R.; Pihajamaki, H.; Ylikomi, T. An association of serum vitamin D concentrations <40 nmol/L with acute respiratory tract infection in young Finnish men. *Am. J. Clin. Nutr.* **2007**, *86*, 714–717.

14. Leow, L.; Simpson, T.; Cursons, R.; Karalus, N.; Hancox, R.J. Vitamin D, innate immunity and outcomes in community acquired pneumonia. *Respirology* **2011**, *16*, 611–616.

15. Ginde, A.A.; Camargo, C.A., Jr.; Shapiro, N.I. Vitamin D insufficiency and sepsis severity in emergency department patients with suspected infection. *Acad. Emerg. Med.* **2011**, *18*, 551–554.

16. Braun, A.B.; Gibbons, F.K.; Litonjua, A.A.; Giovannucci, E.; Christopher, K.B. Low serum 25-hydroxyvitamin D at critical care initiation is associated with increased mortality. *Crit. Care Med.* **2012**, *40*, 63–72.

17. Intermoutain Healthcare Annual Report. Intermountain Healthcare 2010. Available online: http://intermountainhealthcare.org/about/overview/Documents/annualreport2010.pdf (accessed on 12 December 2012).

18. Mehrotra, R.; Kermah, D.A.; Salusky, I.B.; Wolf, M.S.; Thadhani, R.I.; Chiu, Y.W.; Martins, D.; Adler, S.G.; Norris, K.C. Chronic kidney disease, hypovitaminosis D, and mortality in the United States. *Kidney Int.* **2009**, *76*, 977–983.

19. Institute of Medicine. Dietary References Intakes for Calcium and Vitamin D. Available online: http://www.iom.edu/Activities/Nutrition/DRIVitDCalcium/2010-Nov-30.aspx (accessed on 12 December 2012).

20. Anderson, J.L.; May, H.T.; Horne, B.D.; Bair, T.L.; Hall, N.L.; Carlquist, J.F.; Lappé, D.L.; Muhlestein, J.B.; Intermountain Heart Collaborative (IHC) Study Group. Relation of vitamin d deficiency to cardiovascular risk factors, disease status, and incident events in a general healthcare population. *Am. J. Cardiol.* **2010**, *106*, 953–958.

21. Sterling, K.A.; Eftekhari, P.; Girndt, M.; Kimmel, P.L.; Raj, D.S. The immunoregulatory function of vitamin D: Implications in chronic kidney disease. *Nat. Rev. Nephrol.* **2012**, *8*, 403–412.

22. Wu, S.; Ren, S.; Nguyen, L.; Adams, J.S.; Hewison, M. Splice variants of the CYP27b1 gene and the regulation of 1,25-dihydroxyvitamin D3 production. *Endocrinology* **2007**, *148*, 3410–4318.

23. Van Etten, E.; Stoffels, K.; Gysemans, C.; Mathieu, C.; Overbergh, L. Regulation of vitamin D homeostasis: Implications for the immune system. *Nutr. Rev.* **2008**, *66*, S125–S134.

24. Jeng, L.; Yamshchikov, A.V.; Judd, S.E.; Blumberg, H.M.; Martin, G.S.; Ziegler, T.R.; Tangpricha, V. Alterations in vitamin D status and anti-microbial peptide levels in patients in the intensive care unit with sepsis. *J. Transl. Med.* **2009**, *7*, 28.

25. Moller, S.; Laigaard, F.; Olgaard, K.; Hemmingsen, C. Effect of 1,25-dihydroxy-vitamin D_3 in experimental sepsis. *Int. J. Med. Sci.* **2007**, *4*, 190–195.

26. Bukoski, R.D.; Xue, H. On the vascular inotropic action of 1,25-(OH)2 vitamin D3. *Am. J. Hypertens.* **1993**, *6*, 388–396.

27. Walters, M.R.; Wicker, D.C.; Riggle, P.C. 1,25-Dihydroxyvitamin D3 receptors identified in the rat heart. *J. Mol. Cell. Cardiol.* **1986**, *18*, 67–72.

5

Vitamin D Insufficiency and Bone Mineral Status in a Population of Newcomer Children in Canada

Hassanali Vatanparast [1,2,*], Christine Nisbet [3] and Brian Gushulak [4]

[1] Division of Nutrition and Dietetics, College of Pharmacy and Nutrition, University of Saskatchewan, Saskatoon, SK S7N 5A2, Canada

[2] School of Public Health, University of Saskatchewan, Saskatoon, SK S7N 5A2, Canada

[3] Division of Nutrition and Dietetics, College of Pharmacy and Nutrition, University of Saskatchewan, Saskatoon, SK S7N 5A2, Canada; E-Mail: christine.nisbet@usask.ca

[4] Migration Health Consultants, Qualicum Beach, British Columbia, V9K 1S9, Canada; E-Mail: brian.gushulak@gmail.com

* Author to whom correspondence should be addressed; E-Mail: vatan.h@usask.ca;

Abstract: Background: Low levels of circulating vitamin D are more likely to be found in those with darker skin pigmentation, who live in areas of high latitude, and who wear more clothing. We examined the prevalence of vitamin D deficiency and inadequacy in newcomer immigrant and refugee children. Methods: We evaluated circulating vitamin D status of immigrant children at the national level. Subsequently, we investigated vitamin D intake, circulating vitamin D status, and total body bone mineral content (TBBMC) in newcomer children living in Saskatchewan. Results: In the sample of newcomer children in Saskatchewan, the prevalence of inadequacy in calcium and vitamin D intakes was 76% and 89.4%, respectively. Vitamin D intake from food/supplement was significantly higher in immigrants compared to refugees, which accords with the significant difference in serum status. Circulating vitamin D status indicated that 29% of participants were deficient and another 44% had inadequate levels of serum 25(OH)D for bone health. Dietary vitamin D intake, sex, region of origin, and length of stay in Canada were significant predictors of serum vitamin D status. Results for TBBMC revealed that 38.6% were found to have low TBBMC compared to estimated values for age, sex, and ethnicity. In the regression model, after controlling for possible confounders, children who were taller and had greater circulating vitamin D also had greater TBBMC. Nationally, immigrant children, particularly girls, have significantly lower plasma 25(OH)D than non-immigrant children. Interpretation: Newcomer immigrant and refugee children are at a high risk of vitamin D deficiency and inadequacy, which may have serious negative consequences for their health.

Keywords: vitamin D; newcomer immigrant children; bone mineral status

---

1. Introduction

Recent studies report various health benefits for vitamin D along with its important role in bone health [1]. Limited food sources of vitamin D and long winters resulting in reduced sun exposure in Canada have raised concerns, particularly in growing children where vitamin D is needed for bone mineral accrual. National data report a low prevalence of vitamin D deficiency in children aged 6–11 years compared to other age groups [2]. However, the growing proportion of immigrants in Canada, particularly children, may represent communities at greater risk for vitamin D deficiency. Some new arrivals have high skin pigmentation, and social and cultural factors that can result in insufficient vitamin D intake from food [3–6]. From 2002 to 2004, 150 cases of rickets were reported in Canadian children [7]. Darker-skinned individuals represented 89% of cases, while 24% were immigrants [7]. In a cross-sectional study in Edmonton, vitamin D concentrations decreased in children as age increased [8]. The authors speculated that this is possibly due to less consumption of milk fortified with vitamin D and less exposure to the sun [8]. In response to the paucity of information in this area, we evaluated circulating vitamin D status of immigrant and refugee children new to Canada. Additionally, we examined the association between circulating vitamin D with bone mineral status.

2. Methods

Two studies were conducted to address the following research objectives: (i) to obtain a national perspective on vitamin D status of immigrant children in comparison to non-immigrant children; (ii) to evaluate determinants of vitamin D and its association with bone mineral status in children new to Canada.

2.1. Study 1. Vitamin D Status of Canadian Immigrant and Non-Immigrant Children

We used data from the Canadian Health Measures Survey (CHMS), cycle 1, 2007–2009, conducted by Statistics Canada [9]. The CHMS is a nationally representative survey among approximately 5500 Canadians aged 6–79 years, representative of 96.3% of Canadians. Circulating 25-hydroxyvitamin D [25(OH)D] levels were obtained for Canadian non-immigrant and first-generation immigrant children aged 6–11 years. In CHMS data, immigrants are not differentiated from refugees. The information on vitamin D measurement in the CHMS is found elsewhere [2]. Descriptive data are presented as mean ± SEM. A statistically significant difference in vitamin D status among immigrant *versus* non-immigrant children is indicated by no overlap in 95% Confidence Intervals [10]. As per Statistics Canada's recommendation, analyses were weighted and bootstrapped to obtain estimates representative of the Canadian population. Degree of freedom was considered 11 due to sampling structure, and alpha was set at 0.05. Data manipulation, cleaning, and creating new variables were done using SPSS 19. All analyses were conducted by STATA SE 11.

2.2. Study 2. Healthy Immigrant Children (HIC)

2.2.1. Study Design and Participants

In the absence of official data sources that identifies immigration status in Saskatchewan, a convenience sample of study participants ($n = 72$) were recruited with the assistance of several organizations that have regular contact with immigrant and refugees. These organizations include Saskatoon Open Door Society, Saskatchewan Intercultural Association, and ethno-cultural associations. Participant recruitment posters were also placed in accessible public locations including the universities, public libraries, health care facilities and commercial locations. Interpreters were used for 50 (69%) participants while 22 (31%) were able to speak English and, therefore, did not require an interpreter.

In a cross-sectional design (2010–2011), health and nutrition measures were collected from immigrant ($n = 33$) and refugee ($n = 39$) children aged 7–11 years who had been living in Saskatoon, Saskatchewan, Canada for no more than five years. An immigrant is someone who "comes as a permanent resident to a country other than one's native land" [11]. A refugee is someone who "owing to well-founded fear of being persecuted for reasons of race, religion, nationality, membership of a particular social group or political opinion", is unable or unwilling to return to his/her country of birth due to fear for their safety [12]. This age range is an important time for bone acquisition and for establishing healthy dietary habits. Ethics approval was obtained from the University of Saskatchewan Biomedical Research Ethics Board (Bio # 09-197).

2.2.2. Data Collection

Data collection for the study included multiple variables. Demographics and socioeconomic status were evaluated using questionnaires from the Canadian Community Health Survey [13]. Food security status was evaluated using the version of the United States Department of Agriculture questionnaire that was modified by Canada [14].

Anthropometric measurements included height, weight and waist circumference. Values were recorded in centimeters to the nearest millimeter. All measurements were taken twice for consistency to help eliminate human error. Percentile Body Mass Index (BMI) was categorized as normal, overweight, or obese according to World Health Organization (WHO) child classifications [15].

To assess physical activity, we used the CHMS children's physical activity questionnaire (CPA). Another variable was derived to examine sedentary activity in hours per day. Based on the CHMS, two questions on sun exposure were also included [9].

Three 24-h dietary recalls were administered to each child to obtain a usual intake. All 24-h recalls were administered at least three weeks apart and conducted in person. The child's caregiver assisted in the dietary assessments. Diet analyses were performed in "The Food Processor Nutrition and Fitness Software version SQL 10.5", Esha Research, Salem, USA. Foods were categorized into food groups consistent with *Eating Well with Canada's Food Guide* [16]. To examine the overall nutrition status, we used the Canadian version of the Healthy Eating Index (HEIC) [17]. The HEIC has been validated and incorporates recommendations from *Eating Well with Canada's Food Guide* [17]. This index categorizes diets into one of three categories, "poor", "needs improvement", and "good" [17].

2.2.3. Outcome Measures

Blood samples were taken from 1 May to 30 September 2010 using a finger prick on eight 6-mm spots on a filter card. Circulating 25(OH)D was analyzed from dried blood spots, using a standard LC-MS/MS assay by ZRT Laboratory which is widely used for measuring 25-Hydroxy Vitamin D2/D3 [18,19]. The ZRT Laboratory participates in DEQAS, the Vitamin D Quality Assessment Scheme, which provides control samples to ensure assay accuracy [18,19]. Plasma and blood spot determinations were deemed to be equivalent because of the high stability of 25(OH)D in serum or plasma [20]. The blood spot card measurements of vitamin D levels are in agreement with serum and whole blood specimen [21]. Recent recommendations by the Institute of Medicine's dietary reference intake (DRI) panel on vitamin D were used to define vitamin D status including less than 30 nmol/L as deficient, 30–50 nmol/L as inadequate, and more than 50 nmol/L as sufficient [22].

Bone mineral status was assessed using Dual-energy X-ray Absorptiometry (DXA), Hologic Inc., Discovery-Wi, Bedford, USA, Serial #80964. This study focused on Total Body Bone Mineral Content (TBBMC) as the most accurate measure in children [23]. The coefficient of variation for TBBMC in our laboratory is 0.5%. Values obtained for TBBMC were compared to estimated normal values for each child's age, sex, and ethnicity based on data from four longitudinal studies [24].

2.2.4. Statistical Analyses

Descriptive statistics were analyzed by calculating means and standard deviations of variables of interest as well as the distribution of participants in various categories. We used a two-sided independent Student's *t*-test or non-parametric equivalent (Mann Whitney *U*-test) to investigate differences between refugees and immigrants and between males and females. Pearson's Chi square was used to analyze categorical variables. Finally, multivariate analyses (linear and logistic regression) were conducted to examine the association between variables of interest and health outcomes (vitamin D status, TBBMC), controlling for possible confounders. Analyses were conducted using PASW Statistics 18 by Polar Engineering and Consulting, Chicago, USA. In all analyses, alpha was set at 0.05. All data, when possible, was compared to Canadian published data.

3. Results

Descriptive data from CHMS revealed that mean plasma 25(OH)D concentrations in non-immigrant children was significantly higher than in immigrant children. This difference is over 20 nmol/L in immigrant girls (Table 1).

Table 1. Plasma 25-hydroxyvitamin D [25(OH)D] (nmol/L) concentrations in immigrant and non-immigrant children aged 6–11 years in Canada [1].

Children aged 6–11 years	Plasma 25-hydroxyvitamin D [25(OH)D] (Mean ± SEM)
All children (n = 1,817,260)	75.1 ± 2.4
Boys	79.9 ± 2.0
Girls	73.1 ± 3.0
Immigrant children (n = 134,833)	61.1 ± 5.9 *
Immigrant boys	69.0 ± 7.9
Immigrant girls	54.1 ± 4.5 **
Non-immigrant children (n = 1,682,427)	76.2 ± 2.2
Non-immigrant boys	77.5 ± 1.9
Non-immigrant girls	74.7 ± 2.8

[1] Data from the Canadian Health Measures Survey Cycle 1, 2007–2009. * Significantly lower than non-immigrant children. ** Significantly lower than non-immigrant boys and girls.

In the HIC study, the mean ± SD age of participants was 8.9 ± 1.4 years, with no significant difference between immigrants (n = 33) and refugees (n = 39). There was also no significant difference in distribution of males (n = 48) and females (n = 24) according to immigration status. Most immigrant children in the study were from the Middle East (73%), while refugee children were from various regions including South East Asia, Africa, the Middle East and Latin America in descending order. In 2009, approximately 78% of newcomers in Saskatchewan were from Asia and the Pacific (59.9%), Africa and the Middle East (15.4%) and South and Central America (2.5%) [25]. These regions contribute to around 80% of immigrants in Canada [26]. The mean length of stay in Canada was 2.6 ± 1.5 years. Over 55% of families were from the lowest income bracket according to Statistics Canada classification.

Table 2 presents general characteristics of participants. Percentile height (mean ± SD) was lower than the 50th percentile with no significant difference between immigrants and refugees. The majority of children were found to have a normal BMI while 22.2% were overweight and 6.9% were obese. Results showed 87.5% of immigrant and refugee newcomer children were obtaining the recommended number of hours per day of physical activity (≥60 min) according to the Canadian Society for Exercise Physiology [27]. However, many participants were spending too much time (>2 h/day) in sedentary activities such as time spent watching television or movies, playing video games, or using the computer.

Table 2. General characteristics of healthy immigrant children study participants.

Characteristics	Immigrants n = 33 (45.8%)	Refugees n = 39 (54.2%)	All participants n = 72 (100%)
Age (Mean ± SD)	8.9 ± 1.6	8.9 ± 1.3	8.9 ± 1.4
Sex			
Male	22 (66.7%)	26 (66.7%)	48 (66.7%)
Female	11 (33.3%)	13 (33.3%)	24 (33.3%)
Length of stay in Canada in years (Mean ± SD)	2.6 ± 1.5	2.5 ± 1.1	2.5 ± 1.3

Table 2. *Cont.*

Height in cm (Mean ± SD)	132.6 ± 13.2	130.3 ± 10.9	131.4 ± 12.0
Percentile Height (Mean ± SD)	49.7 ± 31.1	42.6 ± 30.8	45.8 ± 31.0
Weight in kg (Mean ± SD)	32.1 ± 10.6	29.9 ± 7.8	30.9 ± 9.2
Percentile Weight (Mean ± SD)	68.8 ± 27.4	64.9 ± 28.8	66.7 ± 28.0
Physical activity in h/week (Mean ± SD)	13.1 ± 5.4	12.0 ± 3.7	12.5 ± 4.6
Recommended level (≥60 min/day)	29 (87.9%)	34 (87.2%)	63 (87.5%)
Less than recommended level (<60 min/day)	4 (12.1%)	5 (12.8%)	9 (12.5%)

Dietary vitamin D and calcium intakes and HEIC are presented in Table 3. Only 24.2% of participants met recommendations for servings per day of milk and alternatives. The prevalence of calcium intake inadequacy was 76%. Vitamin D intake from food and supplement was 213 ± 195 IU (mean ± SD) for all participants with a prevalence of inadequacy of 89.4%. Only two children reported taking a vitamin D supplement regularly. Vitamin D intake from food and supplement was significantly higher in immigrants compared to refugees, which accords with the significant difference in serum status (Table 3). There was a significant difference in mean ± SD HEIC scores between immigrants and refugees at 65.4 ± 7.7 *vs.* 60.4 ± 8.8, respectively ($p = 0.021$). The majority of participants (90.9%) needed to improve their diet. Only one immigrant was classified in "good" quality diet category based on HEIC, while no refugees did. There were also five refugees who had poor diets, while no immigrants did.

Table 3. Nutrient intake related to bone health.

Characteristics	Immigrants n = 33 (45.8%)	Refugees n = 39 (54.2%)	All participants n = 72 (100%)
Vitamin D intake in IU/day (Mean ± SD)	249 ± 247	181 ± 130	213 ± 195
Prevalence of vitamin D intake inadequacy [n (%)]	25 (81%) *	34 (97%)	59 (89%)
Calcium intake in mg	764 ± 393	676 ± 380	718 ± 386
Prevalence of calcium intake inadequacy [n (%)]	23 (74%)	27 (77%)	50 (76%)
Milk and alternatives			
Mean intake (servings/day)	1.9 ± 1.2	1.6 ± 1.1	1.7 ± 1.2
Meeting Canada's Food Guide recommendations	10 (32.3%)	6 (17.1%)	16 (24.2%)
Healthy Eating Index Canada			
Mean Score	65.4 ± 7.7 *	60.4 ± 8.8	62.7 ± 8.6
Good Diet	1 (3.2%)	0 (0.0%)	1 (1.5%)
Diet Needs Improvement	30 (96.8%)	30 (85.7%)	60 (90.9%)
Poor Diet	0 (0.0%)	5 (14.3%)	5 (7.6%)

* Significantly different from refugee children, *t*-test ($P < 0.05$).

Total serum 25(OH)D (nmol/L) was significantly higher in immigrant compared to refugee children ($p = 0.021$) (Table 4). Overall, 29% of participants were vitamin D deficient and another 44% had inadequate levels of serum 25(OH)D for bone health [22]. Children spent 3.6 ± 1.6 h/day (mean ± SD) in the sun in the summer months during peak times (11:00 am–4:00 pm), which was consistent across immigration status. Very few children regularly applied sunscreen, whereas more than half of children never did (Table 4). In linear regression analyses, after controlling for possible confounders including total caloric intake, age, sunscreen use, total hours spent in the sun in the summer months during peak times, and calcium intake; dietary vitamin D intake (Standardized Regression Coefficient: 0.46 ± 0.11, $p < 0.001$), sex (Standardized Regression coefficient: -0.39 ± 0.11, $p < 0.001$), region of origin (Standardized Regression coefficient: 0.24 ± 0.11, $p = 0.027$), and length of stay in Canada (Standardized Regression Coefficient: -0.23 ± 0.11, $p = 0.04$) were found to be significant predictors of serum vitamin D status. Females—those who had been living in Canada longer, those from regions with darker skin pigmentation, and those with lower vitamin D intake—were at greater risk of low circulating vitamin D.

Table 4. Vitamin D status of newcomer children.

Characteristics	Immigrants $n = 33$ (45.8%)	Refugees $n = 39$ (54.2%)	All participants $n = 72$ (100%)
H/day spent in the sun during peak times (Mean ± SD)	3.6 ± 1.7	3.5 ± 1.5	3.6 ± 1.6
Sunscreen use			
always	0 (0.00%)	2 (5.1%)	2 (2.8%)
often	4 (12.1%)	0 (0.00%)	4 (5.6%)
sometimes	5 (15.2%)	10 (25.6%)	15 (20.8%)
rarely	3 (9.1%)	5 (12.8%)	8 (11.1%)
never	21 (63.6%)	22 (56.4%)	43 (59.7%)
Total serum vitamin D in nmol/L (Mean ± SD)	45.7 ± 13.9 *	37.8 ± 15.5	41.2 ± 15.2
Deficient and inadequate <50 nmol/L	19 (63.3%)	31 (79.5%)	50 (72.5%)
Sufficient ≥50 nmol/L	11 (36.7%)	8 (20.5%)	19 (27.5%)
Total body bone mineral content (TBBMC) in grams (Mean ± SD)	984.9 ± 245.0	947.8 ± 208.8	964.6 ± 224.9
Low TBBMC	13 (41.9%)	14 (35.9%)	27 (38.6%)

* Significant difference from refugees; for means a t-test was used and for categorical variables chi square was used.

TBBMC was low in 38.6% of participants compared to estimated values for age, sex, and ethnicity [24]. In the regression model, after controlling for possible confounders, including immigration status; food security; age; sex; region of origin; physical activity level; total caloric intake; and intakes of calcium, magnesium, phosphorus, sodium, and caffeine, height and serum vitamin D status were found to be determinants of TBBMC (Table 5). Children who were taller and had greater serum vitamin D also had greater TBBMC.

Table 5. Factors associated with total body bone mineral content (TBBMC) in regression analysis (using the stepwise procedure) among all subjects ($n = 56$).

Outcome variable	Constant	Regression coefficient		Total R^2
		Height (cm)	Serum vitamin D (nmol/L)	
TBBMC	−1257.33	0.95 ± 0.06	0.13 ± 0.06	0.82
Partial R^2		0.90	0.27	
p-value		<0.001	0.047	

Table 5. *Cont.*

Outcome variable	Excluded variables					
	Sex	Region of origin	Age	Calcium (mg)	Calories (kcal)	Immigration Status
TBBMC	0.01	−0.09	−0.12	0.07	0.07	0.05
Partial R^2	0.03	−0.20	−0.17	0.13	0.14	0.12
p-value	0.832	0.147	0.227	0.353	0.323	0.408
Outcome variable	Excluded variables					
	H/week in physical activities	Food security	Magnesium (mg)	Phosphorous (mg)	Sodium (mg)	Caffeine (mg)
TBBMC	0.02	0.11	0.06	0.06	−0.04	−0.03
Partial R^2	0.03	0.23	0.11	0.11	−0.08	−0.06
p-value	0.805	0.095	0.419	0.434	0.574	0.660

4. Interpretation

The HIC study is the first to evaluate vitamin D status of newcomer immigrant and refugee children aged 7–11 years in Canada. Data from a nationally representative sample showed alarmingly low 25(OH)D levels in immigrant children, particularly girls. HIC also showed a rate of 25(OH)D deficiency among newcomer immigrant and refugee children. Among these growing children, after controlling for biological and environmental co-factors, serum vitamin D was a significant predictor of TBBMC.

Using CHMS data, we previously reported Canadian children 6–11 years had higher 25(OH)D concentrations than adolescents and adults [2]. However, non-White Canadians were less likely to achieve recommended levels. This same study showed first generation immigrant children aged 6–11 years, particularly girls, had significantly lower 25(OH)D compared to their non-immigrant counterparts. Many newcomers have darker skin pigmentation and are, therefore, at greater risk for deficiency as melanin in the skin prevents the body from synthesizing vitamin D [28]. It is likely that females were at greater risk of deficiency than males due to cultural practices associated with greater covering of females causing insufficient skin exposure to the sun even though they may have been outdoors [28].

In the absence of comprehensive data on dietary intakes and other health measures in CHMS, specifically in newcomer children, data from HIC provides more insight into health concerns faced by this population. Many newcomer children, particularly refugees, did not have a good quality diet including dietary sources of vitamin D. However, vitamin D intake was still the main predictor of serum vitamin D. Circulating vitamin D of 75 nmol/L is considered beneficial for multiple health outcome [29]. None of the HIC participants met the 25(OH)D level of 75 nmol/L and over 29% were vitamin D deficient. This occurred even though non-Caucasian immigrant and refugee children spent almost four hours a day outside during peak times in summer months and the majority of participants rarely or never used sunscreen. It is more difficult to get the necessary vitamin D in areas of high latitude, especially during winter months [3–6]. This may explain why those who had been in Canada longer were at greater risk of deficiency; vitamin D stores are depleted each winter and not replenished enough in the summer. Girls, children with low vitamin D intake, those from regions with darker skin, and those with longer duration of stay in Canada were at higher risk of having inadequate/deficient levels of serum vitamin D.

Since bone mineral mass decreases with age, research has emphasized the importance of achieving optimal bone mineral accrual during childhood and adolescence, which will decrease skeletal-related health issues later in life [30–33]. Therefore, meeting requirements for vitamin D and calcium in these critical ages is crucial [34,35]. Most newcomer children in this study were not getting the recommended amounts of vitamin D and dietary calcium for bone health. Low intakes of calcium and vitamin D accord with low intakes of milk and alternatives, the main dietary sources of these two important nutrients [35]. Inadequate levels impede proper bone growth, which can result in stunting and increase the risk of developing osteoporosis in the future [4,5,22]. Serum vitamin D was a significant predictor of TBBMC in this study. TBBMC was lower than predicted values for age, sex and ethnicity in over 38% of participants. A recent Canadian study found significantly higher TBBMC values in Caucasian compared to Asian children [36]. There was no significant difference in TBBMC according to immigration status in HIC. Further research with a larger sample size is needed to examine TBBMC in children according to ethnicity.

The relatively small sample size in the HIC study may limit the conclusions. However, the accordance of HIC findings on serum vitamin D status of immigrant children with those from the CHMS confirms the importance of HIC results. In the absence of a large-scale comprehensive study on the nutrition and health status of newcomer children, our data could provide valuable insight into this area. HIC also distinguishes refugees from immigrants. Self-reported data on dietary intake using a 24-h recall is subject to under-reporting/over-reporting and omission of frequently forgotten items. To maximize accuracy of the data, we used three 24-h recalls where our expert research personnel used proper probing and assessment aids such as food model booklets, measuring cups and spoons, and color pictures for various food items to help recall names of food items. The premise of the study is to investigate and document disparities in and between host and mobile populations that reflect biological, social and behavioral differences between these populations. Defining these differences can lead to greater awareness of their existence in health providers who may appreciate them and assist those developing programs and policies to identify and mitigate preventable outcomes. Once a framework of existing disparities is defined, further investigation to explore and delineate specific co-founding factors can be undertaken.

5. Conclusion

In addition to the beneficial effects of vitamin D on bone, recent data on the association between vitamin D and chronic diseases including certain types of cancers, diabetes, and multiple sclerosis, demonstrate the importance of this nutrient in growing children [34,35]. Although more research is warranted, a considerably high rate of vitamin D intake inadequacy and serum deficiency/inadequacy in newcomer children is already associated with bone mineral mass during pre-adolescence. This, therefore, requires preventive interventions to minimize the risk of serious vitamin D related diseases.

References

1. Wacker, M.; Holick, M.F. Vitamin D—effects on skeletal and extraskeletal health and the need for supplementation. *Nutrients* **2013**, *5*, 111–148.

2. Whiting, S.J.; Langlois, K.A.; Vatanparast, H.; Greene-Finestone, L.S. The vitamin D status of Canadians relative to the 2011 Dietary Reference Intakes: An examination in children and adults with and without supplement use. *Am. J. Clin. Nutr.* **2011**, *94*, 128–135.

3. Grant, W.B.; Holick, M.F. Benefits and requirements of vitamin D for optimal health: A review. *Altern. Med. Rev.* **2005**, *10*, 94–111.

4. Hintzpeter, B.; Scheidt-Nave, C.; Muller, M.J.; Schenk, L.; Mensink, G.B. Higher prevalence of vitamin D deficiency is associated with immigrant background among children and adolescents in Germany. *J. Nutr.* **2008**, *138*, 1482–1490.

5. Mithal, A.; Wahl, D.A.; Bonjour, J.P.; Burckhardt, P.; Dawson-Hughes, B.; Eisman, J.A.; El-Haji Fuleihan, G.; Josse, R.G.; Lips, P.; Morales-Torres, J. Global vitamin D status and determinants of hypovitaminosis D. *Osteoporos. Int.* **2009**, *20*, 1807–1820.

6. Van der Meer, I.M.; Karamali, N.S.; Boeke, A.J.; Lips, P.; Middelkoop, B.J.; Verhoeven, I.; Wuister, J.D. High prevalence of vitamin D deficiency in pregnant non-Western women in The Hague, Netherlands. *Am. J. Clin. Nutr.* **2006**, *84*, 350–353.

7. Ward, L.M.; Gaboury, I.; Ladhani, M.; Zlotkin, S. Vitamin D-decifiency rickets among children in Canada. *CMAJ* **2007**, *177*, 161–166.

8. Roth, D.E. Bones and beyond: An update on the role of vitamin D in child and adolescent health in Canada. *Appl. Physiol. Nutr. Metab.* **2007**, *32*, 770–777.

9. Statistics Canada. Canadian Health Measures Survey (Detailed information for Spring 2007 to Spring 2009 (Cycle 1)), 2010. Available online: http://www.statcan.gc.ca/cgi-bin/imdb/p2SV.pl?Function=getSurvey&SDDS=5071&lang=en&db=imdb&adm=8&dis=2 (accessed on 30 August 2012).

10. Health Canada. Canadian Community Health Survey Cycle 2.2, Nutrition (2004)—A Guide to Accessing and Interpreting the Data. Available online: http://www.hc-sc.gc.ca/fn-an/alt_formats/hpfb-dgpsa/pdf/surveill/cchs-guide-escc-eng.pdf (accessed on 25 August 2012).

11. Immigration. In *Canadian Oxford Dictionary*; Oxford University Press: New York, NY, USA, 2011. Available online: http://www.oxfordreference.com/views/SEARCH_RESULTS.html?y=14&q=immigrate&category=t150&x=4&ssid=865872107&scope=book&time=0.830259983485593 (accessed on 15 August 2012).

12. United Nations High Commissioner for Refugees. Convention Relating to the Status of Refugees Article, 1951. Available online: http://www2.ohchr.org/English/law/refugees.htm#wp1037003 (accessed on 15 August 2012).

13. Statistics Canada. Master and share files derived variables documentation, 2008. Available online: http://www.statcan.gc.ca/imdb-bmdi/document/5049_D11_T9_V1-eng.pdf (accessed on 27 August 2012).

14. Health Canada. Canadian Community Health Survey, Cycle 2.2, Nutrition (2004)—Income-related household food security in Canada. Ottawa (ON): Office of Nutrition Policy and Promotion Health Products and Food Branch, 2007. Available online: http://www.hc-sc.gc.ca/fn-an/ alt_formats/hpfb-dgpsa/pdf/surveill/income_food_sec-sec_alim-eng.pdf (accessed on 19 July 2012).

15. World Health Organization. Growth reference 5–19 years, 2007. Available online: http://www. who.int/growthref/en/ (accessed on 19 July 2012).

16. Health Canada. Eating well with Canada's food guide, 2007. Available online: http://www. hc-sc.gc.ca/fn-an/food-guide-aliment/index-eng.php (accessed on 11 June 2012).

17. Garriguet, D. Diet quality in Canada. *Health Rep.* **2009**, *20*, 41–52.

18. Eyles, D.; Anderson, C.; Ko, P.; Jones, A.; Thomas, A.; Burne, T.; Mortensen, P.B.; Norgaard-Pedersen, B.; Hougaard, D.M.; McGrath, J. A sensitive LC/MS/MS assay of 25OH vitamin D3 and 25OH vitamin D2 in dried blood spots. *Clin. Chim. Acta* **2009**, *403*, 145–151.

19. Newman, M.S.; Brandon, T.R.; Groves, M.N.; Gregory, W.L.; Kapur, S.; Zava, D.T. A liquid chromatography/tandem mass spectrometry method for determination of 25-hydroxi vitamin D2 and 25-hydroxy vitamin D3 in dried blood spots: A potential adjunct to diabetes and cardiometabolic risk screening. *J. Diabetes Sci. Technol.* **2009**, *3*, 156–162.

20. Hollis, B.W. Measuring 25-hydroxyvitamin D in a clinical environment: Challenges and needs. *Am. J. Clin. Nutr.* **2008**, *88*, 507S–510S.

21. Larkin, E.K.; Gebretsadik, T.; Koestner, N.; Newman, M.S.; Liu, Z.; Carroll, K.N.; Minton, P.; Woodward, K.; Hartert, T.V. Agreement of blood spot card measurements of vitamin D levels with serum, whole blood specimen types and a dietary recall instrument. *PLoS One* **2011**, *6*, e16602.

22. Institute of Medicine. *Dietary reference intakes for calcium and vitamin D*; The National Academies Press: Washington, DC, USA, 2010. Available online: http://www.iom.edu/Reports/ 2010/Dietary-Reference-Intakes-for-Calcium-and-Vitamin-D.aspx (accessed on 27 August 2012).

23. Fewtrell, M.S. Bone densitometry in children assessed by dual X ray absorptiometry: Uses and pitfalls. *Arch. Dis. Child.* **2003**, *88*, 795–798.

24. Baxter-Jones, A.D.; Burrows, M.; Bachrach, L.K.; Lloyd, T.; Petit, M.; Macdonald, H.; Mirwald, R.L.; Bailey, D.; McKay, H. International longitudinal pediatric reference standards for bone mineral content. *Bone* **2009**, *46*, 208–216.

25. Government of Saskatchewan. Saskatchewan Statistical Immigration Report 2009, 2008. Available online http://aeel.gov.sk.ca/sk-immigration-statistical-report-2009 (accessed on 23 August 2012).

26. Citizenship and Immigration Canada facts and figures 2011. Available online: http://www. cic.gc.ca/english/pdf/research-stats/facts2011.pdf (accessed on 23 August 2012).

27. Canadian Society for Exercise Physiology, Communique, March Newsletter. Available online: http://www.csep.ca/english/view.asp?x=804 (accessed on 27 August 2012).

28. Nellen, J.F.; Smulders, Y.M.; Frissen, P.H.; Slaats, E.H.; Silberusch, J. Hypovitaminosis D in immigrant women: Slow to be diagnosed. *BMJ* **1996**, *312*, 570–572.

29. Wimalawansa, S.J. Vitamin D in the new millennium. *Curr. Osteoporos. Rep.* **2012**, *10*, 4–15.

30. Caradonna, P.; Rigante, D. Bone health as a primary target in the pediatric age. *Eur. Rev. Med. Pharmacol. Sci.* **2009**, *13*, 117–128.

31. Nichols, D.L.; Sanborn, C.F.; Essery, E.V.; Clark, R.A.; Letendre, J.D. Impact of curriculum-based bone loading and nutrition education program on bone accrual in children. *Pediatr. Exerc. Sci.* **2008**, *20*, 411–425.

32. Vatanparast, H.; Baxter-Jones, A.; Faulkner, R.A.; Bailey, D.A.; Whiting, S.J. Positive effects of vegetable and fruit consumption and calcium intake on bone mineral accrual in boys during growth from childhood to adolescence: The University of Saskatchewan Pediatric Bone Mineral Accrual Study. *Am. J. Clin. Nutr.* **2005**, *82*, 700–706.

33. Bailey, D.A.; Faulkner, R.A.; McKay, H.A. Growth, physical activity, and bone mineral acquisition. *Exerc. Sport Sci. Rev.* **1996**, *24*, 233–266.

34. Whiting, S.J.; Calvo, M.S. Dietary recommendations for vitamin D: A critical need for functional end points to establish an estimated average requirement. *J. Nutr.* **2005**, *135*, 304–309.

35. Holick, M.F. Health benefits of vitamin D and sunlight: A D-bate. *Nat. Rev. Endocrinol.* **2011**, *7*, 73–75.

36. Burrows, M.; Baxter-Jones, A.; Mirwald, R.; Macdonald, H.; McKay, H. Bone mineral accrual across growth in a mixed-ethnic group of children: Are Asian children disadvantaged from an early age? *Calcif. Tissue Int.* **2009**, *84*, 366–378.

6

Calcidiol Deficiency in End-Stage Organ Failure and after Solid Organ Transplantation: *Status quo*

Ursula Thiem *, Bartosz Olbramski and Kyra Borchhardt

Division of Nephrology and Dialysis, Department of Internal Medicine III, Medical University of Vienna, Spitalgasse 23, Vienna 1090, Austria; E-Mails: n0642244@students.meduniwien.ac.at (B.O.); kyra.borchhardt@meduniwien.ac.at (K.B.)

* Author to whom correspondence should be addressed; E-Mail: ursula.thiem@meduniwien.ac.at;

Abstract: Among patients with organ failure, vitamin D deficiency is extremely common and frequently does not resolve after transplantation. This review crystallizes and summarizes existing data on the *status quo* of vitamin D deficiency in patients with organ failure and in solid organ transplant recipients. Interventional studies evaluating different treatment strategies, as well as current clinical practice guidelines and recommendations on the management of low vitamin D status in these patients are also discussed.

Keywords: vitamin D; heart failure; pulmonary disease; liver failure; chronic kidney disease; transplantation; calcidiol; rejection; supplementation; guidelines

1. Introduction

Vitamin D deficiency is a commonly observed phenomenon in patients with organ failure and solid organ transplant recipients. It occurs in patients with different types of solid organ transplant and frequently persists even in the long-term, post-transplant period (reviewed in [1]). The causes of vitamin D deficiency in these patients are diverse. Vitamin D deficiency may be primarily ascribed to lifestyle and environmental factors that result in reduced exposure to sunlight, as the main source of vitamin D is the skin, where it is synthesized from 7-dehydrochoesterol under the influence of ultraviolet light (reviewed in [2]). On the other hand, in patients with end-stage organ disease, there may be additional disease-specific factors that contribute to vitamin D deficiency, such as liver dysfunction [3] or uremia, which reduces the capacity of the skin to synthesize vitamin D [4,5]. After transplantation, the avoidance of sunlight, due to the increased risk of skin cancer in immunosuppressed patients [6], may be the main factor causing vitamin D deficiency [7]. Additional factors might involve the use of glucocorticoids, which were shown to enhance the catabolism of calcidiol [8].

Vitamin D deficiency is also commonly observed in the general population [9]. The National Health and Nutrition Examination Survey (NHANES) between 2002 and 2004, for example, assessed calcidiol levels in a representative sample of more than 20,000 persons in the USA and revealed that calcidiol levels below 20 ng/mL occur in approximately one third of the studied population [10]. In non-institutionalized elderly people across 11 European countries, 36% of men and 47% of women showed calcidiol levels below 12 ng/mL during winter [11]. For the general population, the Institute of Medicine in 2011 released their report on dietary reference intakes for calcium and vitamin D. For optimal bone health, the recommended dietary allowances of 600 International Units of vitamin D for ages up to 70 years and 800 International Units for ages above 70 years are suggested, corresponding to calcidiol levels above 20 ng/mL [12].

Herein, we review the prevalence of vitamin D deficiency in patients with end-stage organ failure and organ transplant recipients, as well as clinical trials on supplementation strategies and current guidelines on the recommendation of vitamin D intake in these patients. In this review, we consider 25-hydroxyvitamin D (calcidiol) levels below 30 ng/mL as insufficiency or hypovitaminosis, below 20 ng/mL as deficiency and below 10 ng/mL as severe deficiency (×2.5 for conversion to nmol/L).

2. Congestive Heart Failure and Cardiac Transplantation

2.1. Vitamin D Status in Patients with End-Stage Heart Failure

Hypovitaminosis D is highly prevalent among patients with congestive heart failure, with 17% to 57% of the patients displaying severe vitamin D deficiency [13,14]. The vitamin D status was reported to be related to the severity of the disease. In particular, patients evaluated for cardiac transplantation and classified United Network of Organ Sharing (UNOS) status 1 (*i.e.*, hospitalization and dependence on intravenous inotropic agents or left ventricular assist devices) had significantly lower calcidiol levels as compared with patients classified UNOS status 2, who were well enough to be managed as outpatients, (19 ng/mL *vs.* 24 ng/mL). While 23% of status 1 patients displayed severe vitamin D deficiency, only 8% of status 2 patients did so [13]. Similarly, mean serum calcidiol levels were reported to be lower in end-stage congestive heart failure patients awaiting cardiac transplantation who were classified as urgent or high urgent candidates according to the Eurotransplant listing criteria as compared with elective candidates (9.3 ng/mL *vs.* 14 ng/mL). None of the urgent or high urgent and only about 5% of the elective transplant candidates had sufficient vitamin D levels. Severe vitamin D deficiency was present in 57% of urgent or high urgent and in 50% of elective transplant candidates [14].

2.2. Vitamin D Status in Cardiac Transplant Recipients

Only one study reported the vitamin D status at the time of cardiac transplantation. Almost 90% of the patients presented with vitamin D insufficiency and 10% were found to be severely deficient [15]. In short-term heart transplant recipients, mean serum calcidiol levels increased from 18.7 ng/mL, analyzed within 12 months pre-transplant, to 24.5 ng/mL at one year post-transplant. Even though intake of 400 to 800 International Units of vitamin D was recommended to all patients, approximately three quarters of the patients displayed vitamin D insufficiency at one year post-transplant [16]. Similar results were obtained from an Iranian cohort of short-term heart transplant recipients, where two thirds were reported to be vitamin D deficient [17]. Even in the long-term post-transplant period, vitamin D deficiency frequently persists. In cardiac transplant recipients with a mean allograft age of approximately four years, more than 90% of the patients were reported to have hypovitaminosis D, with more than one third of patients displaying severe deficiency [18]. A summary of the vitamin D status in patients with end-stage heart failure and cardiac transplant recipients is presented in Table 1.

2.3. Interventional Studies and Guidelines

Despite the high prevalence of vitamin D insufficiency among patients with advanced heart failure and cardiac transplant recipients, interventional studies are sparse or lacking. In a randomized controlled trial in patients with heart failure (New York Heart Association class II and higher), the effect of daily 500 mg calcium and 2000 International Units vitamin D_3 on survival, cytokine profiles and echocardiographic parameters was studied and compared with calcium treatment alone. After nine months, treatment with vitamin D_3 increased the mean serum calcidiol level by 26.8 ng/mL, while an increase of only 3.6 ng/mL was observed in placebo treated patients. Treatment with vitamin D_3 prevented an increase in tumor necrosis factor alpha, as observed in placebo-treated patients, and increased interleukin 10 levels [19]. Moreover, a recent study investigated the effect of vitamin D_3 on biochemical and functional parameters of congestive heart failure in vitamin D insufficient patients with New York Heart Association class I to III heart failure. The treatment consisted of 50,000 International Units per week for eight weeks. Thereafter, the patients received 50,000 International Units every month for two months. Mean serum calcidiol level increased by 17 ng/mL after the four month treatment period. Interestingly, a decrease in pro-brain natriuretic peptide and high-sensitivity C-reactive protein, as well as an improvement in six minute walk distance and New York Heart Association class was observed [20].

Current guidelines for vitamin D intake in heart transplant candidates and cardiac transplant recipients are based on the beneficial effects of vitamin D therapy on corticosteroid-induced bone loss. In particular, based on expert consensus (Level of Evidence C), the International Society of Heart and Lung Transplantation recommends a daily intake of 1000 to 1500 mg of calcium and 400 to 1000 International Units of vitamin D to all heart transplant candidates and recipients. Serum calcidiol levels should be maintained above 30 ng/mL [21].

Table 1. Vitamin D status in congestive heart failure and cardiac transplant patients.

Ref.	Country, State	N	Study design and study population	Time point of calcidiol analysis	Mean ± SD calcidiol (ng/mL)	% insufficient (<30 ng/mL)	% deficient (<20 ng/mL)	% severely deficient (<10 ng/mL)	Supplementation
[13]	USA, New York	101	cross-sectional study; severe heart failure patients (NYHA III, IV) referred for tx		21			17	5% took supplemental calcium or vitamin D
[14]	Germany	383	cross-sectional study; heart failure patients awaiting tx (elective vs. urgent candidates)		14 vs.9.3	95.4 vs. 100	86.2 vs. 94.8	50.2 vs. 56.9	no
[15]	USA, New York	46	randomized controlled trial; heart transplant recipients	10 ± 7 days after tx	19.1 ± 8.3	89	64.5	9.5	800–1000 IU vitamin D once oral medication was tolerated
[16]	Norway	59	randomized controlled trial; heart transplant recipients	pre-transplant vs. 1 year after tx	18.7 vs. 24.6	73.6			400–800 IU vitamin D and 1000 mg calcium daily recommended
[17]	Iran	26	retrospective study; heart transplant recipients	24.8 ± 21 months after tx	17.8 ± 10.5		66.6		no
[18]	Italy	180	cross-sectional study; heart transplant recipients	3.91 years after tx	14.33 ± 8.25	92		35.5	no

tx, transplantation; NYHA, New York Heart Association; IU, International Units.

3. End-Stage Pulmonary Disease and Lung Transplantation

3.1. Vitamin D Status in Patients with End-Stage Pulmonary Disease

In end-stage pulmonary disease patients, varying prevalence of vitamin D deficiency was reported depending on the underlying disease. Severe vitamin D deficiency was seen in 14% to 40% of patients with cystic fibrosis [22–24], 20% to 42% of patients with chronic obstructive pulmonary disease [22,23], 14% of patients with pulmonary fibrosis [23] and 18% of patients with pulmonary hypertension [23]. Even though in one study, the majority of the patients received multivitamin supplements containing 400 to 800 International Units of vitamin D, 40% had severe vitamin D deficiency, and only 25% of the patients showed serum calcidiol levels above 20 ng/mL [24].

3.2. Vitamin D Status in Lung Transplant Recipients

In short-term lung transplant recipients in the United States, the proportion of patients with vitamin D insufficiency decreased from 79% at the time of transplantation to 26% at one year post-transplant. Approximately half of the patients received vitamin D supplements at the time of transplantation, while all of them did so after lung transplantation. Vitamin D deficiency at the time of transplantation was associated with an increased risk of experiencing acute rejection episodes or infections [25]. Similarly, a European study reported an improvement in vitamin D status after one year of lung transplantation. Mean serum calcidiol levels increased from 25.1 ng/mL at the time of transplantation to 29.4 ng/mL at one year post-transplant. Intake of 400 to 800 International Units of vitamin D was recommended to all patients. Still, approximately half of the patients displayed vitamin D insufficiency at one year post-transplant [16].

Table 2. Vitamin D status in end-stage pulmonary disease and lung transplant patients.

Ref.	Country, State	N	Study design and study population	Time point of calcidiol analysis	Mean ± SD calcidiol (ng/mL)	% insufficient (<30 ng/mL)	% deficient (<20 ng/mL)	% severely deficient (<10 ng/mL)	Supplementation
[22]	USA, New York	70	cross-sectional study; lung transplant candidates (COPD/cystic fibrosis/other)		20/17/14			20/36/20	no
[23]	Switzerland	63	cross-sectional study; end-stage lung disease patients		18 ± 11			25	no
[24]	USA, New York	20	cross-sectional study; lung transplant candidates		16		75	40	80% received 400–800 IU vitamin D
[27]	Norway	71	cross-sectional study; lung transplant candidates (normal vs. underweight)		14.9 ± 6.3 vs. 15.2 ± 6.6	100 vs. 97	55 vs. 52 [a]		no
[28]	USA, North Carolina	70	retrospective study; end-stage cystic fibrosis patients referred for tx		20.9 ± 11.9				90% received vitamin D in the form of ADEK
[25]	USA, Illinois	109	retrospective study; lung transplant recipients	near-transplant period vs. 1 year after tx	28.2	79.4 vs. 26.5			1000 IU daily up to 50,000 IU once or twice weekly in 50% before, 100% after tx
[16]	Norway	35	randomized controlled trial; lung transplant recipients	pre-transplant vs. 1 year after tx	25.1 vs. 29.4	vs. 50			400–800 IU vitamin D and 1000 mg calcium daily recommended
[26]	Belgium	131	cross-sectional study; lung transplant recipients	12–48 months after tx		47.3	19.8	4.6	880–1000 IU vitamin D

tx, transplantation; IU, International Units; [a] <12.5 ng/mL.

Data on the vitamin D status in long-term lung transplant recipients is sparse. In a Belgian cohort of 131 prevalent lung transplant recipients with an allograft age ranging from one to four years, approximately half of the patients were reported to have vitamin D insufficiency, despite daily treatment with 880 to 1000 International Units of cholecalciferol for the prevention of osteoporosis. A subgroup-analysis revealed that the proportion of vitamin D insufficient patients was similar between patients with one, two, three or four years of follow-up (ranging from 42% at one and two years post-transplant to 53% at three and four years post-transplant). Interestingly, after multivariate adjustment, vitamin D deficiency was associated with lower FEV_1 (forced expiratory volume in one second), and patients deficient in vitamin D experienced more episodes of moderate to severe B-grade rejection (lymphocytic bronchiolitis) [26]. Details on the vitamin D status in patients with end-stage pulmonary disease and lung transplant recipients are summarized in Table 2.

3.3. Interventional Studies and Guidelines

Based on the finding that vitamin D deficiency in lung transplant recipients is associated with an increased risk of developing rejection episodes, a randomized controlled trial is currently investigating the effect of a two year therapy of monthly 100,000 International Units of vitamin D in incident lung transplant recipients on the development of bronchiolitis obliterans syndrome, a frequent manifestation of chronic rejection (clinicaltrials.gov NCT01212406).

To our knowledge, there are no guidelines on the management of vitamin D deficiency in patients with end-stage pulmonary disease or lung transplant patients.

4. Liver Failure and Liver Transplantation

4.1. Vitamin D Status in Patients with End-Stage Liver Disease

The liver is the main site where hydroxylation of vitamin D at position C-25 takes place. Thus, it is not surprising that the degree of liver dysfunction correlates with calcidiol levels [3] and that the prevalence of vitamin D insufficiency is particularly high in patients with chronic liver disease [29–32]. At the time of transplantation, between 80% and 95% of the patients with end-stage liver failure were reported to have hypovitaminosis D, with varying prevalence of severe vitamin D deficiency (ranging from 3% up to 50%) [15,33–35]. Notably, in one study, more than one fifth of the patients had serum calcidiol below the detection limit of 6.8 ng/mL [15].

4.2. Vitamin D Status in Liver Transplant Recipients

At three months after liver transplantation, Reese and colleagues observed a marked increase in serum calcidiol levels with a median change of 17.8 ng/mL (interquartile range 8.6 to 25.9 ng/mL). The prevalence of vitamin D deficiency dropped from 84% at the time of transplantation to 24% after three months post-transplant. Moreover, serum vitamin D binding protein and albumin substantially increased, which according to the authors, might have contributed to the marked improvement in vitamin D status by facilitating a shift of calcidiol from the adipose tissue to the circulation. Even though the prevalence of vitamin D deficiency was similar in black and non-black patients at the time of transplantation, median calcidiol levels were significantly lower in black patients (4.9 *vs.* 9.6 ng/mL). At three months after transplantation, vitamin D deficiency was more prevalent among black liver transplant recipients as compared with non-black patients (38% *vs.* 20%) [36]. In contrast, in an Iranian cohort of liver transplant recipients, a high prevalence of vitamin D deficiency persisted in the early post-transplant period [17]. In a Spanish study, 45 liver transplant recipients were followed up to three years after transplantation. Before transplantation, severe vitamin D deficiency was present in 62% of the patients, with a mean serum calcidiol of 9.4 ng/mL. In comparison, 40 healthy age-matched controls displayed a mean serum calcidiol of 23.1 ng/mL. Serum calcidiol levels continuously increased over time (9.5 ng/mL at one month, 16.5 ng at three months, 15.9 ng at six months, 19 ng/mL at 12 months, 19.9 ng/mL at 18 months, 18 ng/mL at 24 months and 19.5 ng/mL at 36 months post-transplant). At one year and three years after transplantation, severe vitamin D deficiency was observed in only 14% and 10% of the patients, respectively [37]. In contrast, in an Israelian cohort of long-term liver transplant recipients with a mean allograft age of 7.5 years, more than one third was reported to have severe vitamin D deficiency [38]. Table 3 summarizes the prevalence of vitamin D insufficiency, deficiency and severe deficiency in patients with end-stage liver disease and liver transplant recipients.

4.3. Interventional Studies and Guidelines

Recently, a clinical practice guideline on the evaluation, treatment and prevention of vitamin D deficiency has been published by the Endocrine Society. According to this guideline, patients with hepatic failure are considered at high risk for vitamin D deficiency. Therefore, calcidiol measurements are reasonable, and supplementation in case of calcidiol levels below 20 ng/mL is recommended. For bone health, adults are considered to require at least 600 to 800 International Units daily. For reaching calcidiol levels above 30 ng/mL, however, higher doses may be required (1500 to 2000 International Units). This recommendation is based on lower quality evidence [39]. For the management of liver transplant patients, the American Association for the Study of Liver Disease and the American Society of Transplantation released a practice guideline, which recommends calcidiol levels to be maintained above 30 ng/mL for optimal bone health. This daily use of 400 to 1000 International Units of vitamin D is suggested; however, calcidiol levels should be measured at least annually to check if the treatment regimen is appropriate. Treatment with vitamin D supplements is recommended in osteopenic liver transplant recipients with a Level of Evidence A [40].

5. Chronic Kidney Disease and Kidney Transplantation

5.1. Vitamin D Status in Patients with Chronic Kidney Disease

Vitamin D deficiency is very common in patients with chronic kidney disease (CKD) across all stages. In North America, a prevalence of vitamin D insufficiency of approximately 85% was reported among patients with advanced kidney disease [41,42]. Severe vitamin D deficiency (<15 ng/mL) was more pronounced in patients with CKD stage 5 (56%), as compared with CKD stage 4 (37%) [42], and mean serum calcidiol was reported to be significantly lower in diabetic as compared with non-diabetic patients [43]. Similarly, in a cohort of chronic kidney disease stage 3 and 4 in the UK, hypovitaminosis

D was very common, with 80% of the patients showing vitamin D insufficiency and 37% severe vitamin D deficiency (<15 ng/mL). After exclusion of patients who received vitamin D supplements or other drugs known to interfere with calcidiol levels, mean serum calcidiol remained unchanged. Likewise, the proportional distribution of patients with vitamin D insufficiency and severe deficiency was similar [44]

Table 3. Vitamin D status in end-stage liver disease and liver transplant patients.

Ref.	Country, State	N	Study design and study population	Time point of calcidiol analysis	Mean ± SD calcidiol (ng/mL)	% insufficient (<30 ng/mL)	% deficient (<20 ng/mL)	% severely deficient (<10 ng/mL)	Supplementation
[15]	USA, New York	23	randomized controlled trial; liver transplant recipients	10 ± 7 days after tx	13.8 ± 7	95	83	30	800–1000 IU vitamin D once oral medication was tolerated
[17]	Iran	23	retrospective study; liver transplant recipients	21.6 ± 21.4 months after tx	14.3 ± 9.6		80.9		no
[33]	Italy	93	retrospective study; liver transplant recipients	at the time of tx	12.5 (1.0–48.5) [a]	92.5		49.5 [d]	60% took 800 IU vitamin D, 40% started in the first month after tx
[34]	USA, Wisconsin	63	retrospective study; liver disease patients awaiting tx			81 [b]	75	6.3	10% took vitamin D supplements
[35]	Australia	10 7	prospective cohort study; liver disease patients assessed for tx (cholestatic vs. hepatocellular disease)		46.5 [a] vs. 42		66	15	5% took vitamin D supplements
[36]	USA, Pennsylvania	20 2	prospective cohort study; liver transplant recipients	at the time of tx vs. 3 months after tx	6.7 vs. 27.4 [a]		84 vs. 24		all received 400 IU vitamin D
[37]	Spain	45	prospective study; liver transplant candidates	at the time of tx	9.4			62	no
		39		1 year after tx	19			14	
		34		2 years after tx	18				
		30		3 years after tx	19.5			10	
[38]	Israel	29	cross-sectional study; liver transplant patients	7.5 ± 4.1 years after tx			65.5 [c]	38	0.25 µg alphacalcidol pre-transplant

tx, transplantation; IU, International Units; [a] median (range), [b] <32 ng/mL; [c] <15 ng/mL; [d] <12.5 ng/mL.

5.2. Vitamin D Status in Kidney Transplant Recipients

Only a few studies investigated the vitamin D status at the time of transplantation. Almost 90% of incident kidney transplant recipients were reported to have insufficient calcidiol levels, with a mean serum calcidiol of 16.6 ng/mL and a trend towards higher calcidiol levels in summer as compared with winter. Notably, vitamin D levels of black kidney transplant recipients were significantly lower compared with non-black patients (13.6 ng/mL vs. 17.5 ng/mL) [45]. Similar findings were obtained from another cohort of African American renal transplant recipients in the early post-transplant period, where 95% of the patients presented with calcidiol levels below 30 ng/mL and 58% showed severe vitamin deficiency (<16 ng/mL), even at the end of summer [46].

Even though vitamin D status was reported to improve in the early post-transplant period [47], low vitamin D levels are frequently observed in long-term kidney transplant recipients [7,48,49]. Querings et al. investigated the vitamin D status of 31 long-term kidney transplant recipients with a mean allograft age of seven years at the end of winter and found a mean serum calcidiol of 10.9 ng/mL. Notably, vitamin D sufficiency was observed in one patient only, and almost one third of the patients had serum calcidiol levels below the detection limit (<4 ng/mL) [7].

In contrast, in a Danish cohort of long-term kidney transplant recipients, approximately one fifth of the patients were found to have sufficient vitamin D during the winter months, with a median calcidiol level of 19.8 ng/mL. A subgroup analysis revealed that 60% of these patients received vitamin D supplements at a median dose of 7.8 μg per day (in the form of ergocalciferol or cholecalciferol or alphacalcidol), which might explain the lower prevalence of vitamin D insufficiency in this cohort. In addition, a median alimentary intake of approximately 3.2 μg vitamin D per day was reported [49]. Moreover, clear seasonal variations in serum calcidiol levels were found in long-term kidney transplant recipients, with 3.5-times more patients reaching calcidiol above 30 ng/mL during summer months compared with winter months. Still, the majority of the patients exhibited vitamin D insufficiency, even during summer [50,51]. In Table 4, details on the vitamin D status in CKD patients and renal transplant patients are presented.

Table 4. Vitamin D status in chronic kidney disease and renal transplant patients.

Ref.	Country	N	Study design and Study population	Time point of calcidiol analysis	Mean ± SD calcidiol (ng/mL)	% insufficient (<30 ng/mL)	%deficient (<20 ng/mL)	% severely deficient (<10 ng/mL)	Supplementation
[41]	USA, diverse regions	178	cross-sectional study; patients with CKD 3 vs. 4		23.3 ± 14.5 vs. 18.6 ± 13.3	71 vs. 83		14 vs. 26	no
[42]	Canada	168	prospective study; CKD patients		18.1 [a]		34.5 [b]		active vitamin D analogs
[43]	Japan	76	prospective study; non-dialyzed CKD patients (non-diabetic vs. diabetic)		22.3 ± 9.4 vs. 11.4 ± 5.6				no
[44]	UK	112	cross-sectional study; patients with CKD 3 and 4		20.8 ± 12	80	36 [b]	6 [c]	
[45]	USA, Massachusetts	112	prospective; renal transplant recipients	at the time of transplantation	16.6 ± 9.6	87.5		28.6	active vitamin D analogs
[46]	USA, Virginia	38	cross-sectional study; African American renal transplant recipients	23 ± 20 months after tx	16 ± 7.4	94.7	57.8 [b]		no
[47]	Turkey	161	longitudinal cohort study; renal transplant recipients	pre-transplant vs. 6 months after tx	18.1 ± 4 vs. 22 ± 4.5	65.8			no
[48]	UK	104	cross-sectional study; renal transplant recipients	3.4 (1.9–12) months after tx	13.2 ± 7.6	97	68 [b]	12 [c]	no
		140		6 (1–24) years after tx	16.8 ± 8	94	51 [b]	5 [c]	no

Table 4. *Cont.*

Ref.	Country	N	Study design and Study population	Time point of calcidiol analysis	Mean ± SD calcidiol (ng/mL)	% insufficient (<30 ng/mL)	%deficient (<20 ng/mL)	% severely deficient (<10 ng/mL)	Supplementation
[7]	Germany	31	cross-sectional study; renal transplant recipients vs. age/gender matched controls	7 (0.5–19) years after tx	10.9 vs. 20	96.8 vs. 80.6	80.6 vs. 54.8	35.5 vs. 12.9	no
[49]	Denmark	173	cross-sectional study; renal transplant recipients (female vs. male)	7.4 (3.3–12.7) years after tx	21.6 vs. 18.2 [a]	74 vs. 88	26 vs. 33 [b]	3 vs. 9 [c]	69% of women and 51% of men took a median daily dose of 400 and 200 IU vitamin D, respectively
[50]	UK	266	cross-sectional study; renal transplant recipients (winter vs. summer)	16 (12–23) years after tx	15.6 ± 10.8 vs. 23.6 ± 12.4	91 vs. 68	59 vs. 31 [b]		10%–20% took alphacalcidol
[51]	Switzerland	50	prospective study; renal transplant recipients (winter vs. summer)	11.1 (0.8–33.6) years after tx	12.4 vs. 17.6 [a]	96 vs. 86	90 vs. 60		61% of women and 51% of men took vitamin D

CKD, chronic kidney disease; tx, transplantation; IU, International Units; [a] median (range); [b] <16 ng/mL; [c] <5 ng/mL.

5.3. Interventional Studies and Guidelines

Even though vitamin D deficiency is extremely common among patients with chronic kidney disease, including renal transplant recipients, there is no consensus on how to treat vitamin D deficiency in these patients. Current guidelines of the National Kidney Foundation for patients with chronic kidney disease recommend the measurement of calcidiol in patients with CKD stage 3 or 4 only in case of elevated parathyroid hormone levels. Oral supplementation with ergocalciferol for six months, with 50,000 International Units per week for four weeks in the case of mild (5 to 15 ng/mL) and 12 weeks in the case of severe (below 5 ng/mL) vitamin D deficiency is proposed. Thereafter, a monthly dose of 50,000 International Units is recommended. For vitamin D insufficiency, ergocalciferol at a monthly dose of 50,000 International Units orally for six months is suggested. All of these recommendations are opinion-based [52]. For patients after renal transplantation, Clinical Practice Guidelines for the Care of Kidney transplant recipients (KDIGO) suggest correction of vitamin D deficiency or insufficiency as done for the general population (Level of Evidence C) [53].

A recent meta-analysis of seventeen observational and five randomized controlled trials in patients with various forms of CKD evaluated the effect of vitamin D supplementation and found a significant improvement of the vitamin D status, with a mean difference of 24.1 ng/mL in observational and 14 ng/mL in randomized controlled trials. Treatment regimens ranged from 4000 International Units daily up to 50,000 International Units daily, with an average treatment period of half a year [41].

The few studies available indicate that renal transplant recipients have a higher need for vitamin D to correct insufficiency than what is known from the general population. In particular, in a randomized controlled trial in kidney transplant recipients, Wissing and colleagues evaluated the effect of 400 mg/day calcium and 25,000 International Units of cholecalciferol per month on bone mineral density one year after transplantation. Surprisingly, this dose was not sufficient to correct vitamin D deficiency in these patients [54]. In contrast, Courbebaisse and colleagues used 100,000 International Units of cholecalciferol once every two weeks for two months and, thereafter, treated the patients with 100,000 International Units of cholecalciferol every two months for another six months. After the initial intensive treatment period, more than 90% of the patients showed calcidiol levels above 30 ng/mL, while only 50% were vitamin D sufficient after the maintenance treatment period, indicating that 100,000 International Units of cholecalciferol every two months is still not sufficient to maintain optimal vitamin D levels [55]. Moreover, these studies demonstrated that spontaneous recovery of vitamin D deficiency after kidney transplantation does not occur. In the untreated control groups, calcidiol either remained stable [55], or even decreased further [54], over time. Based on their previous study, the group of Courbebaisse established a pharmacokinetic model that describes calcidiol levels after treatment with cholecalciferol in kidney transplant recipients within the first year after transplantation. According to this model, a treatment regimen with six doses of 100,000 International Units cholecalciferol every two weeks, followed by 100,000 International Units once per month is proposed to maintain calcidiol levels between 30 and 80 ng/mL [56]. Several clinical trials are currently ongoing with different treatment regimens ([57], NCT00752401, NCT00748618, NCT01431430), which will help to identify strategies to maintain optimal vitamin D status.

6. Conclusions

In summary, studies in patients with organ failure consistently show that vitamin D insufficiency or deficiency is widespread among these patients, even in the healthier sub-population of patients awaiting transplantation. After transplantation, calcidiol levels frequently remain low and, in many cases, do not recover in the long-term post-transplant period. Minor discrepancies in the reported prevalence of vitamin D insufficiency or deficiency might result from the different treatment regimens used (if patients received vitamin D supplements or not), different habits and customs of the studied populations (sun protection and nutrition), but also from the different assays used to measure calcidiol.

From the current evidence, it is not clear whether vitamin D deficiency is one of the causative factors or a consequence in the development and progression of organ failure. For example, the active vitamin D metabolite, 1,25-dihydroxyvitamin D, might affect the development and progression of cardiovascular disease by different mechanisms of action, such as regulation of the mineral metabolism, interaction with the renin-angiotensin-aldosterone system or modulation of immune responses (reviewed in [58,59]). Similarly, it might exert renoprotective effects and, thus, delay the progression of CKD, e.g., by inhibition of the renin-angiotensin-aldosterone system, regulation of the immune system or increase of insulin sensitivity (reviewed in [60]). On the other hand, low calcidiol levels might simply reflect poorer health status in patients with advanced stages of organ failure.

At present, there are only a few recommendations on how to manage vitamin D deficiency in these patients; most of them are based on expert consensus and derived from the beneficial effects of vitamin D on the skeleton. However, especially in the setting of organ transplantation, the effects of vitamin D might go beyond bone health. In particular, the active metabolite, 1,25-dihydroxyvitamin D, has immunomodulatory activity, which is supported by extensive experimental research (reviewed in [61,62]). Recent clinical trials indicate that modulation of the immune system can be achieved by administration of nutritional vitamin D [63–69]. These immunomodulatory effects may be exploited in various diseases, including organ tolerance after transplantation. The increase in regulatory T-cells by nutritional vitamin D, as shown in a randomized controlled trial, could be of particular relevance in organ transplant recipients [63]. To date, however, we do not have sufficient evidence to recommend treatment with vitamin D based on its immunomodulatory actions, and further clinical trials are clearly warranted.

Acknowledgments

U.T. is a recipient of a DOC-fFORTE fellowship of the Austrian Academy of Sciences (#23478) at the Division of Nephrology and Dialysis in cooperation with the Institute of Pathophysiology and Allergy Research, Medical University of Vienna, and was funded by the Marie Curie Initial Training Network, "Multifaceted CaSR", FP7-264663.

Conflict of Interest

The authors declare no conflict of interest.

References

1. Stein, E.M.; Shane, E. Vitamin D in organ transplantation. *Osteoporos. Int.* **2011**, doi:10.1007/s00198-010-1523-8.

2. Holick, M.F. Vitamin D deficiency. *N. Engl. J. Med.* **2007**, *357*, 266–281.

3. Putz-Bankuti, C.; Pilz, S.; Stojakovic, T.; Scharnagl, H.; Pieber, T.R.; Trauner, M.; Obermayer-Pietsch, B.; Stauber, R.E. Association of 25-hydroxyvitamin D levels with liver dysfunction and mortality in chronic liver disease. *Liver Int.* **2012**, *32*, 845–851.

4. Nessim, S.J.; Jassal, S.V.; Fung, S.V.; Chan, C.T. Conversion from conventional to nocturnal hemodialysis improves vitamin D levels. *Kidney Int.* **2007**, *71*, 1172–1176.

5. Jacob, A.I.; Sallman, A.; Santiz, Z.; Hollis, B.W. Defective photoproduction of cholecalciferol in normal and uremic humans. *J. Nutr.* **1984**, *114*, 1313–1319.

6. Euvrard, S.; Kanitakis, J.; Claudy, A. Skin cancers after organ transplantation. *N. Engl. J. Med.* **2003**, *348*, 1681–1691.

7. Querings, K.; Girndt, M.; Geisel, J.; Georg, T.; Tilgen, W.; Reichrath, J. 25-hydroxyvitamin D deficiency in renal transplant recipients. *J. Clin. Endocrinol. Metab.* **2006**, *91*, 526–529.

8. Pascussi, J.M.; Robert, A.; Nguyen, M.; Walrant-Debray, O.; Garabedian, M.; Martin, P.; Pineau, T.; Saric, J.; Navarro, F.; Maurel, P.; *et al.* Possible involvement of pregnane X receptor-enhanced CYP24 expression in drug-induced osteomalacia. *J. Clin. Investig.* **2005**, *115*, 177–186.

9. Mithal, A.; Wahl, D.A.; Bonjour, J.P.; Burckhardt, P.; Dawson-Hughes, B.; Eisman, J.A.; El-Hajj Fuleihan, G.; Josse, R.G.; Lips, P.; Morales-Torres, J. Global vitamin D status and determinants of hypovitaminosis D. *Osteoporos. Int.* **2009**, *20*, 1807–1820.

10. Yetley, E.A. Assessing the vitamin D status of the US population. *Am. J. Clin. Nutr.* **2008**, *88*, 558S–564S.

11. Van der Wielen, R.P.; Lowik, M.R.; van den Berg, H.; de Groot, L.C.; Haller, J.; Moreiras, O.; van Staveren, W.A. Serum vitamin D concentrations among elderly people in Europe. *Lancet* **1995**, *346*, 207–210.

12. Ross, A.C.; Manson, J.E.; Abrams, S.A.; Aloia, J.F.; Brannon, P.M.; Clinton, S.K.; Durazo-Arvizu, R.A.; Gallagher, J.C.; Gallo, R.L.; Jones, G.; *et al.* The 2011 report on dietary reference intakes for calcium and vitamin D from the Institute of Medicine: What clinicians need to know. *J. Clin. Endocrinol. Metab.* **2011**, *96*, 53–58.

13. Shane, E.; Mancini, D.; Aaronson, K.; Silverberg, S.J.; Seibel, M.J.; Addesso, V.; McMahon, D.J. Bone mass, vitamin D deficiency, and hyperparathyroidism in congestive heart failure. *Am. J. Med.* **1997**, *103*, 197–207.

14. Zittermann, A.; Schleithoff, S.S.; Gotting, C.; Dronow, O.; Fuchs, U.; Kuhn, J.; Kleesiek, K.; Tenderich, G.; Koerfer, R. Poor outcome in end-stage heart failure patients with low circulating calcitriol levels. *Eur. J. Heart Fail.* **2008**, *10*, 321–327.

15. Stein, E.M.; Cohen, A.; Freeby, M.; Rogers, H.; Kokolus, S.; Scott, V.; Mancini, D.; Restaino, S.; Brown, R.; McMahon, D.J.; *et al.* Severe vitamin D deficiency among heart and liver transplant recipients. *Clin. Transplant.* **2009**, *23*, 861–865.

16. Forli, L.; Bollerslev, J.; Simonsen, S.; Isaksen, G.A.; Kvamsdal, K.E.; Godang, K.; Gadeholt, G.; Pripp, A.H.; Bjortuft, O. Dietary vitamin K2 supplement improves bone status after lung and heart transplantation. *Transplantation* **2010**, *89*, 458–464.

17. Movassaghi, S.; Nasiri Toosi, M.; Bakhshandeh, A.; Niksolat, F.; Khazaeipour, Z.; Tajik, A. Frequency of musculoskeletal complications among the patients receiving solid organ transplantation in a tertiary health-care center. *Rheumatol. Int.* **2012**, *32*, 2363–2366.

18. Dalle Carbonare, L.; Zanatta, M.; Braga, V.; Sella, S.; Vilei, M.T.; Feltrin, G.; Gambino, A.; Pepe, I.; Rossini, M.; Adami, S.; *et al.* Densitometric threshold and vertebral fractures in heart transplant patients. *Transplantation* **2011**, *92*, 106–111.

19. Schleithoff, S.S.; Zittermann, A.; Tenderich, G.; Berthold, H.K.; Stehle, P.; Koerfer, R. Vitamin D supplementation improves cytokine profiles in patients with congestive heart failure: A double-blind, randomized, placebo-controlled trial. *Am. J. Clin. Nutr.* **2006**, *83*, 754–759.

20. Amin, A.; Minaee, S.; Chitsazan, M.; Naderi, N.; Taghavi, S.; Ardeshiri, M. Can Vitamin D supplementation improve the severity of congestive heart failure? *Congest. Heart Fail.* **2013**, doi:10.1111/chf.12026.

21. Costanzo, M.R.; Dipchand, A.; Starling, R.; Anderson, A.; Chan, M.; Desai, S.; Fedson, S.; Fisher, P.; Gonzales-Stawinski, G.; Martinelli, L.; *et al.* The International Society of Heart and Lung Transplantation Guidelines for the care of heart transplant recipients. *J. Heart Lung Transplant.* **2010**, *29*, 914–956.

22. Shane, E.; Silverberg, S.J.; Donovan, D.; Papadopoulos, A.; Staron, R.B.; Addesso, V.; Jorgesen, B.; McGregor, C.; Schulman, L. Osteoporosis in lung transplantation candidates with end-stage pulmonary disease. *Am. J. Med.* **1996**, *101*, 262–269.

23. Tschopp, O.; Boehler, A.; Speich, R.; Weder, W.; Seifert, B.; Russi, E.W.; Schmid, C. Osteoporosis before lung transplantation: Association with low body mass index, but not with underlying disease. *Am. J. Transplant.* **2002**, *2*, 167–172.

24. Donovan, D.S., Jr.; Papadopoulos, A.; Staron, R.B.; Addesso, V.; Schulman, L.; McGregor, C.; Cosman, F.; Lindsay, R.L.; Shane, E. Bone mass and vitamin D deficiency in adults with advanced cystic fibrosis lung disease. *Am. J. Respir. Crit. Care Med.* **1998**, *157*, 1892–1899.

25. Lowery, E.M.; Bemiss, B.; Cascino, T.; Durazo-Arvizu, R.A.; Forsythe, S.M.; Alex, C.; Laghi, F.; Love, R.B.; Camacho, P. Low vitamin D levels are associated with increased rejection and infections after lung transplantation. *J. Heart Lung Transplant.* **2012**, *31*, 700–707.

26. Verleden, S.E.; Vos, R.; Geenens, R.; Ruttens, D.; Vaneylen, A.; Dupont, L.J.; Verleden, G.M.; van Raemdonck, D.E.; Vanaudenaerde, B.M. Vitamin D deficiency in lung transplant patients: Is it important? *Transplantation* **2012**, *93*, 224–229.

27. Forli, L.; Bjortuft, O.; Boe, J. Vitamin D status in relation to nutritional depletion and muscle function in patients with advanced pulmonary disease. *Exp. Lung Res.* **2009**, *35*, 524–538.

28. Aris, R.M.; Renner, J.B.; Winders, A.D.; Buell, H.E.; Riggs, D.B.; Lester, G.E.; Ontjes, D.A. Increased rate of fractures and severe kyphosis: Sequelae of living into adulthood with cystic fibrosis. *Ann. Intern. Med.* **1998**, *128*, 186–193.

29. Arteh, J.; Narra, S.; Nair, S. Prevalence of vitamin D deficiency in chronic liver disease. *Dig. Dis. Sci.* **2010**, *55*, 2624–2628.

30. Malham, M.; Jorgensen, S.P.; Ott, P.; Agnholt, J.; Vilstrup, H.; Borre, M.; Dahlerup, J.F. Vitamin D deficiency in cirrhosis relates to liver dysfunction rather than aetiology. *World J. Gastroenterol.* **2011**, *17*, 922–925.

31. Miroliaee, A.; Nasiri-Toosi, M.; Khalilzadeh, O.; Esteghamati, A.; Abdollahi, A.; Mazloumi, M. Disturbances of parathyroid hormone-vitamin D axis in non-cholestatic chronic liver disease: A cross-sectional study. *Hepatol. Int.* **2010**, *4*, 634–640.

32. Fisher, L.; Fisher, A. Vitamin D and parathyroid hormone in outpatients with noncholestatic chronic liver disease. *Clin. Gastroenterol. Hepatol.* **2007**, *5*, 513–520.

33. Bitetto, D.; Fabris, C.; Falleti, E.; Fornasiere, E.; Fumolo, E.; Fontanini, E.; Cussigh, A.; Occhino, G.; Baccarani, U.; Pirisi, M.; *et al.* Vitamin D and the risk of acute allograft rejection following human liver transplantation. *Liver Int.* **2010**, *30*, 417–444.

34. Venu, M.; Martin, E.; Saeian, K.; Gawrieh, S. High prevalence of vitamin A deficiency and vitamin D deficiency in patients evaluated for liver transplantation. *Liver Transpl.* **2013**, doi:10.1002/lt.23646.

35. Abbott-Johnson, W.J.; Kerlin, P.; Abiad, G.; Clague, A.E.; Cuneo, R.C. Dark adaptation in vitamin A-deficient adults awaiting liver transplantation: Improvement with intramuscular vitamin A treatment. *Br. J. Ophthalmol.* **2011**, *95*, 544–548.

36. Reese, P.P.; Bloom, R.D.; Feldman, H.I.; Huverserian, A.; Thomasson, A.; Shults, J.; Hamano, T.; Goral, S.; Shaked, A.; Olthoff, K.; *et al.* Changes in vitamin D binding protein and vitamin D concentrations associated with liver transplantation. *Liver Int.* **2012**, *32*, 287–296.

37. Monegal, A.; Navasa, M.; Guanabens, N.; Peris, P.; Pons, F.; Martinez de Osaba, M.J.; Ordi, J.; Rimola, A.; Rodes, J.; Munoz-Gomez, J. Bone disease after liver transplantation: A long-term prospective study of bone mass changes, hormonal status and histomorphometric characteristics. *Osteoporos. Int.* **2001**, *12*, 484–492.

38. Segal, E.; Baruch, Y.; Kramsky, R.; Raz, B.; Tamir, A.; Ish-Shalom, S. Predominant factors associated with bone loss in liver transplant patients—After prolonged post-transplantation period. *Clin. Transplant.* **2003**, *17*, 13–19.

39. Holick, M.F.; Binkley, N.C.; Bischoff-Ferrari, H.A.; Gordon, C.M.; Hanley, D.A.; Heaney, R.P.; Murad, M.H.; Weaver, C.M. Evaluation, treatment, and prevention of vitamin D deficiency: An Endocrine Society clinical practice guideline. *J. Clin. Endocrinol. Metab.* **2011**, *96*, 1911–1930.

40. Lucey, M.R.; Terrault, N.; Ojo, L.; Hay, J.E.; Neuberger, J.; Blumberg, E.; Teperman, L.W. Long-term management of the successful adult liver transplant: 2012 practice guideline by the American Association for the Study of Liver Diseases and the American Society of Transplantation. *Liver Transpl.* **2013**, *19*, 3–26.

41. LaClair, R.E.; Hellman, R.N.; Karp, S.L.; Kraus, M.; Ofner, S.; Li, Q.; Graves, K.L.; Moe, S.M. Prevalence of calcidiol deficiency in CKD: A cross-sectional study across latitudes in the United States. *Am. J. Kidney Dis.* **2005**, *45*, 1026–1033.

42. Ravani, P.; Malberti, F.; Tripepi, G.; Pecchini, P.; Cutrupi, S.; Pizzini, P.; Mallamaci, F.; Zoccali, C. Vitamin D levels and patient outcome in chronic kidney disease. *Kidney Int.* **2009**, *75*, 88–95.

43. Ishimura, E.; Nishizawa, Y.; Inaba, M.; Matsumoto, N.; Emoto, M.; Kawagishi, T.; Shoji, S.; Okuno, S.; Kim, M.; Miki, T.; *et al.* Serum levels of 1,25-dihydroxyvitamin D, 24,25-dihydroxyvitamin D, and 25-hydroxyvitamin D in nondialyzed patients with chronic renal failure. *Kidney Int.* **1999**, *55*, 1019–1027.

44. Stavroulopoulos, A.; Porter, C.J.; Roe, S.D.; Hosking, D.J.; Cassidy, M.J. Relationship between vitamin D status, parathyroid hormone levels and bone mineral density in patients with chronic kidney disease stages 3 and 4. *Nephrology (Carlton)* **2008**, *13*, 63–67.

45. Sadlier, D.M.; Magee, C.C. Prevalence of 25(OH) vitamin D (calcidiol) deficiency at time of renal transplantation: A prospective study. *Clin. Transplant.* **2007**, *21*, 683–688.

46. Tripathi, S.S.; Gibney, E.M.; Gehr, T.W.; King, A.L.; Beckman, M.J. High prevalence of vitamin D deficiency in African American kidney transplant recipients. *Transplantation* 2008, *85*, 767–770.

47. Yilmaz, M.I.; Sonmez, A.; Saglam, M.; Yaman, H.; Kilic, S.; Turker, T.; Unal, H.U.; Gok, M.; Cetinkaya, H.; Eyileten, T.; *et al.* Longitudinal analysis of vascular function and biomarkers of metabolic bone disorders before and after renal transplantation. *Am. J. Nephrol.* **2013**, *37*, 126–134.

48. Stavroulopoulos, A.; Cassidy, M.J.; Porter, C.J.; Hosking, D.J.; Roe, S.D. Vitamin D status in renal transplant recipients. *Am. J. Transplant.* **2007**, *7*, 2546–2552.

49. Ewers, B.; Gasbjerg, A.; Moelgaard, C.; Frederiksen, A.M.; Marckmann, P. Vitamin D status in kidney transplant patients: Need for intensified routine supplementation. *Am. J. Clin. Nutr.* **2008**, *87*, 431–437.

50. Penny, H.; Frame, S.; Dickinson, F.; Garrett, G.; Young, A.R.; Sarkany, R.; Chitalia, N.; Hampson, G.; Goldsmith, D. Determinants of vitamin D status in long-term renal transplant patients. *Clin. Transplant.* **2012**, *26*, E617–E623.

51. Burkhalter, F.; Schaub, S.; Dickenmann, M. Preserved circannual rhythm of vitamin D in kidney transplant patients. *Swiss Med. Wkly.* **2012**, *142*, w13672.

52. National Kidney Foundation. K/DOQI clinical practice guidelines for bone metabolism and disease in chronic kidney disease. *Am. J. Kidney Dis.* **2003**, *42*, S1–S201.

53. KDIGO. KDIGO clinical practice guideline for the care of kidney transplant recipients. *Am. J. Transplant.* **2009**, *9* (Suppl. 3), 1–155.

54. Wissing, K.M.; Broeders, N.; Moreno-Reyes, R.; Gervy, C.; Stallenberg, B.; Abramowicz, D. A controlled study of vitamin D3 to prevent bone loss in renal-transplant patients receiving low doses of steroids. *Transplantation* **2005**, *79*, 108–115.

55. Courbebaisse, M.; Thervet, E.; Souberbielle, J.C.; Zuber, J.; Eladari, D.; Martinez, F.; Mamzer-Bruneel, M.F.; Urena, P.; Legendre, C.; Friedlander, G.; *et al.* Effects of vitamin D supplementation on the calcium-phosphate balance in renal transplant patients. *Kidney Int.* **2009**, *75*, 646–651.

56. Benaboud, S.; Urien, S.; Thervet, E.; Prie, D.; Legendre, C.; Souberbielle, J.C.; Hirt, D.; Friedlander, G.; Treluyer, J.M.; Courbebaisse, M. Determination of optimal cholecalciferol treatment in renal transplant recipients using a population pharmacokinetic approach. *Eur J. Clin. Pharmacol.* **2013**, *69*, 499–506.

57. Thiem, U.; Heinze, G.; Segel, R.; Perkmann, T.; Kainberger, F.; Muhlbacher, F.; Horl, W.; Borchhardt, K. VITA-D: Cholecalciferol substitution in vitamin D deficient kidney transplant recipients: A randomized, placebo-controlled study to evaluate the post-transplant outcome. *Trials* **2009**, *10*, 36.

58. Meems, L.M.; van der Harst, P.; van Gilst, W.H.; de Boer, R.A. Vitamin D biology in heart failure: Molecular mechanisms and systematic review. *Curr. Drug Targets* **2011**, *12*, 29–41.

59. Pilz, S.; Tomaschitz, A.; Marz, W.; Drechsler, C.; Ritz, E.; Zittermann, A.; Cavalier, E.; Pieber, T.R.; Lappe, J.M.; Grant, W.B.; *et al.* Vitamin D, cardiovascular disease and mortality. *Clin. Endocrinol. (Oxf.)* **2011**, *75*, 575–584.

60. Shroff, R.; Wan, M.; Rees, L. Can vitamin D slow down the progression of chronic kidney disease? *Pediatr. Nephrol.* **2012**, *27*, 2167–2173.

61. Di Rosa, M.; Malaguarnera, M.; Nicoletti, F.; Malaguarnera, L. Vitamin D3: A helpful immuno-modulator. *Immunology* **2011**, *134*, 123–139.

62. Thiem, U.; Borchhardt, K. Vitamin D in solid organ transplantation with special emphasis on kidney transplantation. *Vitam. Horm.* **2011**, *86*, 429–468.

63. Bock, G.; Prietl, B.; Mader, J.K.; Holler, E.; Wolf, M.; Pilz, S.; Graninger, W.B.; Obermayer-Pietsch, B.M.; Pieber, T.R. The effect of vitamin D supplementation on peripheral regulatory T cells and beta cell function in healthy humans: A randomized controlled trial. *Diabetes Metab. Res. Rev.* **2011**, *27*, 942–945.

64. Hopkins, M.H.; Owen, J.; Ahearn, T.; Fedirko, V.; Flanders, W.D.; Jones, D.P.; Bostick, R.M. Effects of supplemental vitamin D and calcium on biomarkers of inflammation in colorectal adenoma patients: A randomized, controlled clinical trial. *Cancer Prev Res. (Phila.)* **2011**, *4*, 1645–1654.

65. Bucharles, S.; Barberato, S.H.; Stinghen, A.E.; Gruber, B.; Piekala, L.; Dambiski, A.C.; Custodio, M.R.; Pecoits-Filho, R. Impact of cholecalciferol treatment on biomarkers of inflammation and myocardial structure in hemodialysis patients without hyperparathyroidism. *J. Ren. Nutr.* **2012**, *22*, 284–291.

66. Bischoff-Ferrari, H.A.; Dawson-Hughes, B.; Stocklin, E.; Sidelnikov, E.; Willett, W.C.; Edel, J.O.; Stahelin, H.B.; Wolfram, S.; Jetter, A.; Schwager, J.; *et al.* Oral supplementation with 25(OH)D3 versus vitamin D3: Effects on 25(OH)D levels, lower extremity function, blood pressure, and markers of innate immunity. *J. Bone Miner. Res.* **2012**, *27*, 160–169.

67. Barker, T.; Martins, T.B.; Hill, H.R.; Kjeldsberg, C.R.; Henriksen, V.T.; Dixon, B.M.; Schneider, E.D.; Dern, A.; Weaver, L.K. Different doses of supplemental vitamin D maintain interleukin-5 without altering skeletal muscle strength: A randomized, double-blind, placebo-controlled study in vitamin D sufficient adults. *Nutr. Metab (Lond.)* **2012**, *9*, 16.

68. Alvarez, J.A.; Zughaier, S.M.; Law, J.; Hao, L.; Wasse, H.; Ziegler, T.R.; Tangpricha, V. Effects of high-dose cholecalciferol on serum markers of inflammation and immunity in patients with early chronic kidney disease. *Eur J. Clin. Nutr.* **2013**, *67*, 264–269.

69. Hossein-Nezhad, A.; Spira, A.; Holick, M.F. Influence of vitamin d status and vitamin d3 supplementation on genome wide expression of white blood cells: A randomized double-blind clinical trial. *PLoS One* **2013**, *8*, e58725.

7

A Novel Role for a Major Component of the Vitamin D Axis: Vitamin D Binding Protein-Derived Macrophage Activating Factor Induces Human Breast Cancer Cell Apoptosis through Stimulation of Macrophages

Lynda Thyer [1], **Emma Ward** [1], **Rodney Smith** [1], **Maria Giulia Fiore** [2], **Stefano Magherini** [3], **Jacopo J. V. Branca** [3], **Gabriele Morucci** [3], **Massimo Gulisano** [3], **Marco Ruggiero** [2,*] and **Stefania Pacini** [3]

[1] Macro Innovations Ltd., CB4 0DS Cambridge, UK; E-Mails: youcanfindlyn@hotmail.co.uk (L.T.); eward@macroinnovations.co.uk (E.W.); rsmith@macroinnovations.co.uk (R.S.)

[2] Department of Experimental and Clinical Biomedical Sciences, University of Firenze, 50134 Firenze, Italy; E-Mail: giulietz@hotmail.it

[3] Department of Experimental and Clinical Medicine, University of Firenze, 50134 Firenze, Italy; E-Mails: stemaghe@libero.it (S.M.); jacopo.branca@libero.it (J.J.V.B.); gabriele.morucci@unifi.it (G.M.); massimo.gulisano@unifi.it (M.G.); stefania.pacini@unifi.it (S.P.)

* Author to whom correspondence should be addressed; E-Mail: marco.ruggiero@unifi.it;

Abstract: The role of vitamin D in maintaining health appears greater than originally thought, and the concept of the vitamin D axis underlines the complexity of the biological events controlled by biologically active vitamin D (1,25(OH)(2)D3), its two binding proteins that are the vitamin D receptor (VDR) and the vitamin D-binding protein-derived macrophage activating factor (GcMAF). In this study we demonstrate that GcMAF stimulates macrophages, which in turn attack human breast cancer cells, induce their apoptosis and eventually phagocytize them. These results are consistent with the observation that macrophages infiltrated implanted tumors in mice after GcMAF injections. In addition, we hypothesize that the last 23 hydrophobic amino acids of VDR, located at the inner part of the plasma membrane, interact with the first 23 hydrophobic amino acids of the GcMAF located at the external part of the plasma membrane. This allows 1,25(OH)(2)D3 and oleic acid to become sandwiched between the two vitamin

D-binding proteins, thus postulating a novel molecular mode of interaction between GcMAF and VDR. Taken together, these results support and reinforce the hypothesis that GcMAF has multiple biological activities that could be responsible for its anti-cancer effects, possibly through molecular interaction with the VDR that in turn is responsible for a multitude of non-genomic as well as genomic effects.

Keywords: vitamin D; macrophages; breast cancer; human; apoptosis

1. Introduction

The so-called vitamin D axis is involved in various aspects of human breast cancer, the most common human tumor. The vitamin D axis is composed of the biologically active form of vitamin D (1,25(OH)(2)D3), and by two proteins that specifically bind it. These proteins are the vitamin D receptor (VDR) and the vitamin D binding protein that is the precursor of the vitamin D binding protein-derived macrophage activating factor, also termed GcMAF [1]. The role of vitamin D in human breast cancer is witnessed by the number of studies that have been published on the subject [2]. More intriguing, however, is the relative lack of information about GcMAF and human breast cancer; in fact, in the peer-reviewed literature, as of today (May 2013), there are only four studies on this subject. In two of these studies, the effects of GcMAF were observed on the human breast cancer cell line MCF-7 *in vitro* [3,4]. Another study examined the glycosylation status of vitamin D binding protein in cancer patients including breast cancer patients [5], whereas a less recent study reported the effects of administering GcMAF to metastatic breast cancer patients [6].

It is interesting to notice that no studies have, so far, been performed in order to assess whether GcMAF, which is a known powerful activator of macrophages, was indeed capable of activating macrophages that could in turn "attack" human breast cancer cells. There is indirect evidence suggesting that GcMAF activates macrophages that infiltrate experimental tumors in animal models [7,8]. This evidence, however, is indirect and, most important, refers to experimental tumors other than human breast cancer. In addition, since the observations quoted above were performed in experimental animals, the presence of confounding factors associated with the complexity of the responses of the whole organism to the presence of transplanted or advanced tumors, limits the possibility of interpretation of the presented results.

Therefore, in order to fill this gap of knowledge, we performed experiments to provide clear-cut evidence that GcMAF, as part of the vitamin D axis, activates normal macrophages that in turn exert a tumoricidal action against human breast cancer cells without the presence of confounding factors.

2. Experimental Section

Purified, activity-tested GcMAF was obtained from Immuno Biotech Ltd., Guernsey, Channel Islands. Paricalcitol was from Abbott, Roma, Italy. All other reagents were from Sigma Aldrich, Milano, Italy.

2.1. Cell Lines

Human breast cancer cells (cell line MCF-7) were obtained from the Istituto Zooprofilattico Sperimentale della Lombardia e dell'Emilia-Romagna, Brescia, Italy. Cells were routinely maintained at 37 °C in a humidified atmosphere of 5% CO_2 in Eagle's minimum essential medium in Earle's Balanced salt solution, supplemented with 1 mM sodium pyruvate, 10% fetal bovine serum (FBS), 100 U/mL penicillin, and 100 µg/mL streptomycin (Invitrogen, Carlsbad, CA, USA). No 1,25(OH)(2)D3 was present in the culture medium. In experiments of co-cultures, macrophages (cell line Raw 264.7, HPA Culture Collection) were activated by culturing them in the same medium of MCF-7 cells and in the presence of 100 ng/mL GcMAF for 72 h prior to addition to the MCF-7 cell culture. GcMAF concentration was established by preliminary experiments showing a linear dose-response curve. The initial response was observed at 1 ng/mL and a plateau was reached at 100 ng/mL. These concentrations were consistent with the results previously reported [3,4]. Before addition to the MCF-7 cell culture, the macrophages were gently centrifuged and re-suspended in fresh medium in order to avoid transferring GcMAF to the co-culture. In this way, we could rule out direct effects of GcMAF on MCF-7 cells. The macrophages were added at a ratio of 1:1 to the MCF-7 cell culture. The cells were then allowed to settle for 1 h before time-lapse photography. Photography was taken over a 7-day period using an Olympus CK2 microscope and a GXCAM-3 with NCH Debut capture software. In the experiments described in Figures 1A and 2, the cells were fixed and stained as described below 40 h after co-culturing them.

2.2. Study of Cell Morphology

Cell morphology was studied by phase-contrast microscopy using an Optika inverted microscope (Model XDS-2; Optika Microscopes, Bergamo, Italy). This microscope had a positive-phase plate for phase-contrast imaging below a long working distance condenser lens, and an 8 Mp digital camera with LCD Screen (Optika Microscopes, Bergamo, Italy). The light source was a 6 V/30 W halogen pre-centered illuminator, with adjustable intensity. Phase-contrast imaging was performed on living cells without any fixation or treatment. A series of digital images of living cells were recorded for each experimental point and the most representative were chosen.

Haematoxylin-eosin and Papanicolaou staining were also performed. This last staining results in very transparent cells, such that even thicker specimens with overlapping cells could be recorded. Briefly, cells were stained with Harris haematoxylin as nuclear stain. Orange G and EA-65 (Light Green, Bismarck Brown, and Eosin) were used for cytoplasmic staining (Sigma Aldrich, Milano, Italy). Slides were mounted with permanent mounting medium and observed under light microscopy (Nikon Instruments SpA, Milano, Italy). Pictures shown are representative of typical experimental data. Each experiment was performed with quadrupled samples and was replicated three times.

2.3. Study of Cell Proliferation

Assessment of cell proliferation was determined by a Calbiochem Rapid Cell Proliferation Kit (Calbiochem, D.B.A., Milano, Italy) [9]. Each condition was replicated with quadrupled samples and each experiment was replicated three times. Differences between experimental values were evaluated by the Student's *t*-test.

2.4. Study of Amino Acid Alignments and Functions

Analyses were carried out on the nucleotide and amino-acid sequences of the genes coding for vitamin D binding protein/GcMAF (isoform 1 precursor; gi|324021743|ref|NP_001191235.1) and VDR (gi|38511972|gb|AAH60832.1) in Homo sapiens. In reference to the protein alignments, three parameters have been taken into account:

1. sequence identity
2. sequence similarity
3. hydrophobic profile

These criteria were evaluated because they determine the quality of the alignments. In addition, we evaluated the functional value of the amino acids replaced, *i.e.*, the importance that any divergence assumes within the sequence. The values obtained have allowed the scores to be added, rather than multiplied, in the global calculation of alignment scores. Information concerning the selected genes was obtained from the database at the University of California, Santa Cruz [10] referring to the latest published version of the human genome [11]. In particular, we used the table refGene, containing all gene coding and non-coding for proteins. In this way, it was possible to obtain detailed information on human genes, such as: chromosome, position of the start and the end of transcription, position of the start and the end of coding part, and the number and the positions of exons. The annotations for the genes were obtained using the algorithm liftOver [12].

The presence of conserved elements within the alignment was verified by using the information contained in the phastConsElements28way table of the UCSC database. This table contains the predictions of conserved elements produced by the phastCons program. The positions were reported on the alignment. All operations, from the search of genomic information to the creation of the alignments, were made using R Statistical Mathematical Software. Once the sequences were aligned, the columns of residues were taken into consideration. Any lined-up residue is to be considered implicitly related to evolution. The hydrophobic profile was obtained using software on the website [13]. Among the several systems that can be used for the calculation of the index of the amino acid sequence hydrophobicity/hydrophilicity, we selected the Kyte and Doolittle's method [14]. The three-dimensional protein structures of vitamin D-binding protein and VDR were obtained through the use of the PDB archive [15]. Superposition between the two structures was possible through the use of the Swiss Pdb Viewer software [16]. The PDB archive contains information about experimentally-determined structures of proteins, nucleic acids, and complex assemblies. SwissPdb Viewer is an application that provides an interface allowing analysis of several proteins at the same time. The proteins can be superimposed in order to deduce structural alignments and compare their active sites or any other relevant parts. Amino acid mutations, H-bonds, angles, and distances between atoms are easy to obtain thanks to the intuitive graphic and menu interface.

3. Results

When co-cultured with human breast cancer cells in the absence of GcMAF, macrophages did not interact with human breast cancer cells and their characteristically irregular morphology was maintained (Figure 1A). Little or no vacuoles could be observed in macrophage cytoplasm, indirect evidence of a lack of activation. As described before, human breast cancer cells exhibited their typically non-homogeneous morphology, with some cells larger than other. The morphology of the cells was irregularly polygonal. As expected, human breast cancer cells tended to grow, one on top of the other, forming clusters that reflected the characteristic loss of contact inhibition. Figure 1B depicts phase contrast microphotography of a cluster of human breast cancer cells cultured in the absence of macrophages or any other addition. Cancer cells are visible as cords of cells growing in multi-layers in the center of the Figure. At higher magnification (Figure 1C), the cells appeared densely packed, with linear, non-fragmented, margins, and with a clearly recognizable organization of chromatin inside the nucleus, indicating a strong synthetic activity compatible with the high rate of proliferation of these cells. The nucleoli are clearly visible. Figure 1D, shows Papanicolau staining of only human breast cancer cells; a significant cluster can be observed in the left lower side of the image. The nuclei appear heavily stained as expected in growing cancer cells. The perimeter of the cells is linear with no indents or signs of fragmentation. Empty (white) areas in the well are also clearly observable. These represent naked areas of the plastic well that reflect the loss of adherence typical of cancer cells. Loss of adherence is a pre-requisite for cellular detachment, invasiveness, and metastatic potential.

Figure 1. (**A**) Haematoxylin-eosin staining (magnification 300×); in the absence of GcMAF, small macrophages do not appear to interact with MCF-7 human breast cancer cells. The picture refers to 40 h co-culture. (**B**) Phase contrast microphotography (300×) of a cluster of cancer cells in the center. (**C**) At higher magnification (1200×) the cells appear densely packed. (**D**) Papanicolau staining (1200×); a cluster in the left lower side of the image. The nuclei are heavily stained and the perimeter of the cells is linear with no indents or signs of fragmentation.

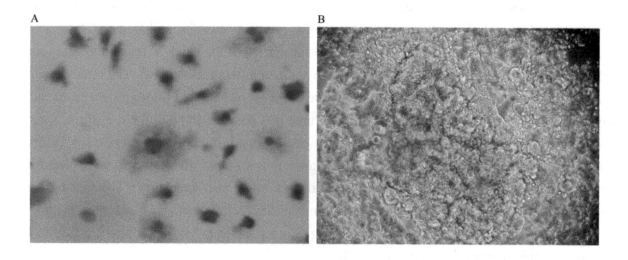

Figure 1. *Cont.*

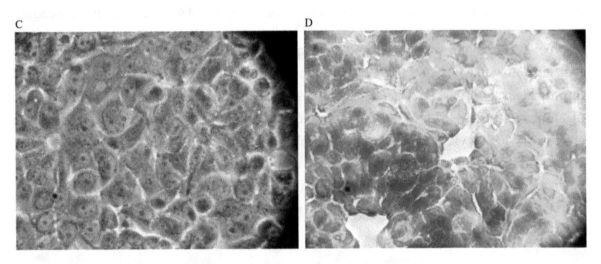

However, when human breast cancer cells were co-cultured with macrophages that had been previously activated by GcMAF (100 ng/mL) for 72 h, the picture was completely different as shown in Figures 2 and 3. The pictures show co-culture of GcMAF-activated macrophages and human breast cancer cells after 40 h incubation. GcMAF-activated macrophages appeared as small cells that surrounded human breast cancer cells. Figure 2A (Papanicolau staining,) clearly shows a group of human breast cancer cell in the center of the image surrounded by hundreds of small macrophages. At higher magnification, (Figure 2B) one human breast cancer cell appears completely surrounded by macrophages that are also observable on top of the cell. The nucleus of the macrophages is well stained, whereas the chromatin in the nucleus of the cancer cell appears fragmented and disorganized. The nucleoli, however, are still recognizable; this phenomenon can be interpreted as an index of remaining synthetic activity as expected in cells undergoing active apoptosis. The cytoplasm of macrophages appears vacuolated thus suggesting active phagocytosis. Figure 2C shows another field where two large human breast cancer cells are surrounded by GcMAF-activated macrophages that appear to emit cytoplasmic extrusions that search for contact with the membrane of cancer cells. The cell in the center of Figure 2C, at higher magnification (Figure 2D), shows a peculiar aspect; the chromatin in the nucleus appears fragmented and, in the lower right corner, the cytoplasm appears to be indented as if the two macrophages in that region were actively deconstructing the cytoplasmic assembly of the cancer cell. A similar phenomenon can be observed on the left where two macrophages indent the cytoplasmic profile of the cancer cell.

It is worth noticing that all these morphological changes are consistent with the induction of apoptosis of human breast cancer cells by activated macrophages [17]. In particular, some of the morphological changes were consistent with the early phases of apoptosis and the morphology of the nucleus of human breast cancer cells shown in Figure 2 is almost superimposable to that represented in Figure 1 (left panel) of Hacker, 2000 [17]. Even the changes in the morphology of the cytoplasm were consistent with the induction of apoptosis by GcMAF-activated macrophages and the cytoplasm of human breast cancer cells showed the typical pattern of disintegration that precedes the formation of apoptotic bodies. In addition, in this case, the morphology of the cytoplasm of the cancer cells appears remarkably similar to that presented in Figure 1 (middle panel) of Hacker, 2000 [17]. Although the morphological features observed here are suggestive of active apoptosis, further studies using ELISA tests to quantify the level of human active caspase-3 protein, the major executioner protease in apoptosis, will determine quantitatively the degree of apoptosis induced by GcMAF-activated macrophages.

Figure 2. Co-culture of GcMAF-activated macrophages and human breast cancer cells; Papanicolau staining. (**A**) Cancer cells in the center are surrounded by hundreds of small macrophages (100×). (**B**) One human breast cancer cell is completely surrounded by macrophages that are also observable on top of the cell (200×). (**C**) Two large cancer cells are surrounded by GcMAF-activated macrophages (100×). (**D**) The same cell (200×); the chromatin in the nucleus is fragmented and, in the lower right corner, the cytoplasm is to be indented as if the two macrophages in that region were actively deconstructing the cytoplasm of the cancer cell.

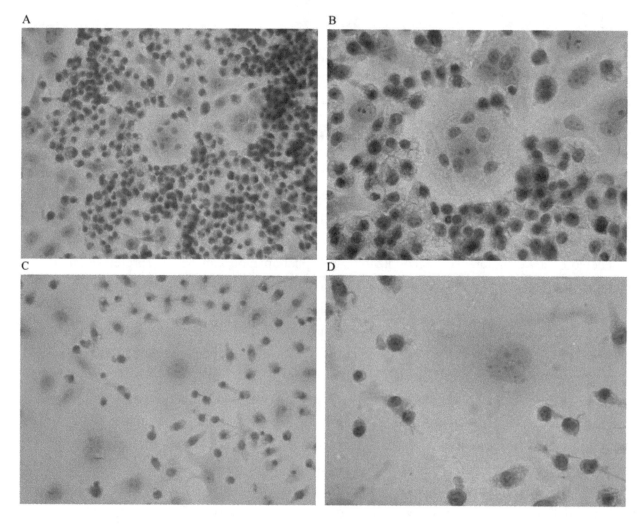

Time-lapse micro-photography shows that after about seven days of co-culture of GcMAF-activated macrophages with human breast cancer cells, the irregular growth of the breast carcinoma cells was arrested and the large protruding cell biomass was reduced. Figure 3A shows the human breast cancer cells and the GcMAF-activated macrophages at day one; the cancer cells, as expected, form an irregular layer that covers the field of observation. Individual cancer cells can be recognized as well as the naked areas of the plate as described above. GcMAF-activated macrophages appear as small cells that are attached to the cancer cells, in most cases, above them. It is interesting to notice that almost no macrophages can be observed in the naked areas of the plate, thus confirming the observation that

GcMAF-activated macrophages seek for contact with the cancer cells. After seven days of co-incubation (Figure 3B), no individual cancer cell can be recognized. After macrophage-induced apoptosis, their apoptotic bodies are all grouped together in the center of the field of observation, and most of the field is empty of cancer cells. Most GcMAF-activated macrophages surround and infiltrate the mass of cancer cell debris in the center.

Figure 3. Phase contrast microphotography from time-lapse recording of co-culture of GcMAF-activated macrophages and human breast cancer cells. (**A**) Day one of co-culture; the cancer cells form an irregular layer. Individual cancer cells can be recognized. GcMAF-activated macrophages appear as small cells that are attached to the cancer cells, in most cases above them. (**B**) Day seven of co-culture. No individual cancer cell can be recognized. Their apoptotic bodies are grouped together in the center of the field, and most of the field is empty of cancer cells. Most GcMAF-activated macrophages surround and infiltrate the mass of cancer cell debris in the center.

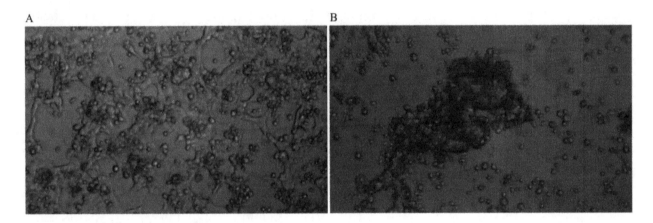

Taken together these results demonstrate for the first time that GcMAF-activated macrophages induce human breast cancer cell apoptosis and the subsequent reduction of the cancer cell mass following phagocytosis of apoptotic cancer cells by macrophages.

4. Discussion

It is long considered that the role of vitamin D in maintaining health is much greater than originally supposed, up to the point that some authors jokingly wonder whether "does vitamin D make the world go 'round'?" [18]. The emergence of the concept of the vitamin D axis [1,19] further underlines the complexity of the biological events controlled by 1,25(OH)(2)D3 through its two binding proteins (VDR and vitamin D-binding protein/GcMAF) that interfere with a growing number of events at the cellular and molecular level. In this study we focused our attention on the product of deglycosylation of the vitamin D-binding protein that is GcMAF, probably one of the most potent macrophage activators so far discovered [20]. Our results demonstrate that GcMAF stimulates macrophages that in turn attack human breast cancer cells, possibly induce their apoptosis and eventually phagocytise them. These results are consistent with the observation that macrophages infiltrated experimental tumors implanted in severely immunodeficient mice after GcMAF injections [8]. However, at variance with the observation reported above, in our experiments we could rule out indirect effects due to the adaptive response of the whole organism to the presence of an advanced tumor and to the GcMAF-induced inhibition of angiogenesis with consequent tumor hypoxia and necrosis [8]. A limitation of the present study is represented by the use of only two cell lines, which are human breast cancer cell line MCF-7, and mouse Raw 264.7 macrophages. It should be noticed, however, that GcMAF exerted qualitatively superimposable effects on primary human mononuclear cells [21] and in the human monocytoid cell line, MonoMac 6 [22]. Future experiments will elucidate whether the effects observed in this study can be extrapolated to other human breast cancer cell lines challenged with GcMAF-activated human macrophages.

The observation that GcMAF, a component of the vitamin D axis, exerts tumoricidal effects on human breast cancer cells through macrophage activation raises the question of whether there is any interaction between GcMAF and the VDR. Such a type of interaction would be critical to understand the effects of 1,25(OH)(2)D3 and GcMAF at the molecular level. This question might appear odd at first, as, for many years, it had been thought that VDR was localized in the cytoplasm and in the nucleus, and GcMAF could not cross the plasma membrane and therefore had to be recognized by a surface receptor, possibly a lectin-type receptor [23]. However, the observation of an association between the polymorphisms of the gene coding for VDR, and differential responses to GcMAF in human monocytes [21], as well as with metastatic breast cancer [24], raises the apparently odd issue of a molecular interaction between GcMAF and the VDR. In support for this hypothesis there is the observation that the VDR translocates to the plasma membrane [25], and plasma membrane associated VDR is responsible for the rapid, non-genomic effects of vitamin D [26]. Thus, in order to verify the possibility of a molecular interaction between GcMAF and VDR, we compared the amino acid sequences corresponding to their respective 1,25(OH)(2)D3 binding sites. There are 23 hydrophobic amino acids near the amino terminus of GcMAF (-----MKRVLVLLLAVAFGHALERGRDY) and 23 amino acids near the carboxyl terminus of the VDR (SFQPECSMKLTPLVLEVFGNEIS-----). If these two sequences are aligned (Figure 4A), it is possible to observe, not only that in both proteins there is a long stretch [21,24] of hydrophobic amino acids (highlighted in green in Figure 4A, upper insert), but that four hydrophobic amino acids are identical (L L FG; indicated in yellow and in green above and under the alignment. The sequence of GcMAF is above). In addition, 11 amino acids have similar functional valence as indicated by the conventional symbols (*), (.) and (:). Therefore, in the 1,25(OH)(2)D3 binding domains of GcMAF and VDR there are in total 11 out of 23 amino acids that show functional identity or similarity and 13–14 that are hydrophobic. A molecular interaction between the two proteins can therefore be proposed (Figure 4A). According to this model, the last 23 hydrophobic amino acids of VDR (VDR is on the right of Figure 4A), located at the inner part of the plasma membrane (represented as a dotted line), could interact with the first 23 hydrophobic amino acids of the GcMAF (GcMAF is on the left of the Figure 4A) located at the external part of the plasma membrane, with 1,25(OH)(2)D3 (represented in yellow) sandwiched between the two vitamin D-binding proteins. Oleic acid, taken as an example of an unsaturated fatty acid bound to GcMAF [27], could stabilize the complex at the level of the plasma membrane. In fact, both 1,25(OH)(2)D3 and oleic acid in GcMAF are located in a shallow cleft of the GcMAF protein that makes them accessible to the plasma membrane. In addition to the mode of interaction proposed in Figure 4A, there could be further additional interaction that takes into consideration just the fact that vitamin D binding-protein (and therefore also GcMAF) binds unsaturated fatty acids as demonstrated by Williams *et al.*, 1998 [27]. The fatty acid binding site is located between domains II and III, which is between positions 304 and 387. When we aligned the 23 hydrophobic amino acids of the VDR quoted above (represented in the insert in Figure 4B; also in this case, the sequence of GcMAF is represented above that of VDR) and the corresponding hydrophobic amino acids of the unsaturated fatty acid binding site of GcMAF (in particular, those in position 356–386), we observed that there was a significant degree of functional homology; in fact there are eight amino acids with similar functional valence in a long stretch of hydrophobic amino acids (highlighted in blue).

Figure 4. Amino acid alignments and three-dimensional protein structures of vitamin D-binding protein/GcMAF and VDR. (**A**) 23 hydrophobic amino acids of VDR (on the right), located at the inner part of the plasma membrane (dotted line), interact with 23 hydrophobic amino acids of the GcMAF (on the left of the Figure) located at the external part of the plasma membrane. In the insert the hydrophobic amino acids are highlighted in green and the four hydrophobic amino acids that are identical (L L FG) are highlighted in yellow and in green above and under the alignment. Vitamin D indicates 1,25(OH)(2)D3. (**B**) 23 hydrophobic amino acids of the VDR interact with a stretch of hydrophobic amino acids of the unsaturated fatty acid binding site of GcMAF. In the insert, eight amino acids with similar functional valence in a long stretch of hydrophobic amino acids highlighted in blue.

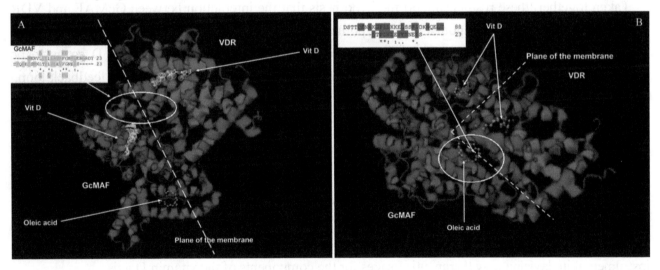

Therefore, it can be hypothesized that GcMAF and the VDR have multiple sites of interaction at the level of the plasma membrane. According to this model, the presence of 1,25(OH)(2)D3, in the culture medium should increase the effects of GcMAF by facilitating the interaction between GcMAF and VDR. Consistent with this model, we previously demonstrated that the effects of 1,25(OH)(2)D3 and GcMAF were synergistic in inhibiting MCF-7 cell proliferation [4], and the preliminary results reported in Table 1 indicate that GcMAF and paricalcitol, a non-hypercalcemic VDR agonist, also have synergistic effects. In the experiment described in Table 1, we chose to use paricalcitol instead of 1,25(OH)(2)D3 in order to determine whether the synergism between 1,25(OH)(2)D3 and GcMAF that we had previously observed [4], was to be ascribed exclusively to 1,25(OH)(2)D3, or could also be obtained with other VDR agonists. From the results presented in Table 1, it appears that paricalcitol, and, possibly, other VDR agonists, could fit the molecular model proposed in Figure 4.

Table 1. Effects of GcMAF and paricalcitol on Raw 264.7 macrophages. Raw 264.7 cells were incubated for 30 min with indicated additions. The effects of GcMAF on macrophage activation were assessed by determining cell proliferation. In fact, it was demonstrated that monocytes/macrophages activated by GcMAF administration immediately stop DNA replication and rapidly synthesize a large amount of Fc-receptors as well as an enormous variation of receptors [28]. Paricalcitol was added at the concentration of 300 fg/mL. At this concentration, paricalcitol did not exert any effect. In the presence of paricalcitol (300 fg/mL), the effect of 4 ng/mL GcMAF was identical to that of 40 ng/mL GcMAF in the absence of paricalcitol. These results demonstrate that the presence of a selective VDR agonist at a concentration that is not sufficient to activate VDR *per se* increases by an order of magnitude the response to GcMAF. Data are presented as means ± S.E.M. ($n = 12$). * $p < 0.02$ *vs.* control.

Treatment	Absorbance units ($\times 10^3$)
Control (no addition)	390 ± 11
Paricalcitol	450 ± 10
GcMAF 40 ng/mL	379 ± 9 *
GcMAF 4 ng/mL + paricalcitol	327 ± 10 *

Taken together, these results support the hypothesis that the interaction between GcMAF and VDR might be facilitated by VDR agonists. This hypothesis is further strengthened by the recent observation that activated macrophages are able to generate enough biologically active vitamin D so as to be detectable in the general circulation [29], thus suggesting a paracrine/autocrine positive feedback loop.

5. Conclusions

The results presented in this study suggest that the role of vitamin D in physiology and pathology is far more complex than previously envisaged. Thus, in addition to 1,25(OH)(2)D3 itself, at least another component of the vitamin D axis, GcMAF, exerts significant effects at the cellular level and it appears that the effects of GcMAF are interconnected with VDR activation. Therefore, it can be hypothesized that these interconnections between 1,25(OH)(2)D3, GcMAF and VDR will be instrumental in devising new therapeutic usages for the components of the vitamin D axis.

Acknowledgments

Marco Ruggiero, Stefania Pacini and Massimo Gulisano received grants from the University of Firenze and the Project PRIN 2009.

Conflict of Interest

All authors declare no conflicts of interest.

References

1. Ruggiero, M.; Pacini, S. The vitamin D axis in chronic kidney disease—State of the art and future perspectives. *Eur. Nephrol.* **2011**, *5*, 15–19.
2. Shao, T.; Klein, P.; Grossbard, M.L. Vitamin D and breast cancer. *Oncologist* **2012**, *17*, 36–45.
3. Pacini, S.; Morucci, G.; Punzi, T.; Gulisano, M.; Ruggiero, M. Gc protein-derived macrophage-activating factor (GcMAF) stimulates cAMP formation in human mononuclear cells and inhibits angiogenesis in chick embryo chorionallantoic membrane assay. *Cancer Immunol. Immunother.* **2011**, *60*, 479–485.
4. Pacini, S.; Punzi, T.; Morucci, G.; Gulisano, M.; Ruggiero, M. Effects of vitamin D-binding protein-derived macrophage-activating factor on human breast cancer cells. *Anticancer Res.* **2012**, *32*, 45–52.
5. Rehder, D.S.; Nelson, R.W.; Borges, C.R. Glycosylation status of vitamin D binding protein in cancer patients. *Protein Sci.* **2009**, *18*, 2036–2042.
6. Yamamoto, N.; Suyama, H.; Yamamoto, N.; Ushijima, N. Immunotherapy of metastatic breast cancer patients with vitamin D-binding protein-derived macrophage activating factor (GcMAF). *Int. J. Cancer* **2008**, *122*, 461–467.
7. Toyohara, Y.; Hashitani, S.; Kishimoto, H.; Noguchi, K.; Yamamoto, N.; Urade, M. Inhibitory effect of vitamin D-binding protein-derived macrophage activating factor on DMBA-induced hamster cheek pouch carcinogenesis and its derived carcinoma cell line. *Oncol. Lett.* **2011**, *2*, 685–691.
8. Nonaka, K.; Onizuka, S.; Ishibashi, H.; Uto, Y.; Hori, H.; Nakayama, T.; Matsuura, N.; Kanematsu, T.; Fujioka, H. Vitamin D binding protein-macrophage activating factor inhibits HCC in SCID mice. *J. Surg. Res.* **2012**, *172*, 116–122.
9. Hayon, T.; Dvilansky, A.; Shpilberg, O.; Nathan, I. Appraisal of the MTT-based assay as a useful tool for predicting drug chemosensitivity in leukemia. *Leuk. Lymphoma* **2003**, *44*, 1957–1962.
10. UCSC Genome Bioinformatics. Available online: http://genome.ucsc.edu (accessed on 22 January 2013).
11. Index of/goldenPath/hg18. Available online: http://hgdownload.cse.ucsc.edu/goldenPath/hg18 (accessed on 25 January 2013).
12. Lift Genome Annotations. Available online: http://genome.ucsc.edu/cgi-bin/hgLiftOver (accessed on 26 January 2013).
13. ProtScale. Available online: http://web.expasy.org/protscale/ (accessed on 6 February 2013).
14. ProtScale Tool. Available online: http://web.expasy.org/protscale/pscale/Hphob.Doolittle.html (accessed on 6 February 2013).
15. Biological Macromolecular Resource. Available online: http://www.rcsb.org/pdb/home/home.do (accessed on 11 February 2013).
16. DeepView—Swiss-PdbViewer. Available online: http://spdbv.vital-it.ch/ (accessed on 13 February 2013).
17. Häcker, G. The morphology of apoptosis. *Cell Tissue Res.* **2000**, *301*, 5–17.
18. Wagner, C.L.; Taylor, S.N.; Hollis, B.W. Does vitamin D make the world go "round"? *Breastfeed. Med.* **2008**, *3*, 239–250.

19. Chishimba, L.; Thickett, D.R.; Stockley, R.A.; Wood, A.M. The vitamin D axis in the lung: A key role for vitamin D-binding protein. *Thorax* **2010**, *65*, 456–462.

20. Uto, Y.; Yamamoto, S.; Mukai, H.; Ishiyama, N.; Takeuchi, R.; Nakagawa, Y.; Hirota, K.; Terada, H.; Onizuka, S.; Hori, H. β-Galactosidase treatment is a common first-stage modification of the three major subtypes of Gc protein to GcMAF. *Anticancer Res.* **2012**, *32*, 2359–2364.

21. Pacini, S.; Morucci, G.; Punzi, T.; Gulisano, M.; Ruggiero, M.; Amato, M.; Aterini, S. Effect of paricalcitol and GcMAF on angiogenesis and human peripheral blood mononuclear cell proliferation and signaling. *J. Nephrol.* **2012**, *25*, 577–581.

22. Pacini, S.; Branca, J.J.V.; Morucci, G.; Gulisano, M.; Ruggiero, M. Effects of GcMAF on monocyte-macrophage cells. 2013, to be submitted for publication.

23. Iida, S.; Yamamoto, K.; Irimura, T. Interaction of human macrophage C-type lectin with *O*-linked *N*-acetylgalactosamine residues on mucin glycopeptides. *J. Biol. Chem.* **1999**, *274*, 10697–10705.

24. Ruggiero, M.; Pacini, S.; Aterini, S.; Fallai, C.; Ruggiero, C.; Pacini, P. Vitamin D receptor gene polymorphism is associated with metastatic breast cancer. *Oncol. Res.* **1998**, *10*, 43–46.

25. Capiati, D.; Benassati, S.; Boland, R.L. 1,25(OH)2-vitamin D3 induces translocation of the vitamin D receptor (VDR) to the plasma membrane in skeletal muscle cells. *J. Cell. Biochem.* **2002**, *86*, 128–135.

26. Ceglia, L.; Harris, S.S. Vitamin d and its role in skeletal muscle. *Calcif. Tissue Int.* **2013**, *92*, 151–162.

27. Williams, M.H.; van Alstyne, E.L.; Galbraith, R.M. Evidence of a novel association of unsaturated fatty acids with Gc (vitamin D-binding protein). *Biochem. Biophys. Res. Commun.* **1988**, *153*, 1019–1024.

28. Yamamoto, N.; Ushijima, N.; Koga, Y. Immunotherapy of HIV-infected patients with Gc protein-derived macrophage activating factor (GcMAF). *J. Med. Virol.* **2008**, *81*, 16–26.

29. Adams, J.S.; Hewison, M. Extrarenal expression of 25-hydroxyvitamin D-1-hydroxylase. *Arch. Biochem. Biophys.* **2012**, *523*, 95–102.

8

Vitamin D: Deficiency, Sufficiency and Toxicity

Fahad Alshahrani [1] and Naji Aljohani [2,3,4,]*

[1] Department of Medicine, King Abdulaziz Medical City, Riyadh 14611, Saudi Arabia;
   E-Mail: fahad_alshahrani@yahoo.com

[2] Specialized Diabetes and Endocrine Center, King Fahad Medical City, Riyadh 59046,
   Saudi Arabia; E-Mail: najijohani@gmail.com

[3] Faculty of Medicine, King Saud bin Abdulaziz University for Health Sciences, Riyadh 22490,
   Saudi Arabia

[4] Prince Mutaib Chair for Biomarkers of Osteoporosis, College of Science, King Saud University,
   Riyadh 11451, Saudi Arabia

* Author to whom correspondence should be addressed; E-Mail: najijohani@gmail.com;

Abstract: The plethora of vitamin D studies over the recent years highlight the pleomorphic effects of vitamin D outside its conventional role in calcium and bone homeostasis. Vitamin D deficiency, though common and known, still faces several challenges among the medical community in terms of proper diagnosis and correction. In this review, the different levels of vitamin D and its clinical implications are highlighted. Recommendations and consensuses for the appropriate dose and duration for each vitamin D status are also emphasized.

Keywords: vitamin D; vitamin D deficiency; vitamin D toxicity

1. Introduction

Vitamin D plays an essential role in the regulation of metabolism, calcium and phosphorus absorption of bone health. However, the effects of vitamin D are not limited to mineral homeostasis and skeletal health maintenance. The presence of vitamin D receptors (VDR) in other tissue and organs suggest that vitamin D physiology extends well above and beyond bone homeostasis [1]. Additionally, the enzyme responsible for the conversion of 25[OH] D to its biologically active form [Vitamin D (1,25[OH]$_2$ D)] has been identified in other tissues aside from kidneys [2,3], and that extra renal synthesis of 1,23[OH]$_2$D may be equally important in regulating cell growth and differentiation via paracrine or autocrine regulatory mechanisms [4].

The mechanism of action of vitamin D$_3$ through its hormonal form, dihydroxyvitaminD$_3$, involves a nuclear VDR that regulates the transcription of several target genes in a variety of vitamin D target cells that are primarily involved in the calcium homeostasis of cell differentiation [5]. Hypervitaminosis D occurs when pharmacologic doses of vitamin D are consumed for prolonged periods of time or from a single megadose translating to a large increase in circulating 25[OH]D concentrations [6].

2. Vitamin D Metabolism

Vitamin D has two distinct forms: vitamins D$_2$ and D$_3$. Vitamin D$_2$ is a 28-carbon molecule derived from ergosterol (a component of fungal cell membranes), while vitamin D$_3$ is a 27-carbon derived from cholesterol [7]. UV-B irradiation of skin triggers photolysis of 7-dehydrocholesterol (pro-vitamin D$_3$) to pre-vitamin D$_3$, which is rapidly converted to vitamin D$_3$ by the skin's temperature. Vitamin D (D$_2$ and D$_3$) from the skin and diet undergo two sequential hydroxylations: first in the liver (25[OH]D) and then in the kidney, leading to its biologically active form 1,25-dihydroxyvitamin D (1,25[OH]$_2$D) [8]. Table 1 shows the nomenclature for vitamin D precursors and metabolites.

Table 1. Nomenclature of vitamin D precursors and metabolites.

Common Name	Clinical Name	Abbreviation	Comments
7-Dehydrocholesterol	Pro-vitamin D$_3$	7DHC	Lipid in cell membranes
Cholecalciferol	Pre-vitamin D$_3$		Photosynthesized in skin or diet
Ergocalciferol	Pre-vitamin D$_2$		Obtained from diet. Equivalent to vitamin D$_3$ as precursor for active vitamin D
Calcidiol	25-Hydroxyvitamin D	25[OH]D	Best reflects vitamin D status
Calcitriol	1,25-Dihydroxvitamin D	1,25[OH]D$_2$	Active form of vitamin D, tightly regulated

The 1,25 [OH]$_2$D ligand binds with high affinity to vitamin D receptors (VDRs), which then increases intestinal absorption of both calcium and phosphorus. In addition, vitamin D is actively involved in bone formation, resorption, mineralization, and in maintenance of neuromuscular function. Circulating 1,25[OH]$_2$D inhibits serum parathyroid hormone (PTH) levels by negative feedback mechanism and by increased serum calcium levels. It also regulates bone metabolism through activation of the VDRs found in osteoblasts, releasing biochemical signals and leading to the formation of mature osteoclasts [9].

In a low vitamin D state, the small intestine can absorb approximately 10%–15% of dietary calcium. When adequate however, intestinal absorption of dietary calcium rises to approximately 30%–40% [9,10]. Hence, low vitamin D levels (25[OH]D) may lead to insufficient calcium absorption, and this has clinical implications not only for bone health but also for most metabolic functions. The increase in PTH restores calcium homeostasis by increasing tubular reabsorption of calcium in the kidney, increasing bone calcium mobilization and enhancing $1,25[OH]_2D$ production [10].

3. Optimum 25[OH]D Levels

The vitamin D level needed to optimize intestinal calcium absorption (34 ng/mL) is lower than the level needed for neuromuscular performance (38 ng/mL) [11,12]. Experts however believe that the lower limit of adequate 25[OH]D levels should be 30 ng/mL [13]. Still others recommend a lower limit of 40 ng/mL, since impaired calcium metabolism due to low serum 25[OH]D levels may trigger secondary hyperparathyroidism, increased bone turnover and progressive bone loss [14,15].

The proposed 25[OH]D cut-off for optimum skeletal health is the level that reduces PTH to a minimum and increases calcium absorption to its maximum [11,16]. Several studies have shown that PTH levels plateau at a minimum steady-state level as serum 25[OH]D levels approach and rise above approximately 30 ng/mL (75 nmol/L) [16–18]. The established consensus of several vitamin D cut-offs is presented in Table 2 [18–20]. It is noteworthy, however, that there is a continued debate and exchange of knowledge with respect to the optimum cut-off for 25(OH)D.

Table 2. Diagnostic Cut-Offs of levels of serum 25[OH]D.

25[OH] Level (ng/mL)	25[OH]D Level (nmoL/L)	Laboratory Diagnosis
<20	<50	Deficiency
20–32	50–80	Insufficiency
54–90	135–225	Normal in sunny countries
>100	>250	Excess
>150	>325	Intoxication

4. Measurements of 25[OH]D *versus* 1,25[OH]$_2$D$_3$

The clinical advantages of choosing 25[OH]D instead of calcitriol as a marker for vitamin D status has been listed by Rajasree *et al.* [21]. First, 25[OH]D has the highest concentration of all vitamin D metabolites. Second, its levels remain stable for almost two weeks. Lastly, vitamin D toxicity is thought to be a function of 25[OH]D instead of calcitriol. It has been observed that serum 25[OH]D is the best indicator of vitamin D status among individuals without kidney disease [22]. Furthermore, 25[OH]D in large amounts can replace calcitriol to stimulate bone calcium metabolism [23]. Although nephrectomy abolishes a response to physiological dose of 25[OH]D, a large dose (1000 fold) of 25[OH]D can stimulate intestinal calcium absorption and bone calcium metabolism in nephrectomized rats [24]. Hughes *et al.*, studied vitamin D intoxication in two human patients with normal kidney function and showed that both patients had 16-fold above normal concentrations of plasma 25[OH]D levels (500–600 ng/mL), while 1,25[OH]D$_2$D$_3$ plasma concentrations were only modestly elevated (40–56 pg/mL) [25]. Differences in calcidiol *versus* calcitriol are presented in Table 3.

Table 3. Calcidiol *versus* Calcitriol.

Metabolite function	25[OH]D	1,25[OH]$_2$D$_3$
Nutritional Status	Best indicator	Does not indicate nutritional status
Half life	>15 days	<15 h
Stability in serum	Stable	Unstable
Hypovitaminosis D	Indicative (low)	Non-indicative (normal to elevated)
Hypervitaminosis D	Indicative (elevated)	Non-indicative (low to normal or mild elevated)
Calcium regulation	Possible under non-physiological conditions	Tight under physiological conditions
PTH regulation	Depends on vitamin D status	Tight
DBP binding	High affinity (releases the free metabolite once DBP is saturated	Low affinity to exert the physiological function
VDR binding	Strongest among metabolite other than calcitriol	High affinity to elicit the biological function

Note: VDR: vitamin D receptor; DBP: vitamin D binding protein; PTH: parathyroid hormone.

5. Supplementation of Vitamin D$_2$ *versus* Vitamin D$_3$

Multiple preparations of vitamin D and its metabolites are commercially available for supplement use. The two most common supplements are ergocalciferol (vitamin D$_2$) and cholecalciferol (vitamin D$_3$). Some studies [26,27], but not all [28], suggest that vitamin D$_3$ increases serum 25[OH]D more efficiently than vitamin D$_2$. A large, single dose of vitamin D$_2$ does not last longer than a large dose of D$_3$. In a study conducted by Armas *et al.*, [27], subjects were given one dose of 50,000 IU of either vitamin D$_2$ or vitamin D$_3$. Vitamin D$_2$ was absorbed just as well as vitamin D$_3$, yet blood levels of 25[OH]D started dropping rapidly after 3 days among subjects given vitamin D$_2$ whereas those on vitamin D$_3$ sustained high levels for two weeks before dropping gradually.

A daily dose of 4000 IU of vitamin D$_3$ for two weeks was observed to be 1.7 times more effective in raising 25[OH]D levels than 4000 IU of vitamin D$_2$ [26]. On the other hand, Holick *et al.* found that a daily dose of 1000 IU of vitamin D$_2$ over 11 weeks duration increased 25[OH]D levels from 42 to 67 nmoL/L (16.9 to 26.8 ng/mL) [28]. Consequently, vitamin D$_3$ levels also increased from 49 to 72 nmoL/L (19.6 to 28.9 ng/mL). It took 6 weeks for 25[OH]D levels to plateau on that regimen. In another study, Glendenning *et al.* compared 1000 IU of D$_2$ *versus* D$_3$ in patients who had vitamin D insufficiency with subsequent hip fractures. After three months, those who were supplemented with D$_3$ had a 31%–52% greater increase in 25[OH]D levels than those supplemented with D$_2$. However, parathyroid hormone levels did not differ between groups [29].

In children, Gordon *et al.*, assigned 40 infants and toddlers with vitamin D deficiency to one of three regimens (2000 IU oral vitamin D$_2$ daily, 50,000 IU vitamin D$_2$ weekly or 2000 IU vitamin D$_3$ daily) for 6 weeks. At the end of the trial, 25[OH]D levels increased from 42.5 to 90 nmoL/L and there were no significant differences between treatment groups [30].

In terms of bioavailability, Biancuzzo *et al.*, tested changes in 25[OH]D status from a daily dose of 1000 IU of vitamin D$_2$ or D$_3$ from either calcium-fortified orange juice with vitamin D or supplement capsules for 11 weeks. The average 25[OH]D levels of all groups (D_2 from orange juice, D_2 from capsules, D_3 from orange juice, D_3 from capsules) went up to about 25 nmoL/L with no significant differences between groups [31].

Treatment for most studies found D_2 to be less effective than D_3, whereas in studies finding them equally effective, the treatment was daily amounts between 400 and 2000 IU [32]. Houghton and Vieth indicated that vitamin D_3 is the most potent form of vitamin D in all primate species, including humans, owing to the diminished binding of vitamin D_2 metabolites to DBP in plasma [33]. They also confirmed the finding of Hollick [34], which indicated that the difference in binding capacity is potentially explained by the presence of a methyl group at carbon-24 position on the D_2 molecule. The different hydroxylation sites of two forms of vitamin D leads to the production of unique biologically active metabolites. Based on this, the 24-hydroxylation after the 25-hydroxylation results in the formation of $1,24,25[OH]_3D_2$ and the deactivation of vitamin D_2 molecule. On the other hand, the vitamin D_3 metabolite $1,24,25[OH]_3D_3$ must undergo an additional side chain oxidation to be biologically deactivated [35]. Interestingly, $1,24,25[OH]_3D_3$ has the ability to bind VDR with ~40% capacity higher than with $1,25[OH]_2D_3$ [36].

6. Candidates for Calcidiol (25-OHD) Measurements

The best indicator of vitamin D status is 25-OHD because it reflects cutaneous and dietary intake, not to mention it is the major circulating form of vitamin D [37]. While there are many established causes of vitamin D deficiency, as listed in Table 4, screening for the general population warrants further investigation. The United States Preventive Services Task Force (USPSTF) did not comment for or against routine screening for vitamin D deficiency. One approach is to consider serum testing in patients at high risk for vitamin D deficiency, and treating without testing those at a lower risk [38]. Just recently, a statement from Osteoporosis Canada suggested that based on clinical suspicion for vitamin D insufficiency and its complications the clinical approach can take into account three settings (Table 5).

Table 4. Major causes of vitamin D deficiency [13].

Causes	Example
Reduced skin synthesis	Sunscreen, skin pigment, season/time of day, aging
Decreased absorption	Cystic fibrosis, celiac disease, Crohn's disease, gastric bypass, medications that reduce cholesterol absorption
Increased sequestration	Obesity (BMI > 30)
Increased catabolism	Anti-convulsant, glucocorticoid
Breastfeeding	Exclusively without vitamin D supplementation
Decreased synthesis of 25-hydroxyvitamin D	Hepatic failure
Increased urinary loss of 25-hydroxyvitmain D	Nephrotic proteinuria
Decreased synthesis of 1,25-dihydroxyvitmain D	Chronic renal failure
Inherited disorders	Vitamin D resistance

Table 5. Approach to vitamin D correction [39].

Risk Category	Action	Level of Evidence
Low: Adult < 50 years Without comorbid conditions affecting vitamin D absorption or action	400–1000 IU No calcidiol measurement required	Level 3 Evidence grade D
Moderate: Adult > 50 years With or without osteoporosis but without comorbid conditions that affect vitamin D absorption or action	800–2000 IU Calcidiol measurement in initial assessment but if therapy for osteoporosis is prescribed, calcidiol should be measured after three to four months, of an adequate dose.	Level 2 Evidence grade B Level 3 Evidence grade D
High: Co-morbid conditions that affect vitamin D absorption or action and/or recurrent fractures or bone loss despite osteoporosis treatment	Calcidiol should be measured and supplementation based on the measured value.	Grade B Recommendation

7. Vitamin D Correction

In patients with normal absorptive capacity, for every 40 IU/day (1 μg/day) of vitamin D_3, serum 25(OH)D concentrations increase by approximately 0.3 to 0.4 ng/mL (0.7 to 1.0 nmol/L) [40]. Largest increments are seen in patients with the lowest starting 25(OH)D level, but subsequently declines as 25(OH)D concentration reaches 40 ng/mL (100 nmol/L) [41]. Nutritional deficiency (25OHD < 50 nmol/L) requires initial treatment with 50,000 units of vitamin D_2 or vitamin D_3 orally once per week for 6–8 weeks, and then 800 to 1000 IU of vitamin D_3 orally thereafter [42]. Intramuscular cholecalciferol (300,000 IU) in one or two doses per year is also an option for increasing serum 25 OHD level [43].

Nutritional insufficiency (25 OHD 50–75 nmol/L) requires treatment with 800 to 1000 IU of vitamin D_3 daily. This intake will bring the average adult's vitamin D status to 7 nmol/L higher over a three-month period. Still, many individuals might need higher doses. In malabsorptive states, oral dosing and duration of treatment is dependent on the individual patient's on vitamin D absorptive capacity. High doses of vitamin D (10,000 to 50,000 IU daily) may be necessary for patients who had gastrectomy or malabsorption history. Patients who remain deficient or insufficient on such doses need to be treated with hydroxylated vitamin D metabolites, since they are more readily absorbed than with ordinary sun or sun camp exposure. All patients should maintain a daily calcium intake of at least 1000 mg (for ages 31 to 50 years) to 1200 mg (for ages 51 and older) per day [44].

8. Vitamin D Toxicity

Vitamin D as a fat-soluble vitamin raised concerns about toxicity from excessive supplementation. Widespread vitamin D fortification of foods and drinks from the 1930s to 1950s in the United States and Europe led to reported cases of toxicity [45]. Hypercalcemia is responsible for producing most of the symptoms of vitamin D toxicity. Early symptoms of vitamin D toxicity include gastrointestinal disorders like anorexia, diarrhea, constipation, nausea, and vomiting. Bone pain, drowsiness, continuous headaches, irregular heartbeat, loss of appetite, muscle and joint pain are other symptoms that are likely to appear within a few days or weeks; frequent urination, especially at night, excessive thirst, weakness, nervousness and itching; kidney stones [46].

There are three major hypotheses for vitamin D toxicity [47]:

(i) **Raised plasma 1,25[OH]D concentrations lead to increased intracellular 1,24[OH]D concentrations.** This hypothesis is not widely supported as many studies revealed that vitamin D toxicity is associated with normal or marginally elevated 1,25[OH]D [23]. It was only Mawer *et al.* who reported elevated 1,25[OH]D with vitamin D toxicity [48].

(ii) **Vitamin D intake raises plasma 25[OH]D levels to concentrations that exceed DBP binding capacity, and free 25[OH]D has direct effects on gene expression once it enters target cells.** High dietary vitamin D intake alone increases plasma 25[OH]D. The low affinity of 1,25[OH]D for the transport protein DBP and its high affinity for VDR dominate normal physiology. This makes it the only ligand with access to the transcriptional signal transduction machinery. However, in vitamin D intoxication, overloading by various vitamin D metabolites significantly compromises the capacity of the DBP by allowing other metabolites to enter the cell nucleus. Of all the inactive metabolites, 25[OH]D has the strongest affinity for the VDR, and thus at sufficiently high concentrations, could stimulate transcription [47].

(iii) **Vitamin D intake raises the concentrations of many vitamin D metabolites**, including vitamin D itself and 25[OH]D, and these concentrations exceed the DBP binding capacity and release of "free" 1,25[OH]D which enters target cells [47].

The amount of UVB radiation required for vitamin D sufficiency can be calculated from the amount of vitamin D produced from one minimal erythemal dose (MED), or 10,000–25,000 IU of oral vitamin D [9].The MED can be defined as the amount of time needed to cause skin to turn pink. The length of time varies with geographical location, skin pigmentation, percent of body fat, and age. Excessive exposure to sunlight will not cause vitamin D intoxication because sunlight degrades any excess vitamin D [48].

The highest recorded individual serum 25[OH]D concentration obtained from sunshine was from a farmer in Puerto Rico with a level of 225 nmol/L [49]. On the other hand, the highest recorded individual 25[OH]D achieved from artificial ultraviolet light treatment sessions was 275 nmol/L [50]. Vieth reported that vitamin D toxicity probably begins to occur after chronic consumption of approximately 40,000 IU/day (100 of the 400 IU capsules) [6]. Reports in which pharmacologic doses of vitamin D were given for a prolonged time, the indications why it was given and in which the final serum 25[OH]D concentrations are provided and summarized in Table 6.

9. Hypersensitivity to Vitamin D

Vitamin D hypersensitivity syndromes are often mistaken for vitamin D toxicity. The most common is primary hyperparathyroidism. Granulomatous diseases, such as sarcoidosis, granulomatous TB and some cancers also cause vitamin D hypersensitivity, as the granuloma or the tumor may make excessive amounts of calcitriol, thus raising serum calcium levels [6].

Table 6. Studies reporting elevated vitamin D status and associated diseases.

Reference, year, and daily dosage (µg)	Duration	Final 25[OH]D concentration (nmoL/L)	Indication
Mason et al., [51], 1980 1250	>52 weeks	717	Hypoparathyroidism
Haddock et al., [49], 1982 1875	>100 weeks	1707.5	Hypoparathyroidism
Gertner and Domenech [52], 1977 500–2000	12–52 weeks	442–1022	Various
Counts et al., [53], 1975 2500	12 weeks	1550	Anephric
Hughes et al., [25], 1976 2500–6250 n = 3	>52 weeks	1000–1600	Not stated
Streck et al., [54], 1979 2500	3.8 years	707.5	Hypoparathyroidism
Davies and Adams [55], 1978			
3750	364 weeks	1125	Paget disease
2500	520 weeks	1000	Thyroidectomy
Mawer et al., [48], 1985			Hypoparathyroidism
1875	520 weeks	568	Hypophosphatemic
5000	520 weeks	1720	rickets
2500	520 weeks	995	Carpal tunnel
1250	1248 weeks	632	syndrome
4285	26 weeks	908	Celiac disease
2500	520 weeks	856	Chilblain
2500	312 weeks	778	Thyroidectomy
1250	1040 weeks	903	Arthritis
			Hypoparathyroidism
Allen and Skah [56], 1992			
1875	19 years	267	Hypoparathyroidism
Rizzoli et al., [57], 1994			
15,000	96 weeks	221	
7500	3 weeks	801	Osteoporosis
7500	74 weeks	1692	Osteoporosis
1075	12 weeks	374	Hypoparathyroidism
7500	4 weeks	650	Osteoporosis
7500	4 weeks	621	Osteoporosis
250	390 weeks	608	Osteomalacia
Pettifor et al., [58] 1995			Not stated
50,000 (n = 11)	10 days	847–1652	
Jacobus et al., [59] 1992			Not stated
725–4364 (n = 8)	6 years	"mean" 731	

10. Conclusions

The present review discussed current knowledge on vitamin D physiology, its clinical relevance and evidence-based treatment options on vitamin D status correction. Caution should still be practiced by clinicians in providing vitamin D supplementation among vitamin D deficient populations, with proper monitoring using approved and certified methods. Indications for vitamin D supplementation outside the conventional calcium homeostasis should also be considered to maximize extra-skeletal benefits of vitamin D correction.

Conflicts of Interest

The authors declare no conflict of interest.

References

1. DeLuca, H. Overview of General physiological tenures and function of vitamin D. *Am. J. Clin. Nutr.* **2004**, *80*, 16895–16965.
2. Mawer, E.B.; Hayes, M.E.; Heys, S.E.; Davies, M.; White, A.; Stewart, M.F.; Smith, G.N. Constitutive synthesis of 1,25 dihydroxy vitamin D_3 by a human small cell lung cancer cell line. *J. Clin. Endocrinol. Metab.* **1994**, *79*, 554–560.
3. Schwartz, G.G.; Whitlutch, L.W.; Chen, T.C.; Lokeshwar, B.L.; Holick, M.F. Human prostate cells synthesize 1,25 dihydroxyvitamin D_3. *Cancer Epidemiol. Biomark. Prev.* **1998**, *7*, 391–395.
4. Holick, M.F. Sunlight, vitamin D and health: A D-lightful story. *Nor. Acad. Sci. Lett.* **2008**, *2008*, 147–166.
5. Jones, G.; Strugnell, S.; DeLuca, H.F. Current understanding of the molecular action of vitamin D. *Physiol. Rev.* **1998**, *78*, 1193–1231.
6. Vieth, R. Vitamin D supplementation, 25 hydroxy-vitamin D concentrations, and safety. *Am. J. Clin. Nutr.* **1999**, *69*, 842–856.
7. Ahmed, M.S.; Shoker, A. Vitamin D metabolites; protective *versus* toxic properties: Molecular and cellular perspectives. *Nephrol. Rev.* **2010**, *2*, 19–26.
8. Holick, M.F. High prevalence of vitamin D inadequacy and implications for health. *Mayo Clin. Proc.* **2006**, *81*, 353–373.
9. Holick, M.F. Sunlight and vitamin D for bone health and prevention of autoimmune diseases, cancers and cardiovascular disease. *Am. J. Clin. Nutr.* **2004**, *80*, 1678S–1688S.
10. Holick, M.F. Vitamin D: the underappreciated D-lightful hormone that is important for skeletal and cellular health. *Curr. Opin. Endocrinol. Diabetes* **2002**, *9*, 87–98.
11. Heaney, R.P.; Dowell, M.S.; Hale, C.A.; Bendich, A. Calcium absorption varies within the reference range for serum 25-hydroxyvitamin D. *J. Am. Coll. Nutr.* **2003**, *22*, 142–146.
12. Bischoff-Ferrari, H.A.; Dietrich, T.; Orav, E.J.; Hu, F.B.; Zhang, Y.; Karlson, E.W.; Dawson-Hughes, E.B. Higher 25 hydroxy-vitamin D concentration are associated with better lower-extremity function in both active and inactive persons aged > 60 yrs. *Am. J. Clin. Nutr.* **2004**, *80*, 752–758.
13. Holick, M.F. Vitamin D deficiency. *N. Engl. J. Med.* **2007**, *357*, 266–281.

14. Cannell, J.J.; Hollis, B.W.; Zasloff, M.; Heaney, R.P. Diagnosis and treatment of vitamin D deficiency. *Expert Opin. Pharmacother.* **2008**, *9*, 107–118.

15. Lips, P. Vitamin D deficiency of secondary hyperparathyroidism in the elderly: Consequences for bone loss and fractures and therapeutic implications. *Endocr. Rev.* **2001**, *22*, 477–501.

16. Chapuy, M.C.; Preziosi, P.; Maamer, M.; Arnaud, S.; Galan, P.; Hercberg, S.; Meunier, P.J.; Prevalence of vitamin D insufficiency in an adult normal population. *Osteopros. Int.* **1997**, *7*, 439–443.

17. Holick, M.F.; Siris, E.S.; Binkley, N.; Beard, M.K.; Khan, A.; Katzer, J.T.; Petruschke, R.A.; Chen, E.; de Papp, A.E. Prevalence of vitamin D inadequacy among postmenopausal North American women receiving osteoporosis therapy. *J. Clin. Endocrinol. Metab.* **2005**, *90*, 3215–3224.

18. Heaney, P.R. Functional indices of vitamin D status and ramifications of vitamin D deficiency. *Am. J. Clin. Nutr.* **2004**, *80*, 1706S–1709S.

19. Hanley, D.A.; Davison, K.S. Vitamin D insufficiency in North America. *J. Nutr.* **2005**, *135*, 332–337.

20. Hollis, B.W.; Wagner, C.L. Assessment of dietary vitamin D requirements during pregnancy and lactation. *Am. J. Clin. Nutr.* **2004**, *79*, 717–726.

21. Rajasree, S.; Rajpal, K.; Kartha, C.C.; Sarma, P.S.; Kutty, V.R.; Iyer, C.S.; Girija, G. Serum 25-dihyroxyvitamin D_3 levels are elevated in South Indian patients with ischemic heart disease. *Eur. J. Epidemiol.* **2001**, *17*, 567–571.

22. Wang, T.J.; Pencina, M.J.; Booth, S.L.; Jacques, P.F.; Ingelsson, E.; Lanier, K.; Benjamin, E.J.; DÁgostino, R.B.; Wolf, M.; Vasan, R.S. Vitamin D deficiency and risk of cardiovascular disease. *Circulation* **2008**, *117*, 503–511.

23. Shepard, M.R.; Deluca, H.F. Plasma concentrations of vitamin D_3 and its metabolites in the rat as infused by vitamin D_3 intake. *Arch. Biochem. Biophys.* **1980**, *202*, 43–53.

24. Paulovitch, H.; Gurabedian, M.; Bulsan, S. Calcium mobilizing effect of large doses of 25-dyroxycalciferol ion anephric rats. *J. Clin. Investig.* **1973**, *52*, 2656–2659.

25. Hughes, M.R.; Baylink, D.J.; Jones, P.J.; Haussler, M.R. Radioligand receptor assay for 25-hydroxvitamin D_2/D_3 and 1 alpha,25-hydroxyvitamin. *J. Clin. Investig.* **1976**, *58*, 61–70.

26. Trang, H.M.; Cole, D.E.; Rubin, L.A.; Pierratos, A.; Siu, S.; Vieth, R. Evidence that vitamin D_3 increases serum 25-hydroxyvitamin D more efficiently than does vitamin D_2. *Am. J. Clin. Nutr.* **1998**, *68*, 854–858.

27. Armas, L.A.; Hollis, B.W.; Heaney, R.P. Vitamin D_2 is much less effective than vitamin D_3 in humans. *J. Clin. Endocrinol. Metab.* **2004**, *89*, 5387–5391.

28. Holick, M.F.; Biancuzzo, R.M.; Chen, T.C.; Klein, E.K.; Young, A.; Bibuld, D.; Reitz, R.; Salameh, W.; Ameri, A.; Tannenbaum, A.D. Vitamin D_2 is as effective as vitamin D_3 in maintaining circulating concentrations of 25-hydroxyvitamin D. *J. Clin. Endocrinol. Metab.* **2008**, *93*, 677–681.

29. Glendenning, P.; Chew, G.T.; Seymour, M.J.; Goldswain, P.R.; Inderjeeth, C.A.; Vasikaran, S.D.; Toronto, M.; Musk, A.A.; Fraser, W.D. Serum 25 hydroxyvitamin D levels in vitamin D insufficient hip fracture patients after supplementation wit ergocalciferol and cholecalciferol. *Bone* **2009**, *45*, 870–875.

30. Gordon, C.M.; Williams, A.L.; Feldman, H.A.; May, J.; Sinclair, L.; Vasquez, A.; Coz, J.E. Treatment of hypovitaminosis D in infants and toddlers. *J. Clin. Endocrinol. Metab.* **2008**, *93*, 2716–2721.

31. Biancuzzo, R.M.; Young, A.; Bibuld, D.; Cai, M.H.; Winter, M.R.; Klein, E.K.; Ameri, A.; Reitz, R.; Salameh, W.; Chen, T.C.; *et al.* Fortification of orange juice with vitamin D_2 or vitamin D_3 is as effective as an oral supplement in maintaining vitamin D status in an adult. *Am. J. Clin. Nutr.* **2010**, *91*, 162–166.

32. Chan, J. Vitamin D update for nutrition professionals. *Veget. Nutr.* **2009**, *18*, 1–2.

33. Houghton, A.L.; Vieth, R. The case against ergocalciferol (vitamin D_2 as a vitamin supplement). *Am. J. Clin. Nutr.* **2006**, *84*, 694–697.

34. Hollis, B.W. Comparison of equilibrium and disequilibrium assay conditions of ergocalciferol and cholicalciferol and their metabolites. *J. Steroid Biochem.* **1989**, *21*, 81–86.

35. Horst, R.L.; Reinhardt, T.A.; Ramberg, C.F.; Koszewski, N.J.; Napoli, J.L. 24-Hydroxylation of 1,25-dihydroxyergocalciferol: An unambiguous deactivation process. *J. Biol. Chem.* **1986**, *261*, 9250–9256.

36. Jones, G. *Analog Metabolism in Vitamin D*; Feldman, D., Glorieux, F., Pike, J.W., Eds.; Elsevier Academic Press: Melville, NY, USA, 1997; pp. 73–94.

37. Institute of Medicine Standing Committee on the Scientific Evaluation of Dietary Reference Intakes. *Dietary Reference Intakes for Calcium, Phosphorus, Magnesium, Vitamin D, and Fluoride*; National Academy Press: Washington, DC, USA, 1997.

38. Teresa, K.; Amy, G.; Jackie, R.; Jennie, H.; Sarina, S. Vitamin D: An evidence based review. *J. Am. Board. Fam. Med.* **2009**, *22*, 698–706.

39. Hanley, D.A.; Cranney, A.; Jones, G.; Whiting, S.J.; Leslie, W.D. Guidelines Committee of the Scientific Advisory Council of Osteoporosis of Canada. Vitamin D in adult health and disease; a review and guideline statement from Osteoporosis Canada (summary). *Can. Med. Assoc. J.* **2010**, *182*, 1315–1319.

40. Dawson-Hughes, B. Treatment of Vitamin D Deficient States, 2010. Wolters Kluwer Health Website. Available online: http://www.update.com/contents/treatment-of-vitamin-d-deficiency-in-adults (accessed on 11 September 2013).

41. Vieth, R. Critique of the consideration for establishing the tolerable upper intake level for vitamin D: Critical need for revision upwards. *J. Nutr.* **2006**, *136*, 1117–1122.

42. Dawson-Hughes, B.; Heaney, R.P.; Holick, M.F.; Lips, P.; Meunier, P.J.; Vieth, R. Estimates of optimal vitamin D status. *Osteoporos. Int.* **2005**, *16*, 713–716.

43. De Torrente de la Jara, G.; Pecoud, A.; Favrat, B. Female asylum seekers with musculoskeletal pain; the importance of diagnosis and treatment of hypovitaminosis D. *BMC Fam. Pract.* **2006**, *7*, 4.

44. Institute of Medicine (US) Standing Committee on the Scientific Evaluation of Dietary Reference Intakes. *Dietary Reference Intakes for Calcium, Phosphorus, Magnesium, Vitamin D, and Fluoride*; National Academies Press: Washington, DC, USA, 1997.

45. Holick, M.F. Vitamin D deficiency: What a pain it is. *Mayo Clin. Proc.* **2003**, *78*, 1457–1459.

46. Schwalfenberg, G. Not enough vitamin D: health consequences for Canadians. *Can. Fam. Phys.* **2007**, *53*, 841–854.

47. Jones, G. Pharmacokinetics of vitamin D toxicity. *Am. J. Clin. Nutr.* **2008**, *88*, 5825–5865.

48. Mawer, E.B.; Hann, J.T.; Berr, J.L.; Davies, M. Vitamin D metabolism in patients intoxicated with ergocalciferol. *Clin. Sci. (Lond.)* **1985**, *68*, 135–141.

49. Haddock, L.; Corcino, J.; Vazquez, M.D. 25 OHD serum level in the normal Puerto Rican population and in subject with tropical sprue and parathyroid disease. *Puerto Rico Health Sci. J.* **1982**, *1*, 85–91.

50. Krause, R.; Buhring, M.; Hopfenmuller, W.; Holick, M.F.; Sharma, A.M. Ultraviolet B and blood pressure. *Lancet* **1998**, *352*, 709–710.

51. Mason, R.S.; Lissner, D.; Grunstein, H.S.; Posen, S. A simplified assay for dihydroxylated vitamin D metabolites in human serum: Application to hyper- and hypovitaminosis D. *Clin. Chem.* **1980**, *26*, 444–450.

52. Gertner, J.M.; Domenech, M. 25-Hydroxyvitamin D levels in patients treated with high-dosage ergo- and cholecalciferol. *Clin. Pathol.* **1977**, *30*, 144–150.

53. Counts, S.J.; Baylink, D.J.; Shen, F.H.; Sherrard, D.J.; Hickman, R.O. Vitamin D intoxication in an anephric child. *Ann. Intern. Med.* **1975**, *82*, 196–200.

54. Streck, W.F.; Waterhouse, C.; Haddad, J.G. Glucocorticoid effects in vitamin D intoxication. *Arch. Intern. Med.* **1979**, *139*, 974–977.

55. Davies, M.; Adams, P.H. The continuing risk of vitamin-D intoxication. *Lancet* **1978**, *2*, 621–623.

56. Allen, S.H.; Shah, J.H. Calcinosis and metastatic calcification due to vitamin D intoxication. A case report and review. *Horm. Res.* **1992**, *37*, 68–77.

57. Rizzoli, R.; Stoermann, C.; Ammann, P.; Bonjour, J.P. Hypercalcemia and hyperosteolysis in vitamin D intoxication: Effects of clodronate therapy. *Bone* **1994**, *15*, 193–198.

58. Pettifor, J.M.; Bikle, D.D.; Cavaleros, M.; Zachen, D.; Kamdar, M.C.; Ross, F.P. Serum levels of free 1,25-dihydroxyvitamin D in vitamin D toxicity. *Ann. Intern. Med.* **1995**, *122*, 511–513.

59. Jacobus, C.H.; Holick, M.F.; Shao, Q.; Chen, T.C.; Holm, I.A.; Kolodny, J.M.; Fuleihan, G.E.; Seely, E.W. Hypervitaminosis D associated with drinking milk. *N. Engl. J. Med.* **1992**, *326*, 1173–1177.

9

Urban-Rural Differences Explain the Association between Serum 25-Hydroxyvitamin D Level and Insulin Resistance in Korea

Bo Mi Song [1,2], **Yumie Rhee** [3], **Chang Oh Kim** [3], **Yoosik Youm** [4], **Kyoung Min Kim** [5], **Eun Young Lee** [3], **Ju-Mi Lee** [2,6], **Young Mi Yoon** [2] and **Hyeon Chang Kim** [2,6,*]

[1] Department of Public Health, Yonsei University Graduate School, Seoul 120-752, Korea;
E-Mail: sbm1396@yuhs.ac

[2] Cardiovascular and Metabolic Disease Etiology Research Center, Yonsei University College of Medicine, Seoul 120-752, Korea; E-Mails: jmlee01@yuhs.ac (J.-M.L.); yun3416@yuhs.ac (Y.M.Y.)

[3] Department of Internal Medicine, Yonsei University College of Medicine, Seoul 120-752, Korea;
E-Mails: yumie@yuhs.ac (Y.R.); cokim@yuhs.ac (C.O.K.); leyme@yuhs.ac (E.Y.L.)

[4] Department of Sociology, Yonsei University College of Social Sciences, Seoul 120-752, Korea;
E-Mail: yoosik@yonsei.ac.kr

[5] Department of Internal Medicine, Seoul National University Bundang Hospital, Seongnam 463-707, Korea; E-Mail: kyoungmin02@gmail.com

[6] Department of Preventive Medicine, Yonsei University College of Medicine, Seoul 120-752, Korea

* Author to whom correspondence should be addressed; E-Mail: hckim@yuhs.ac;

Abstract: An increasing number of studies report associations between low serum 25-hydroxyvitamin D [25(OH)D] level and insulin resistance; however, whether low vitamin D levels directly contribute to increased insulin resistance is unclear. We investigated the impact of residential area on the association between 25(OH)D and insulin resistance in elderly Koreans. Using data from the Korean Urban Rural Elderly study, we conducted cross-sectional analyses in 1628 participants (505 men and 1123 women). Serum 25(OH)D was analyzed as both continuous and categorized variables. Homeostasis model assessment for insulin resistance (HOMA-IR) was calculated using fasting blood glucose and insulin levels. In men, 25(OH)D level was inversely associated with HOMA-IR (standardized $\beta = -0.133$, $p < 0.001$) after adjustment for age, body mass index, waist circumference, smoking, alcohol intake, exercise, and study year. However, we noted significant urban-rural differences in 25(OH)D level (43.4 *versus* 65.6 nmol/L; $p < 0.001$) and HOMA-IR (1.2 *versus* 0.8 mmol·pmol/L^2; $p < 0.001$). When we additionally adjusted for residential area, the association between 25(OH)D and HOMA-IR was attenuated (standardized $\beta = -0.063$, $p = 0.115$). In women, the association between 25(OH)D and HOMA-IR was not significant before or after adjustment for residential area. Environmental or lifestyle differences in urban and rural areas may largely explain the inverse association between serum 25(OH)D and insulin resistance.

Keywords: vitamin D; insulin resistance; elderly; Korean; residential area

---

1. Introduction

Vitamin D plays important roles in calcium and phosphate absorption in the intestine, sustaining sufficient concentrations thereof in the blood. Access to these minerals at bone-forming sites makes normal mineralization of bone possible [1,2]. Reports from across the world indicate that vitamin D deficiency is widespread and is re-emerging as a major health problem globally [3]. Studies from Asian countries, with a few exceptions, have reported a high prevalence of vitamin D deficiency in both sexes and all age groups [4–10].

Increasing evidence suggests that vitamin D deficiency may also be an important cause in a variety of nonskeletal disorders including impaired glucose metabolism [11–14]. Several studies have reported that low serum 25-hydroxyvitamin D [25(OH)D] may be significantly associated with increased insulin resistance [1,15,16]. On the other hand, other studies have failed to detect a significant relationship between circulating vitamin D levels and insulin resistance [17–21]. Therefore, whether or not low serum vitamin D concentrations directly contribute to the development of insulin resistance remains controversial.

In relation to differences in sunlight exposure and physical activity, residential area and one's occupation can affect serum 25(OH)D levels, as well as insulin sensitivity. However, the impact of residential area or occupation on the association between serum 25(OH)D level and insulin resistance has not been appropriately assessed. Thus, we attempted to investigate the association between serum 25(OH)D and insulin resistance, as well as the impact of residential area thereon, in an elderly cohort recruited from urban and rural communities.

2. Experimental Section

2.1. Study Population

This study used data from the Korean Urban Rural Elderly (KURE) study, an ongoing community-based cohort study. The KURE study planned to recruit 4000 participants aged 65 years or older from urban and rural communities of South Korea. During the summer seasons (June to September) of 2012 and 2013, a total of 2025 participants from urban communities (Seodaemun-gu, Eunpyeong-gu, and Mapo-gu, Seoul, Korea) and rural communities (Yangsa-myeon and Hajeom-myeon, Gangwha-gun, Incheon, Korea) were enrolled. All participants completed a health questionnaire and health examinations following an identical protocol. The sampling and data collection procedures have been described in detail elsewhere [22]. We finally conducted a cross-sectional analysis in 1628 participants (505 men and 1123 women) aged 65 to 95 years old, after excluding those undergoing treatment with insulin injection or diabetes medication (n = 397). All participants provided written informed consent forms at the beginning of the study, which was approved by the Institutional Review Board of Severance Hospital at Yonsei University College of Medicine (approval number: 4-2012-0172; approval date: 3 May 2012).

2.2. Questionnaire Data

All participants were individually interviewed using standardized questionnaires to obtain information on their demographics, medical history, medication use, and health behaviors. Trained interviewers carried out the questionnaire surveys according to the predefined protocol, and double-checked whether responses were inappropriate or missing. Occupations were classified as managers; professionals; technicians and associated professionals; clerical support workers; service workers; sales workers; agricultural, forestry, and fishery workers; craft and related trades workers; plant and machine operators and assemblers; elementary workers; soldiers; housewives; and the unemployed, according to the Korea Standard Classification of Occupations [23]. Smoking status was classified into two groups: current smokers or current nonsmokers (past smokers or those who had never smoked). Alcohol intake was categorized as regular alcohol drinking or other (participants who drink less than once a week or not at all). Physical activity was investigated on a regular basis regardless of indoor or outdoor exercise and categorized as regular exercise or other.

2.3. Physical Examination

Study participants wore lightweight hospital gowns for convenient and reliable examinations. Standing height was measured up to 0.1 cm with a stadiometer (DS-102, JENIX, Seoul, Korea) and body weight was measured up to 0.1 kg with a digital scale (DB-150, CAS, Yangju, Korea) according to the pre-developed protocol. Body mass index (BMI) was calculated as weight in kilograms divided by the square of height in meters (kg/m^2). Waist circumference was measured up to 0.1 cm at the midpoint between the lower borders of the rib cage and the iliac crest with an ergonomic circumference measuring tape (SECA 201, SECA, Hamburg, Germany). Participants were seated for at least five min before undergoing blood pressure measurement; two measurements at a five-min interval were obtained using an automatic sphygmomanometer (Omron HEM-7111, Omron Healthcare Co., Ltd., Kyoto, Japan). If the two measurements differed by $\geq$10 mmHg for either systolic or diastolic blood pressure, an extra measurement was conducted after five minutes, and the last two measurements were averaged for analyses.

2.4. Laboratory Assays

Overnight fasting blood samples from all participants were collected from the antecubital vein. Serum 25(OH)D, currently considered a reliable indicator of vitamin D store [24], was measured by an automated chemiluminescence immunoassay (Liaison, Diasorin, Dietzenbach, Germany). This assay is widely available and offers higher throughput capacity, lower sample volume requirement, and reduced operator error [25]. The intra-assay coefficient of variation thereof was 5.5% at 18.0 nmol/L and 4.8% at 319.5 nmol/L; the inter-assay coefficient of variation thereof was 12.9% at 18.0 nmol/L and 7.3% at 319.5 nmol/L. Fasting glucose level was measured using the colorimetry method. Fasting insulin level was measured in accordance with a chemiluminescence immunoassay, with an intra-assay coefficient of variation of 4.6% at 102.0 pmol/L and 3.3% at 864.7 pmol/L, and an inter-assay coefficient of variation of 5.9% at 102.0 pmol/L and 4.8% at 864.7 pmol/L. Insulin resistance was estimated by Homeostasis Model Assessment for Insulin Resistance (HOMA-IR), the product of fasting glucose level (mmol/L) and insulin level (pmol/L) divided by 135 [26].

2.5. Statistical Analysis

We evaluated differences in general characteristics and variables of interest between men and women. Continuous variables were described as mean and standard deviation (for normally distributed variables) or as median and interquartile range (for skewed variables), and tested by independent t-test and Wilcoxon rank sum test, respectively. Categorical variables were described as numbers (percentages) and tested by chi-square tests. General characteristics and concentrations of selected biomarkers were also analyzed according to three categories of serum 25(OH)D concentrations [2]. One-way analysis of variance was used for continuous variables and a chi-square test was used for categorical variables. As serum 25(OH)D, triglycerides, fasting glucose, insulin, and HOMA-IR were right-skewed, they were log-transformed for parametric tests. The relationships between serum 25(OH)D levels and other variables were evaluated using partial correlation coefficients while controlling for age. Multiple linear regression analyses were used to assess the independent association between serum 25(OH)D and HOMA-IR in three adjusted models: (1) adjusting for study year and age; (2) additional adjustment for BMI, waist circumference, smoking status, alcohol intake, and regular exercise; and (3) additional adjustment for residential area. All statistical analyses were performed using SAS version 9.2 (SAS Institute, Cary, NC, USA), and statistical significance was defined as a two-sided p-value less than 0.05.

3. Results

The general characteristics of the study participants are presented in Table 1. This study comprised 505 men with a mean age of 72.8 years and 1123 women with a mean age of 71.4 years. Mean BMI was significantly lower in men than in women; however, mean waist circumference was significantly higher in men than in women. The median serum 25(OH)D level was significantly higher in men than in women (49.4 *vs.* 39.9 nmol/L). Fasting glucose level was not significantly different between men and women. However, fasting insulin (29.4 *vs.* 35.4 pmol/L) and HOMA-IR (1.1 *vs.* 1.3 mmol·pmol/L^2) were lower in men than in women. Cigarette smoking and alcohol drinking were more frequently reported in men than in women. Meanwhile, frequency of regular exercise was similar between men and women.

Table 1. General characteristics of the study participants.

Variables	Men (n = 505)	Women (n = 1123)	p-value
Age, year	72.8 ± 4.9	71.4 ± 4.7	<0.001
Height, cm	164.6 ± 5.4	152.2 ± 5.6	<0.001
Weight, kg	64.3 ± 8.9	56.3 ± 8.0	<0.001
Body mass index, kg/m^2	23.7 ± 2.9	24.3 ± 3.0	<0.001
Waist circumference, cm	85.7 ± 8.6	82.7 ± 8.7	<0.001
Systolic blood pressure, mmHg	129.5 ± 14.5	127.4 ± 15.7	0.008
Diastolic blood pressure, mmHg	74.1 ± 8.8	72.7 ± 8.6	0.004
Total cholesterol, mmol/L	4.5 ± 0.8	5.0 ± 0.9	<0.001
HDL cholesterol, mmol/L	1.2 ± 0.3	1.4 ± 0.3	<0.001
LDL cholesterol, mmol/L	2.7 ± 0.7	2.9 ± 0.8	<0.001
Triglycerides, mmol/L	1.3 [0.3–1.7]	1.3 [1.0–1.8]	0.040
25(OH)D, nmol/L	49.4 [35.4–61.9]	39.9 [28.2–54.9]	<0.001
Fasting glucose, mmol/L	5.1 [4.8–5.5]	5.1 [4.8–5.4]	0.364
Fasting insulin, pmol/L	29.4 [19.8–43.8]	35.4 [24.6–53.4]	<0.001
HOMA-IR, mmol·pmol/L^2	1.1 [0.7–1.7]	1.3 [0.9–2.1]	<0.001
HOMA-IR ≥ 2.5, n (%)	56 (11.1)	190 (16.9)	0.003
Impaired fasting glucose, n (%)	116 (23.0)	218 (19.4)	0.115
Hypertension, n (%)	293 (58.0)	694 (61.8)	0.165
Dyslipidemia, n (%)	243 (48.1)	627 (55.8)	0.005
Current smoker, n (%)	81 (16.0)	17 (1.5)	<0.001
Regular alcohol drinker, n (%)	195 (38.6)	58 (5.2)	<0.001
Regular exercise, n (%)	282 (55.8)	663 (59.0)	0.248

Data are expressed as mean ± standard deviation, median [inter quartile range], or number (percent). LDL cholesterol levels were calculated for 499 men and 1119 women. Abbreviations: HDL, high-density lipoprotein; LDL, low-density lipoprotein; HOMA-IR, homeostasis model assessment for insulin resistance.

Table 2 presents the characteristics of the study population according to 25(OH)D concentration: <50 (deficient), 50 to 75 (insufficient), and ≥75 nmol/L (sufficient) [2]. The majority of the participants (52% of men and 69% of women) were 25(OH)D deficient, while an additional 36% of men and 25% of women were 25(OH)D insufficient. Men and women with higher 25(OH)D concentrations tended to have lower BMI and waist circumference. Participants with higher 25(OH)D concentrations were also associated with lower fasting insulin and HOMA-IR levels, although the association was statistically significant only in men. Table 3 presents the linear correlations between serum 25(OH)D and indices of obesity and glucose metabolism. After controlling for age, serum 25(OH)D level was negatively correlated with fasting insulin and HOMA-IR but not with fasting glucose.

Table 2. Characteristics of the study participants by vitamin D concentration.

Variables	Men (n = 505)				Women (n = 1123)			
	<50 (n = 264, 52.3%)	50–75 (n = 184, 36.4%)	≥75 (n = 57, 11.3%)	p for Trend	<50 (n = 771, 68.7%)	50–75 (n = 280, 24.9%)	≥75 (n = 72, 6.4%)	p for Trend
Age, year	72.7 ± 4.8	72.9 ± 4.7	72.8 ± 5.7	0.937	71.5 ± 4.7	71.2 ± 4.5	71.6 ± 4.9	0.907
Height, cm	164.4 ± 5.4	165.0 ± 5.2	163.9 ± 6.1	0.517	152.2 ± 5.6	152.2 ± 5.8	152.5 ± 4.8	0.625
Weight, kg	64.8 ± 8.4	64.4 ± 9.5	61.8 ± 9.1	0.021	56.8 ± 8.2	55.4 ± 7.6	54.3 ± 7.2	0.012
Body mass index, kg/m^2	24.0 ± 2.8	23.6 ± 3.0	22.9 ± 2.6	0.014	24.5 ± 3.1	23.9 ± 2.8	23.4 ± 2.9	0.002
Waist circumference, cm	86.3 ± 8.4	85.5 ± 8.8	83.3 ± 8.5	0.017	83.2 ± 8.8	81.9 ± 8.4	79.9 ± 7.6	0.002
Systolic BP, mmHg	129.1 ± 15.9	130.2 ± 13.1	129.2 ± 11.3	0.978	127.7 ± 16.1	127.2 ± 14.6	125.7 ± 15.7	0.316
Diastolic BP, mmHg	74.0 ± 9.4	74.1 ± 8.1	74.3 ± 8.5	0.867	72.8 ± 9.0	72.7 ± 8.1	71.8 ± 7.4	0.350
Total cholesterol, mmol/L	4.63 ± 0.83	4.48 ± 0.82	4.35 ± 0.71	0.019	5.04 ± 0.92	4.82 ± 0.93	4.56 ± 0.83	<0.001
HDL cholesterol, mmol/L	1.22 ± 0.33	1.25 ± 0.29	1.32 ± 0.33	0.038	1.35 ± 0.34	1.38 ± 0.33	1.34 ± 0.32	0.688
LDL cholesterol, mmol/L	2.72 ± 0.76	2.61 ± 0.72	2.47 ± 0.66	0.019	2.99 ± 0.82	2.81 ± 0.81	2.62 ± 0.71	<0.001
Triglycerides, mmol/L	116 [84–161]	103 [79–152]	102 [90–123]	0.021	120 [90–165]	113 [82–152]	102 [76–140]	0.014
Fasting glucose, mmol/L	91 [86–99]	91 [86–98]	92 [87–98]	0.596	91 [86–98]	90 [85–95]	90 [86–97]	0.471
Fasting insulin, pmol/L	5.3 [3.7–7.9]	4.7 [3.2–7.1]	3.5 [2.5–5.1]	<0.001	6.2 [4.3–9.2]	5.2 [3.7–8.4]	5.5 [4.2–7.6]	0.059
HOMA-IR, mmol·pmol/L^2	1.20 [0.80–1.88]	1.04 [0.71–1.66]	0.83 [0.56–1.30]	<0.001	1.41 [0.97–2.16]	1.20 [0.79–1.93]	1.24 [0.92–1.80]	0.060
HOMA-IR ≥ 2.5, n (%)	36 (13.6)	19 (10.3)	1 (1.8)	0.013 *	140 (18.2)	42 (15.0)	8 (11.1)	0.070 *
Current smoker, n (%)	44 (16.7)	29 (15.8)	8 (14.0)	0.620 *	13 (1.7)	3 (1.1)	1 (1.4)	0.565 *
Regular alcohol drinker, n (%)	88 (33.3)	78 (42.4)	29 (50.9)	0.005 *	49 (6.4)	8 (2.9)	1 (1.4)	0.008 *
Regular exercise, n (%)	166 (62.9)	91 (49.5)	25 (43.9)	<0.001 *	459 (59.5)	161 (57.5)	43 (59.7)	0.738 *

Data are expressed as mean ± standard deviation, median [inter quartile range], or number (percent). p for trend was derived from a general linear model using contrast coefficients or from the Cochran-Armitage trend test *. Abbreviations: BP, blood pressure; HDL, high-density lipoprotein; LDL, low-density lipoprotein; HOMA-IR, homeostasis model assessment for insulin resistance.

Table 3. Pearson's correlation coefficients between serum 25(OH)D * and other variables.

Variables	Men (*n* = 505)		Women (*n* = 1123)	
	Partial Correlation Coefficient [†]	*p*-value	Partial Correlation Coefficient [†]	*p*-value
Body mass index	−0.152	0.005	−0.126	<0.001
Waist circumference	−0.117	0.009	−0.107	<0.001
Fasting glucose *	−0.071	0.110	−0.035	0.245
Fasting insulin *	−0.211	<0.001	−0.096	0.001
HOMA-IR *	−0.207	<0.001	−0.095	0.001

* Analyzed with log-transformed values. [†] Age-adjusted. Abbreviation: HOMA-IR, homeostasis model assessment for insulin resistance.

We compared the distributions of serum 25(OH)D level and HOMA-IR according to residential area (Table 4). Urban-living male participants exhibited lower serum 25(OH)D levels (43.4 *vs.* 65.6 nmol/L) but higher HOMA-IR (1.2 *vs.* 0.8 mmol·pmol/L^2), compared to their rural-living counterparts. Similarly, urban-living female participants had lower serum 25(OH)D levels (38.2 *vs.* 49.9 nmol/L) but higher HOMA-IR (1.4 *vs.* 1.2 mmol·pmol/L^2), compared to their rural-living counterparts.

Table 4. Serum 25(OH)D and HOMA-IR according to residential area.

Region	Men (*n* = 505)		Region	Women (*n* = 1123)	
	25(OH)D	HOMA-IR		25(OH)D	HOMA-IR
Urban (*n* = 371)	43.4 [32.7–55.2]	1.2 [0.8–1.8]	Urban (*n* = 948)	38.2 [27.2–51.9]	1.4 [0.9–2.1]
Rural (*n* = 134)	65.6 [54.2–76.1]	0.8 [0.5–1.3]	Rural (*n* = 175)	49.9 [36.7–61.7]	1.2 [0.8–1.8]
p-value	<0.001	<0.001	*p*-value	<0.001	0.002

Data are expressed as median [inter quartile range]. Abbreviation: HOMA-IR, homeostasis model assessment for insulin resistance.

Table 5 presents the association between serum 25(OH)D level and HOMA-IR after multiple linear regression analyses. In men, serum 25(OH)D levels showed a significant inverse association with HOMA-IR (standardized $\beta = -0.203$, $p < 0.001$) when adjusted for age and study year. The association remained significant (standardized $\beta = -0.133$, $p < 0.001$) after additionally adjusting for BMI, waist circumference, smoking, alcohol intake, and exercise. However, the association was markedly attenuated after additional adjustment for residential area (standardized $\beta = -0.063$, $p = 0.115$). In women, serum 25(OH)D was significantly associated with HOMA-IR (standardized $\beta = -0.092$, $p < 0.001$) when adjusted for age and study year. However, the association disappeared after additional adjustment for BMI, waist circumference, smoking, alcohol intake, and exercise ($p = 0.187$). When we additionally assessed the association between serum 25(OH)D and HOMA-IR, stratified by residential area, we found no significant association for either urban or rural participants (Table 6). When we controlled occupation instead of residential area, similar results were observed (data presented in Supplemental Table 1 and 2). However, we did not differentiate the effects of residential area and occupation, because they are too closely correlated.

Table 5. Association between log-transformed serum 25(OH)D and log-transformed HOMA-IR in men and women.

Variables	Men (n = 505)						Women (n = 1123)					
	std. β	p-value	std. β	p-value	std. β	p-value	std. β	p-value	std. β	p-value	std. β	p-value
25(OH)D, nmol/L	−0.203	<0.001	−0.133	<0.001	−0.063	0.115	−0.092	<0.001	−0.035	0.187	−0.022	0.415
Study year, year	0.057	0.193	0.054	0.148	0.067	0.067	0.057	0.055	0.074	0.007	0.076	0.006
Age, year	−0.018	0.689	0.042	0.264	0.056	0.130	0.031	0.301	0.026	0.341	0.035	0.201
Body mass index, kg/m²			0.318	<0.001	0.321	<0.001			0.257	<0.001	0.264	<0.001
Waist circumference, cm			0.249	<0.001	0.225	<0.001			0.231	<0.001	0.222	<0.001
Current smoker (vs. others)			−0.074	0.045	−0.071	0.049			−0.006	0.825	−0.008	0.751
Regular alcohol drinker (vs. others)			−0.001	0.981	0.001	0.978			−0.010	0.718	−0.011	0.685
Regular exercise (vs. none)			0.027	0.468	−0.012	0.751			−0.003	0.920	−0.021	0.456
Rural (vs. urban)					−0.183	<0.001					−0.074	0.008
Coefficient of determination	adj. R^2 = 0.041		adj. R^2 = 0.336		adj. R^2 = 0.360		adj. R^2 = 0.011		adj. R^2 = 0.219		adj. R^2 = 0.223	

Abbreviation: HOMA-IR, homeostasis model assessment for insulin resistance.

Table 6. Association between log-transformed serum 25(OH)D and log-transformed HOMA-IR in men and women according to residential area.

Variables	Urban (n = 1319)				Rural (n = 309)			
	Men (n = 371)		Women (n = 948)		Men (n = 134)		Women (n = 175)	
	std. β	p-value	std. β	p-value	std. β	p-value	std. β	p-value
25(OH)D, nmol/L	−0.052	0.263	−0.008	0.785	−0.084	0.217	−0.084	0.224
Study year, year	0.101	0.035	0.046	0.129	0.035	0.582	0.180	0.011
Age, year	0.141	0.003	0.060	0.044	−0.120	0.090	−0.084	0.236
Body mass index, kg/m²	0.281	<0.001	0.304	<0.001	0.422	0.002	0.116	0.308
Waist circumference, cm	0.224	0.003	0.178	<0.001	0.221	0.094	0.369	0.001
Current smoker (vs. others)	−0.054	0.240	−0.003	0.910	−0.114	0.091	−0.072	0.285
Regular alcohol drinker (vs. others)	0.037	0.433	−0.021	0.464	−0.105	0.120	0.080	0.231
Regular exercise (vs. none)	−0.033	0.480	−0.010	0.747	0.007	0.918	−0.018	0.790
Coefficient of determination	adj. R^2 = 0.241		adj. R^2 = 0.215		adj. R^2 = 0.467		adj. R^2 = 0.250	

Abbreviation: HOMA-IR, homeostasis model assessment for insulin resistance.

4. Discussion

The current study was designed to examine the impact of residential area or occupation on the association between serum 25(OH)D level and insulin resistance. Herein, we observed a significant association between serum 25(OH)D and HOMA-IR in men; however, the association was markedly attenuated after adjusting for residential area or occupation.

Several studies, including a few reports from the Korean population, have revealed inverse associations between vitamin D and insulin resistance [1,15,16,27,28]. A random sample of the general population of Copenhagen, Denmark, demonstrated that low 25(OH)D level is not significantly related to incident type 2 diabetes mellitus after adjusting for confounders; however, it was significantly associated with adverse longitudinal changes in continuous markers of glucose homeostasis [27]. In a nested case-control study performed on US military service members, participants with a low serum 25(OH)D level exhibited a substantially higher risk of developing insulin-requiring diabetes mellitus than those with a higher level [15]. In a Thai population study, low vitamin D level was shown to be modestly associated with a small increase in risk of type 2 diabetes mellitus in urban elderly residents only [28]. In the Fourth Korea National Health and Nutrition Examination Survey (KNHANES), a low serum 25(OH)D level was associated with fasting insulin, HOMA-IR, and diabetes [1,16].

Meanwhile, other studies have shown that serum 25(OH)D level is not significantly correlated to glucose metabolism [17–21,29]. Our previous study suggested that vitamin D is not independently associated with insulin resistance among middle-aged Korean men and women [29]. In the Third U.S. National Health and Nutrition Examination Survey, serum 25(OH)D level was inversely associated with insulin resistance and diabetes mellitus only in Mexican Americans and non-Hispanic whites, but not in non-Hispanic blacks [17]. In the Hoorn study, which comprised participants aged 50 to 75 years, no significant relationship was revealed between 25(OH)D, postprandial or fasting glucose concentrations, and incident diabetes [18]. In a healthy Cree community in Quebec, Canada, no association between vitamin D and insulin homeostasis indices (HOMA-IR and HOMA-Beta) was detected [19]. In a cross-sectional study of Pan-European subjects with metabolic syndrome, no correlations were recorded between vitamin D and intravenous glucose tolerance test (IVGTT)-based estimates of insulin secretion and action [20]. Additionally, a Turkish study of children and adolescents found no correlation between insulin measurements during an oral glucose tolerance test and vitamin D deficiency [21].

Compared with previous studies, ours is distinct in that we investigated the gender and residential area-specific association between low 25(OH)D level and insulin resistance in general elderly Koreans, while other Korean studies were carried out indiscriminately on all participants aged 19 years or older with statistical adjustments for gender and residential area [1,16]. Previous studies that set out to investigate the inverse association between vitamin D and insulin resistance also might not have appropriately controlled for residential area and other socio-demographic characteristics. In fact, many previous studies categorized residential areas into rural and urban areas simply based on administrative district, which may not reflect actual urban-rural differences.

The KURE study recruited participants from urban and rural areas. All participants from the two areas resided in the midwestern region of the Korean peninsula, and were of the same ethnic and racial origin, Korean. Total cholesterol, HDL cholesterol, LDL cholesterol, and triglyceride levels were similar between the urban dwellers and the rural dwellers. Distribution of smoking status and alcohol intake were also similar between the two communities. However, there were some differences between the urban and rural residents: in the urban area, only 0.1% of participants worked in the agricultural, forestry, or fishery industry, whereas in the rural area, 60.8% of participants were agricultural, forestry, or fishery workers; people working in these industries typically spend a lot more time working outdoors. Also, urban dwellers were more obese than the rural dwellers (BMI, 24.2 *vs.* 23.5 kg/m², $p < 0.001$; waist circumference, 84.0 *vs.* 82.1 cm, $p < 0.001$). Thus, it was possible for us to take into account residential area as a potential confounder. To compare the effect of residential area *versus* the effect of individual characteristics on the association between serum 25(OH)D and insulin resistance in men, we constructed an additional model that included adjustment for residential area in addition to study year and a participant's age. Adjusting for residential area resulted in greater attenuation of the effect size (std. $\beta = -0.100$, $p = 0.035$) than adjusting for individual characteristics, such as BMI, waist circumference, smoking, alcohol intake, and exercise (std. $\beta = -0.133$, $p < 0.001$). These results implied that urban-rural differences exert a greater influence on the association between serum 25(OH)D and insulin resistance than other measurable variables: we suspect that urban-rural differences are reflective of any number of combinations of environmental and socioeconomic factors, such as dissimilarities in outdoor activity related to one's occupation and physical activity related to traveling to and from work. Nonetheless, our findings suggest that vitamin D itself does not exert major influences on insulin resistance and that residential area largely explains the association between 25(OH)D and insulin resistance.

The study has a few limitations that warrant consideration. First, this study was conducted as a cross-sectional study in which all information was collected at the same point in time; therefore, the causal association between serum 25(OH)D and insulin resistance is uncertain and residual confounders might not be totally removed. Second, we did not examine intake of vitamin D supplements and outdoor activity, which may influence vitamin D concentrations in the body, and thus we could not adjust for them. Third, we did not utilize the euglycemic clamp method, known as a gold standard examination for assessing insulin resistance. Instead, we utilized HOMA-IR as a surrogate marker of insulin resistance. Most epidemiological studies widely support the use of HOMA-IR on the basis of a high correlation between estimates of insulin resistance derived from HOMA and from the glucose clamp [30]. Lastly, serum 25(OH)D level was not measured by tandem-mass spectrometry, the reference method, but by chemiluminescence immunoassay. This immunoassay is intended for quantitative determination of total 25(OH)D and does not distinguish between 25(OH)D2 and 25(OH)D3 [31]. Also, serum 25(OH)D level was measured mainly in the summer and cannot represent annual mean concentrations. Nevertheless, the principal purpose of the current study was to examine the relationship between serum 25(OH)D and insulin resistance in a general elderly population and not to report absolute levels of 25(OH)D over the year. Thus, our findings would not be critically distorted by the single measurement of serum 25(OH)D levels.

5. Conclusions

In conclusion, lower concentrations of vitamin D are associated with increased insulin resistance in elderly Korean men. However, the inverse association between serum 25(OH)D and insulin resistance was largely explained by environmental or lifestyle differences in urban and rural areas. Our findings do not support a causal relationship between serum 25(OH)D and type 2 diabetes, although they cannot rule out a weak causal effect.

Acknowledgments

The study was supported by grants from the Korea Centers for Disease Control and Prevention (2012-E63001-001, 2013-E63007-00). The authors would also like to thank Anthony Thomas Milliken (Editing Synthase, Seoul, Korea) for his help with the editing of this manuscript.

Author Contributions

Yumie Rhee, Chang Oh Kim, Yoosik Youm, and Hyeon Chang Kim designed this research. Kyoung Min Kim and Eun Young Lee supervised the study and acquired data. Young Mi Yoon managed the data. Bo Mi Song analyzed the data and wrote the paper. Ju-Mi Lee and Hyeon Chang Kim provided critical revision of the manuscript for important intellectual content. Hyeon Chang Kim had primary responsibility for final content. All authors read and approved the final manuscript.

Conflicts of Interest

The authors declare no conflicts of interest.

References

1. Choi, H.S.; Kim, K.A.; Lim, C.Y.; Rhee, S.Y.; Hwang, Y.C.; Kim, K.M.; Kim, K.J.; Rhee, Y.; Lim, S.K. Low serum vitamin D is associated with high risk of diabetes in Korean adults. *J. Nutr.* **2011**, *141*, 1524–1528.

2. Holick, M.F. Vitamin D deficiency. *N. Engl. J. Med.* **2007**, *357*, 266–281.

3. Mithal, A.; Wahl, D.A.; Bonjour, J.P.; Burckhardt, P.; Dawson-Hughes, B.; Eisman, J.A.; el-Hajj Fuleihan, G.; Josse, R.G.; Lips, P.; Morales-Torres, J. Global vitamin D status and determinants of hypovitaminosis D. *Osteoporos. Int.* **2009**, *20*, 1807–1820.

4. Harinarayan, C.V.; Ramalakshmi, T.; Prasad, U.V.; Sudhakar, D.; Srinivasarao, P.V.; Sarma, K.V.; Kumar, E.G. High prevalence of low dietary calcium, high phytate consumption, and vitamin D deficiency in healthy south Indians. *Am. J. Clin. Nutr.* **2007**, *85*, 1062–1067.

5. Islam, M.Z.; Akhtaruzzaman, M.; Lamberg-Allardt, C. Hypovitaminosis D is common in both veiled and nonveiled Bangladeshi women. *Asia Pac. J. Clin. Nutr.* **2006**, *15*, 81–87.

6. Chailurkit, L.O.; Rajatanavin, R.; Teerarungsikul, K.; Ongphiphadhanakul, B.; Puavilai, G. Serum vitamin D, parathyroid hormone and biochemical markers of bone turnover in normal Thai subjects. *J. Med. Assoc. Thai.* **1996**, *79*, 499–504.

7. Lim, S.K.; Kung, A.W.; Sompongse, S.; Soontrapa, S.; Tsai, K.S. Vitamin D inadequacy in postmenopausal women in eastern Asia. *Curr. Med. Res. Opin.* **2008**, *24*, 99–106.

8. Wat, W.Z.; Leung, J.Y.; Tam, S.; Kung, A.W. Prevalence and impact of vitamin D insufficiency in southern Chinese adults. *Ann. Nutr. Metab.* **2007**, *51*, 59–64.

9. Nakamura, K. Vitamin D insufficiency in Japanese populations: From the viewpoint of the prevention of osteoporosis. *J. Bone Miner. Metab.* **2006**, *24*, 1–6.

10. Choi, H.S.; Oh, H.J.; Choi, H.; Choi, W.H.; Kim, J.G.; Kim, K.M.; Kim, K.J.; Rhee, Y.; Lim, S.K. Vitamin D insufficiency in Korea—A greater threat to younger generation: The Korea National Health and Nutrition Examination Survey (KNHANES) 2008. *J. Clin. Endocrinol. Metab.* **2011**, *96*, 643–651.

11. Pittas, A.G.; Lau, J.; Hu, F.B.; Dawson-Hughes, B. The role of vitamin D and calcium in type 2 diabetes. A systematic review and meta-analysis. *J. Clin. Endocrinol. Metab.* **2007**, *92*, 2017–2029.

12. Mitri, J.; Muraru, M.D.; Pittas, A.G. Vitamin D and type 2 diabetes: A systematic review. *Eur. J. Clin. Nutr.* **2011**, *65*, 1005–1015.

13. Chiu, K.C.; Chu, A.; Go, V.L.; Saad, M.F. Hypovitaminosis D is associated with insulin resistance and beta cell dysfunction. *Am. J. Clin. Nutr.* **2004**, *79*, 820–825.

14. Pittas, A.G.; Chung, M.; Trikalinos, T.; Mitri, J.; Brendel, M.; Patel, K.; Lichtenstein, A.H.; Lau, J.; Balk, E.M. Systematic review: Vitamin D and cardiometabolic outcomes. *Ann. Int. Med.* **2010**, *152*, 307–314.

15. Gorham, E.D.; Garland, C.F.; Burgi, A.A.; Mohr, S.B.; Zeng, K.; Hofflich, H.; Kim, J.J.; Ricordi, C. Lower prediagnostic serum 25-hydroxyvitamin D concentration is associated with higher risk of insulin-requiring diabetes: A nested case-control study. *Diabetologia* **2012**, *55*, 3224–3227.

16. Rhee, S.Y.; Hwang, Y.C.; Chung, H.Y.; Woo, J.T. Vitamin D and diabetes in Koreans: Analyses based on the Fourth Korea National Health and Nutrition Examination Survey (KNHANES), 2008–2009. *Diabet. Med.* **2012**, *29*, 1003–1010.

17. Scragg, R.; Sowers, M.; Bell, C. Serum 25-hydroxyvitamin D, diabetes, and ethnicity in the Third National Health and Nutrition Examination Survey. *Diabetes Care* **2004**, *27*, 2813–2818.

18. Pilz, S.; van den Hurk, K.; Nijpels, G.; Stehouwer, C.D.; van't Riet, E.; Kienreich, K.; Tomaschitz, A.; Dekker, J.M. Vitamin D status, incident diabetes and prospective changes in glucose metabolism in older subjects: The Hoorn study. *Nutr. Metab. Cardiovasc. Dis.* **2012**, *22*, 883–889.

19. Del Gobbo, L.C.; Song, Y.; Dannenbaum, D.A.; Dewailly, E.; Egeland, G.M. Serum 25-hydroxyvitamin D is not associated with insulin resistance or beta cell function in Canadian Cree. *J. Nutr.* **2011**, *141*, 290–295.

20. Gulseth, H.L.; Gjelstad, I.M.; Tierney, A.C.; Lovegrove, J.A.; Defoort, C.; Blaak, E.E.; Lopez-Miranda, J.; Kiec-Wilk, B.; Riserus, U.; Roche, H.M.; *et al.* Serum vitamin D concentration does not predict insulin action or secretion in European subjects with the metabolic syndrome. *Diabetes Care* **2010**, *33*, 923–925.

21. Erdonmez, D.; Hatun, S.; Cizmecioglu, F.M.; Keser, A. No relationship between vitamin D status and insulin resistance in a group of high school students. *J. Clin. Res. Pediatr. Endocrinol.* **2011**, *3*, 198–201.

22. Lee, E.Y.; Kim, H.C.; Rhee, Y.; Youm, Y.; Kim, K.M.; Lee, J.M.; Choi, D.P.; Yun, Y.M.; Kim, C.O. The Korean urban rural elderly cohort study: Study design and protocol. *BMC Geriatr.* **2014**, *14*, 33, doi:10.1186/1471-2318-14-33.

23. National Statistical Office of Korea. Statistics Korea. Available online: http://kssc.kostat. go.kr/ksscNew_web/index.jsp (accessed on 4 December 2014).

24. Hollis, B.W. Assessment of vitamin D nutritional and hormonal status: What to measure and how to do it. *Calcif. Tissue Int.* **1996**, *58*, 4–5.

25. Wagner, D.; Hanwell, H.E.; Vieth, R. An evaluation of automated methods for measurement of serum 25-hydroxyvitamin D. *Clin. Biochem.* **2009**, *42*, 1549–1556.

26. Matthews, D.R.; Hosker, J.P.; Rudenski, A.S.; Naylor, B.A.; Treacher, D.F.; Turner, R.C. Homeostasis model assessment: Insulin resistance and beta-cell function from fasting plasma glucose and insulin concentrations in man. *Diabetologia* **1985**, *28*, 412–419.

27. Husemoen, L.L.; Thuesen, B.H.; Fenger, M.; Jorgensen, T.; Glumer, C.; Svensson, J.; Ovesen, L.; Witte, D.R.; Linneberg, A. Serum 25(OH)D and type 2 diabetes association in a general population: A prospective study. *Diabetes Care* **2012**, *35*, 1695–1700.

28. Chailurkit, L.O.; Aekplakorn, W.; Ongphiphadhanakul, B. The association between vitamin D status and type 2 diabetes in a Thai population, a cross-sectional study. *Clin. Endocrinol. (Oxf.)* **2012**, *77*, 658–664.

29. Song, B.M.; Kim, H.C.; Choi, D.P.; Oh, S.M.; Suh, I. Association between serum 25-hydroxyvitamin D level and insulin resistance in a rural population. *Yonsei Med. J.* **2014**, *55*, 1036–1041.

30. Levy, J.C.; Matthews, D.R.; Hermans, M.P. Correct homeostasis model assessment (HOMA) evaluation uses the computer program. *Diabetes Care* **1998**, *21*, 2191–2192.

31. Moon, H.W.; Cho, J.H.; Hur, M.; Song, J.; Oh, G.Y.; Park, C.M.; Yun, Y.M.; Kim, J.Q. Comparison of four current 25-hydroxyvitamin D assays. *Clin. Biochem.* **2012**, *45*, 326–330.

10

Vitamin D and the Athlete: Risks, Recommendations and Benefits

Dana Ogan * and Kelly Pritchett

Department of Nutrition, Exercise and Health Science, Central Washington University, 400 E. University Way, Ellensburg, WA 98926, USA; E-Mail: kkerr@cwu.edu

* Author to whom correspondence should be addressed; E-Mail: danastorlie@yahoo.com;

Abstract: Vitamin D is well known for its role in calcium regulation and bone health, but emerging literature tells of vitamin D's central role in other vital body processes, such as: signaling gene response, protein synthesis, hormone synthesis, immune response, plus, cell turnover and regeneration. The discovery of the vitamin D receptor within the muscle suggested a significant role for vitamin D in muscle tissue function. This discovery led researchers to question the impact that vitamin D deficiency could have on athletic performance and injury. With over 77% of the general population considered vitamin D insufficient, it's likely that many athletes fall into the same category. Research has suggested vitamin D to have a significant effect on muscle weakness, pain, balance, and fractures in the aging population; still, the athletic population is yet to be fully examined. There are few studies to date that have examined the relationship between vitamin D status and performance, therefore, this review will focus on the bodily roles of vitamin D, recommended 25(OH)D levels, vitamin D intake guidelines and risk factors for vitamin D insufficiency in athletes. In addition, the preliminary findings regarding vitamin D's impact on athletic performance will be examined.

Keywords: vitamin D; athletic performance; 25(OH)D; supplementation; insufficiency; athlete

1. Introduction

As research has progressed, the importance and versatility of vitamin D in the body has become quite evident, therefore the prevalence of vitamin D insufficiency has been heavily examined in recent years. Research suggests vitamin D's active role in immune function, protein synthesis, muscle function, inflammatory response, cellular growth and regulation of skeletal muscle [1–4]. In addition, a common symptom of clinical vitamin D deficiency is muscle weakness. Due to the many essential roles of vitamin D within the body, it has been suggested that physical performance may be influenced by serum vitamin D status, especially in those who are clinically deficient.

Vitamin D insufficiencies are estimated to affect over one billion people worldwide [5]. The Third National Health and Nutrition Examination Survey (NHANES III) data showed a significant increase in vitamin D insufficiency in the USA over the last 30 years, with over 77% of Americans considered vitamin D insufficient [6]. The alarming rates of insufficiency and the vast metabolic properties of vitamin D have led researchers to examine the influence of vitamin D, not only on disease prevention, but also on physical performance and injury. Vitamin D has been identified in most tissues within the body, including skeletal muscle, which has led to further examination of vitamin D's influence on athletes and physical performance.

Because athletes and sports medicine physicians are primarily concerned with performance, the risk of vitamin D insufficiency among athletes has received growing interest and is under current examination by many researchers. In the last decade, researchers have examined 25(OH)D levels among various groups of athletes, ranging from gymnasts to runners to jockeys. Some findings have suggested that vitamin D levels in athletes are comparable to those of the general population; however, results depended largely on geographical location and type of sport (indoor *vs.* outdoor). It is apparent that the athlete is at an equal risk for vitamin D insufficiency, therefore the potential impact of vitamin D status on performance is now under examination. There are few studies to date that have examined the relationship between vitamin D status and performance, therefore, this review will focus on the bodily roles of vitamin D, recommended serum 25(OH)D level, vitamin D intake guidelines and risk factors for vitamin D insufficiency in athletes. In addition, the preliminary findings regarding vitamin D's impact on athletic performance will be examined.

2. Physiology & Bone Health

Vitamin D functions in two distinct ways within the body, through endocrine and autocrine mechanisms. The first, and most well-known, mechanism is the endocrine function, which enhances intestinal calcium absorption and osteoclast activity [1]. Vitamin D is essential for bone growth, density and remodeling, and without adequate amounts, bone loss or injury will occur [7]. When vitamin D is low, parathyroid hormone (PTH) increases to activate bone resorption in order to satisfy the body's demand for calcium [8]. Low vitamin D increases bone turnover, which increases the risk for a bone injury, like a stress fracture.

A study examining male Finnish military recruits found vitamin D status to be a significant determinant of maximal peak bone mass and also discovered that 25(OH)D levels below 30 ng/mL significantly increased the risk of stress fractures in this subject group [9]. In a large (n = 3700) vitamin D supplementation trial using female navy recruits, subjects receiving 800 IU/day of vitamin D for eight weeks, had a 20% lower incidence in stress fractures than the placebo group [8]. These studies in active populations, such as military recruits, display the critical role that vitamin D plays in optimal bone health. These findings also suggest that sufficient vitamin D status may prevent injuries, such as stress fractures. Stress fractures are quite common among athletes; most commonly seen among track and field sports, in up to 10%–31% of athletes [8]. Stress fractures can significantly influence performance due to debilitating pain and even cause permanent disability [8].

Vitamin D's other pathway is the autocrine pathway. It is less recognized, but many essential metabolic processes take place in this pathway. On a daily basis, over 80% of the vitamin D within the body is utilized through the autocrine pathway [10]. The autocrine pathway is involved in essential body processes like signaling gene response/expression, synthesizing proteins, hormone synthesis, immune/inflammatory response, plus, cell turnover and synthesis [10]. "Without vitamin D, the ability of the cell to respond adequately to pathologic and physiologic signals is impaired" [10].

3. Vitamin D and Muscle Tissue

The autocrine pathway appears to be of utmost importance and has recently received a great deal of attention in regards to vitamin D's influence on skeletal muscle function [11]. Vitamin D receptor (VDR) sites have been identified in virtually every tissue within the body [12]. VDR regulates expression in hundreds of genes that perform essential bodily functions. The discovery of VDR within the muscle suggested a significant role for vitamin D in muscle tissue and has since been identified as a regulator of skeletal muscle [3,11,13–16]. There are two proposed mechanisms by which vitamin D status may influence muscular strength. One possible explanation involves the direct role of 1,25-dihydroxyvitamin D [1,25(OH)$_2$D] on VDRs within the muscle cells [11,17,18]. A second explanation suggests that vitamin D modifies the transportation of calcium in the sarcoplasmic reticulum by increasing the efficiency or number of calcium binding sites involved in muscle contraction. This indirect mechanism however, has only been examined in rat models [11]. On the contrary, one study disputes the evidence for the presence of VDRs within the skeletal muscle cells and suggests that the immunocytochemical staining to detect VDR may be responsible for the false positives results in previous studies [18,19].

Furthermore, it has been suggested that vitamin D supplementation in individuals with low vitamin D status may improve muscle strength. This is believed to be due to an increase in the size and amount of type II (fast twitch) muscle fibers associated with vitamin D supplementation [11,20]. It should be noted that type II fibers are predominant in power and anaerobic activities, and are recruited first to prevent falls, associated with muscle strength in the aging population [11].

Various researchers have found vitamin D to have a significant effect on muscle weakness, pain, balance and fractures in aging individuals [3,4]. It is difficult, however to compare the results given the variety of outcome measures and differences in populations used in the studies [14]. Several observational studies have suggested that vitamin D status influences muscular strength and function in the elderly [11,21]. Contrary to these findings, Chan *et al.*, (2012) found no association between baseline vitamin D status and changes in performance measures over a four year period [14,22].

Replacing vitamin D stores in the elderly population may be protective against fall risk and declining physical function [11,14].

Few studies to date have examined this relationship in the adolescent population. Foo *et al.* (2009) examined the relationship between 25(OH)D status and bone mass, bone turnover, and muscle strength in Chinese adolescent females (*n* = 301) and found that poor vitamin D status (<20 ng/mL) was associated with reduced forearm strength, (using a handgrip dynanmometer) when compared to individuals with adequate vitamin D levels (>20 ng/mL) [17]. Ward *et al.* (2004) suggested that 25(OH)D levels were positively associated with muscle power, and jump height in postmenarchal females (*n* = 91), however physical activity levels were not taken into consideration [11,23].

These findings in regard to muscle tissue and function suggest that vitamin D status may have a significant effect on muscle performance and injury prevention, therefore possibly influencing athletic performance. However, further research is warranted to determine the magnitude of effect of vitamin D on muscle strength and performance.

4. Vitamin D Recommendations (Intake and Desirable Levels)

Although the sun is the most plentiful source of vitamin D, there are also some dietary sources. Some common foods contain significant levels of vitamin D, naturally, including salmon, fatty fish, egg yolks, plus, fortified products also exist, such as, milk, cereal and orange juice [24]. While these dietary sources may appear significant, the process of absorbing dietary vitamin D is only about 50% efficient; therefore, much of the nutrient value is lost in digestion [25]. The lack of dietary vitamin D is yet another factor that increases the risk of vitamin D insufficiency. Most experts agree that a higher intake of vitamin D, through dietary sources, ultraviolet B (UVB) exposure, and supplementation, is necessary to obtain optimal serum vitamin D levels [10,26–28].

In November of 2010, the Institute of Medicine (IOM) released new recommendations for dietary intake of vitamin D, 400–600 IU/day for children & adults (0–70 years), 800 IU/day for older adults (>70 years) [29]. These values are only slightly higher than past recommendations [29]. Many experts argue that while IOM intake recommendations may adequately prevent clinical vitamin D deficiency, they are significantly lower than the level necessary to achieve optimal vitamin D status [5,6,10,26]. The Recommended Dietary Allowance (RDA) for Vitamin D, according to the National Institute of Medicine (IOM) [29] is compared to the Endocrine Society's [30] recommended intake in Table 1. Many believe that the RDA is grossly underestimated [5,6,10,26], including the Endocrine Society, who released vitamin intake guidelines that are significantly higher [30]. The Endocrine Society recommends 400–1000 IU/day for infants, 600–1000 IU/day in children (1–18 years) and 1500–2000 IU/day in adults, in addition to sensible sun exposure [30].

Another area of debate among vitamin D researchers is the terminology and reference values used to define optimal vitamin D status, deficiency, and insufficiency. Optimal serum 25(OH)D concentrations have yet to be defined; however, most researchers have similar reference values [31]. Vitamin D deficiency is often defined as <20 ng/mL (50 nmol/L), and insufficiency defined as 20–32 ng/mL (50–80 nmol/L) and optimal levels are >40 ng/mL (100 nmol/L) [5,10,12,32]. The term insufficiency "appears to be the currently favored term for the range of marginal deficiency and is the theoretical serum concentration that is not high enough to protect against certain chronic diseases" [32].

Table 1. Recommended vitamin D intake levels of the Institute of Medicine *vs.* Endocrine Society [29,30].

Age	Recommended Intake (IU/day)	Upper Limit (IU/day)
National Institute of Medicine		
Children (0–18 years)	400–600	2500 (1–3 years) 3000 (4–8 years) 4000 (13–18 years)
Adults (19–70 years)	600	4000
Older Adults (>70 years)	800	4000
Pregnancy/Lactation	600	4000
The Endocrine Society		
Children (0–18 years)	400–1000	2000–4000
Adults (19–70 years)	1500–2000	10,000
Older Adults (>70 years)	1500–2000	10,000
Pregnancy/Lactation	600–1000 (14–18 years) 1500–2000 (19–50 years)	10,000

Optimal levels of serum 25(OH)D are no exception to the controversy. When serum levels reach >32 ng/mL, parathyroid hormone (PTH) levels become stable and reduce the risk of secondary hypoparathyroidism, which is commonly associated with low vitamin D status. In addition, intestinal calcium absorption is enhanced, reducing the risk of secondary bone disease [5,28]. These basic vitamin D functions are efficiently demonstrated at 25(OH)D levels >32 ng/mL; however, superior benefits are observed at even greater levels. For example, only at 25(OH)D levels >40 ng/mL, does vitamin D begin to be stored in the muscle and fat for future use [20,28]. Therefore, at levels <40 ng/mL, the body relies on a daily replenishment of vitamin D to directly satisfy its daily requirements, which is not likely to be present in the common diet. At levels <40 ng/mL, there appears to be just enough circulating 25(OH)D available for all of the immediate metabolic needs; however, stored vitamin D is not likely available for the advanced processes involved in the critical autocrine pathways [20].

It is estimated that the body requires 3000–5000 IU of vitamin D per day to meet the needs of "essentially every tissue and cell in the body" [12]. The IOM recommends 600 IU of vitamin D for most adults (18–70 years of age) to prevent clinical vitamin D deficiency, defined as 25(OH)D ≤ 20 ng/mL [29]. In contrast, most expert's recommendations are much higher than 600 IU per day, because their recommendations are designed to help reach optimal 25(OH)D levels of at least 40 ng/mL. Intake levels recommended by most experts not only allow support for daily metabolic requirements, but also allow for vitamin D storage and increased availability, which appears to reduce the risk of many diseases and possibly enhance performance. The recommended daily vitamin D intake, according to most experts, is at least 1000 IU per day to maintain optimal 25(OH)D status; however, more is required if levels begin suboptimal [5,10,28]. With over 77% of Americans considered insufficient in vitamin D, it is apparent that the current recommendations are suboptimal [5,6,10,26].

Intake recommendations increase with age, pregnancy, and lactation. In addition, experts recommend much higher initial dosages if 25(OH)D levels begin deficient, ranging from 2000 to 200,000 IU, until optimal 25(OH)D levels are met, then 1000–2000 IU/day for maintenance [5,28,32]. A commonly prescribed treatment to quickly correct vitamin D deficiency is a weekly dose of 50,000 IU of vitamin D for eight weeks [12].

The tolerable upper limit for vitamin D has been set by the IOM at 4000 IU for adults, compared to 10,000 IU/day by the Endocrine Society [29,30] (Table 1). Leading experts have claimed that a daily intake of 10,000 IU would take months, or even years to manifest symptoms of toxicity [28]. A recent publication found no cases of toxicity with daily intakes of 30,000 IU per day for an extended period of time [10]. Regardless of the current dietary intake value, the amount of vitamin D produced from 15 min of unprotected sun exposure is 10,000 to 20,000 IU, in a light-skinned individual, making most experts believe toxicity to be a rare and unlikely event [10,12]. During the months that UVB rays are available from the sun, five to 15 min of unprotected sun exposure between the hours of 10 a.m. and 3 p.m. appear to provide adequate amounts of vitamin D [12].

There have never been any reported cases of vitamin D toxicity from over exposure to the sun; however, symptoms of intoxication, such as hypercalcemia, have been observed when 25(OH)D levels are greater than 150 ng/mL [12]. Serum 25(OH)D levels in individuals living close to the equator and working outdoors are often around 50 ng/mL, supporting the theory that vitamin D toxicity from the sun is extremely unlikely, and suggesting that any toxicities would result only from over supplementation [28]. Regardless, many experts agree than 1000 IU/day in the absence of proper sun exposure can maintain 25(OH)D levels of at least 32 ng/mL [12].

5. Vitamin D Status of Athletes

The distance from the equator, season, and time of day dictate whether vitamin D is available from the sun. Production of vitamin D from the sun is also dictated by cloud cover, pollution, sunblock, skin pigment and age. During the summer months, UVB radiation from the sun can be absorbed in adequate amounts to synthesize vitamin D [5]. However, during winter months, the angle of the sun prevents UVB radiation from reaching latitudes greater than 35–37 degrees, therefore, vitamin D cannot be synthesized from in these areas [5,20].

Research has suggested that low levels of vitamin D are widespread in populations living south of the 35th parallel [26]. Even if one spends ample time in the sun, sunscreen with a sun protection factor (SPF) of 15 results in a 99% decrease in vitamin D absorption [5]. Individuals who spend ample time outdoors may still need vitamin D supplementation to maintain adequate levels during the winter [33,34]. Many outdoor athletes avoid peak sunlight hours, opting to practice early in the morning or late at night, which greatly reduces UVB exposure, putting them at considerable risk of vitamin D insufficiency. Various studies have found many athletes to be at high risk for vitamin D insufficiencies. Table 2 displays prevalence of vitamin D insufficiencies among diverse athletic groups.

Hamilton et al. (2009) revealed that 90% of Middle Eastern sportsmen were vitamin D deficient between April and October [33]. Although these sportsmen were training at favorable latitudes, Qatar (25.4°N), they averaged less than 30 min of sun exposure per day. Another study conducted at favorable latitude (Israel 31.8°N), suggested that 73% of athletes were vitamin D insufficient [35]. The majority (83%) of female, Australian indoor athletes were also found to be vitamin D insufficient [36]. In contrast, a study conducted at less favorable latitude (Laramie, WY 41.3°N), revealed vitamin D insufficiency in 63% of indoor/outdoor athletes during winter, compared to the fall (12%) and spring

(20%) in indoor and outdoor athletes [37]. Finally, a study conducted even further from the equator (Ellensburg, WA 46.9°N), using exclusively outdoor athletes, found 25%–30% with vitamin D insufficiency from fall to winter [38]. Storlie *et al.* suggested that 1000 IU/day of vitamin D was not enough to prevent seasonal decline of vitamin D status in this cohort [38]. Although the results are variable, geographical location (latitude) and gender do not appear to be the major risk factors for vitamin D insufficiency in athletes. Lack of sun exposure appears to be the main risk factor, putting indoor athletes and those who avoid peak daylight hours, regardless of latitudinal location, at the greatest risk for vitamin D insufficiency [2,9,33,35–38].

Table 2. Prevalence of Vitamin D deficiency (<20 ng/mL) and insufficiency (<32 ng/mL) in various athletic populations.

Type of Athlete	Indoor/Outdoor	Gender	Vitamin D Status	Reference
Finnish military recruits	Combination	Male	39% deficient	Valimaki *et al.* [8]
UK professional athletes (jockeys, rugby, soccer)	Combination	Male	62% deficient	Close *et al.* [39]
UK athletes (football, rugby)	Combination	Male	57% deficient	Close *et al.* [40]
Middle Eastern sportsman	Combination	Male	32% insufficient 58% deficient	Hamilton *et al.* [33]
Australian gymnasts	Indoor	Female	33% insufficient	Lovell [36]
Israeli athletes & dancers	Indoor	Male & Female	73% insufficient	Constantini *et al.* [35]
USA indoor/outdoor athletes	Combination	Male & Female	12% insufficient	Halliday *et al.* [37]
USA endurance athletes (runners)	Outdoor	Male & Female	42% insufficient 11% deficient	Willis *et al.* [2]
USA outdoor athletes (rugby, football, track, cross country)	Outdoor	Male	25% insufficient	Storlie *et al.* [38]

6. Vitamin D and Athletic Performance

Original research concerning vitamin D and athletic performance dates back to the early twentieth century, but current performance trials are quite limited and inconclusive. Russian and German researchers were the first to report the convincing effects of ultraviolet light irradiation for improving athletic performance and decreasing chronic sports related pain [20]. These early European researchers suggested significant improvements in time trials, cardiovascular fitness, and strength with treatment of UVB irradiation prior to performance [20]. German Olympic officials considered these effects significant enough for UVB radiation (vitamin D) to be considered an ergogenic aid. In support of this concept, many athletes claim to peak in physical fitness during the time of year that vitamin D (UVB) levels are at their highest, summer and fall [20].

Unfortunately, there are limited experimental studies available and even fewer that demonstrate a performance enhancement from vitamin D supplementation. However, research examining the aging population (>65 years of age) suggests benefits from vitamin D supplementation. Multiple performance studies in older adults have related low vitamin D levels to decreased reaction time, poor balance, and an increased risk of falling [3]. Furthermore, vitamin D supplementation (800 IU/ day) in older adults showed improvements in strength, and walking distance, and a decrease in general discomfort [3]. These favorable results in older adults support the need for further research on athletic performance and vitamin D.

The current research available to support vitamin D's influence on performance is quite limited. An (n = 39), unpublished thesis examined 25(OH)D and maximal oxygen uptake (VO$_2$max) to determine vitamin D's effect on aerobic fitness in physically active college males [41]. Higher 25(OH)D levels were associated with an increased VO2max, compared to those with lower vitamin D levels (p < 0.01) [41]. These findings suggest that a favorable vitamin D status may improve aerobic performance.

Close $et\ al.$ (2013) examined, young, United Kingdom (UK, 53°N) based athletes (n = 30), and examined the effects that vitamin D supplementation (20–40,000 IU/week for 12 weeks) had on muscle performance (1-RM bench press, leg press and vertical jump height) [39]. Subjects were assigned to a placebo, 20,000 IU/week or 40,000 IU/week of vitamin D for 12 weeks. Muscle performance and 25(OH)D was measured at six and 12 weeks, revealing that six weeks of supplementation was enough to correct vitamin D deficiency, however, it was not enough to obtain optimal vitamin D levels >40 ng/mL [39]. Contrary to the findings in the elderly population, no significant improvements in muscle performance were observed after 6 or 12 weeks of vitamin D supplementation, although serum 25(OH)D levels significantly increased over this time, from an average of 20.43 ng/mL to 31.65–39.26 ng/mL [39]. In this study, lower baseline concentrations appeared to respond greater to supplementation, therefore, future studies may find more substantial results by dividing subjects into groups based on their baseline levels.

Although final 25(OH)D concentrations obtained by the athletes were no longer considered deficient (>20 ng/mL), researchers hypothesized that higher total serum levels may be necessary to document enhanced muscle performance in young athletes [8,39]. According to Close $et\ al.$ (2013), higher 25(OH)D levels may be necessary to induce a physiological response within skeletal muscle [39]. To explain the lack of response, the author suggested that skeletal muscle may require higher serum concentrations for a response, compared to other tissues [39]. The significant response shown in elderly subjects, however, may be explained by sarcopenia. If the elderly were actively losing muscle mass, they may have a more sensitive response to vitamin D supplementation in the skeletal muscle [39]. The authors suggested that more convincing results may be observed by giving supplemental doses of vitamin D to increase serum 25(OH)D above 40 ng/mL.

A larger (n = 61 athletes, n = 31 healthy control subjects) UK-based vitamin D supplementation trial resulted in higher mean 25(OH)D levels, as a result of 5000 IU/day of vitamin D3 for eight weeks and found promising muscle performance results [40]. This supplementation regime significantly increased mean 25(OH)D levels from (mean ± SD) 11.62 ± 10.02 ng/mL to 41.27 ± 10.02 ng/mL, whereas a placebo group showed no significant changes. The supplementation group also displayed significant improvements (p = 0.008) in 10-meter sprint times and vertical jump (with no improvements in 1-RM bench and squat tests) compared to the placebo group [40]. One athlete's 25(OH)D levels increased from 22.40 ng/mL to 55.69 ng/mL and showed improvements in all performance areas, this is only one athlete however. These findings support the aforementioned hypothesis that higher serum 25(OH)D levels (>40 ng/mL) may generate more convincing performance improvements [40]. Findings also suggest that a daily dose of vitamin D (5000 IU/day) may be superior in raising 25(OH)D levels when compared to a weekly dose (40,000 IU/week) [39,40]. Based off of these two preliminary studies and guidelines from leading experts, 25(OH)D levels above 40 ng/mL are likely necessary to significantly improve anaerobic athletic performance. There are no studies available that have examined the effect of vitamin D on aerobic or endurance athletic performance.

To maintain 25(OH)D levels of 40 ng/mL, vitamin D supplementation, especially during the winter months, is warranted [20,28,39,40]. The 25(OH)D goal of 40 ng/mL is recommended for athletes because at this level, vitamin D begins to be stored in the muscle and fat for future use. Furthermore, at levels below 32 ng/mL, vitamin D is not likely to be readily available for the advanced processes involved in the autocrine pathways, which is the pathway that is most likely to influence performance [20,25]. This level is also supported by the two comparable Close et al. studies, where the study achieving 25(OH)D levels greater than 40 ng/mL showed significant effects on performance [39,40].

Besides the two UK based performance trials [39,40], recent research on vitamin D and athletes has focused on the prevalence of vitamin D insufficiency among athletes, not the effects on performance. Although performance trials are limited, various other studies have resulted in alternative findings to support vitamin D's positive impact on performance. Willis et al. (2012) revealed that decreased vitamin D was associated with an increased marker for inflammation in endurance athletes [2]. These results call for future investigation to determine whether decreased vitamin D may increase the risk for inflammatory-related injuries [2]. Razavi et al. (2011) found that vitamin D and aerobic exercise improved exercise tolerance in asthmatic patients (compared to a control, only aerobic exercise or only vitamin D supplementation groups), suggesting that vitamin D and aerobic exercise together, may provide anti-inflammatory effects within the lungs [42].

As previously mentioned, the body requires an estimated 3000–5000 IU/day of vitamin D and the high levels of physical activity in athletes may result in increased physiological demands for vitamin D [12]. Since vitamin D is actively used in many metabolic pathways, it is possible that the athlete may require increased intake of vitamin D to assure adequate availability and storage for optimal performance [32]. This hypothesis may explain the lack of response observed from Close et al., when 25(OH)D levels above 40 ng/mL were not achieved and may also support increased vitamin D intake recommendations for athletes [40]. At this point, the appropriate vitamin D supplementation regime for athletes appears to depend on current 25(OH)D levels, season and sun exposure, with the goal of >40 ng/mL in mind. Considering these factors, many athletes, especially indoor athletes and those who are insufficient, will require up to 5000 IU of vitamin D/day for eight weeks, to reach 40 ng/mL, then 1000–2000 IU/day for maintenance.

Although the results of performance trials are not yet convincing enough to support vitamin D as a direct performance enhancer, obtaining optimal 25(OH)D levels can reduce the risk of debilitating stress fracture among athletes, which may indirectly influence performance through prevention of injury [8,9]. In addition, because of its active role in muscle, resolution of vitamin D insufficiency has the potential to impact performance [11,14].

7. Conclusion

Vitamin D is established as a major factor in preventing stress factors and optimizing bone health, both of which are of great importance to the athlete [8,9]. Rates of vitamin D insufficiency in athletes vary among studies, but most researchers agree that athletes should be evaluated regarding vitamin D status and given intake recommendations to maintain optimal 25(OH)D levels >40 ng/mL. Not only does vitamin D assist in growth and maintenance of the bone, but it also aids in regulation of electrolyte metabolism, protein synthesis, gene expression, and immune function [10,28]. These vital functions are essential for all individuals, especially the elite and recreational athlete. Therefore, regardless of the limited literature available in support of a positive effect from vitamin D on performance, obtaining optimal 25(OH)D levels should be a goal for all athletes.

The data are not conclusive to support vitamin D supplementation as a direct performance enhancer, however, research supports the role of vitamin D in the prevention of chronic and acute diseases, such as: cancer, cardiovascular disease, type 2 diabetes, autoimmune diseases and infectious diseases [18]. Athlete or not, optimal vitamin D status is essential to countless fundamental body functions, making it important for all individuals to obtain appropriate levels. Further research is warranted to appropriately define supplementation regimes for specific populations (elderly, athletes, those who are deficient, altering levels for the seasons), establish definite serum 25(OH)D goals, and investigate the effect of vitamin D on physical performance, especially endurance training.

While there is still limited evidence to support vitamin D as a performance enhancer, sports physicians should consider the importance of optimal vitamin D status to prevent stress fractures and muscle injury. Further research is warranted to determine the magnitude of effect from vitamin D on muscle strength and performance. Based off of the prevalence data, high-risk athletes, such as indoor athletes and those who avoid peak daylight hours, should have 25(OH)D levels assessed annually.

Conflict of Interest

The authors declare no conflict of interest.

References

1. Larsen-Meyer, D.E.; Willis, K.S. Vitamin D and athletes. *Curr. Sports Med. Rep.* **2010**, *9*, 220–226.
2. Willis, K.S.; Smith, D.T.; Broughton, K.S.; Larson-Meyer, D.E. Vitamin D status and biomarkers of inflammation in runners. *Open Access J. Sports Med.* **2012**, *3*, 35–42.
3. Campbell, P.M.F.; Allain, T.J. Muscle strength and vitamin D in older people. *Gerontology* **2006**, *52*, 335–338.
4. Ceglia, L. Vitamin D and skeletal muscle tissue and function. *Mole Aspects Med.* **2008**, *29*, 407–414.
5. Holick, M.F. Vitamin D: A D-lightful health perspective. *Nutr. Rev.* **2008**, *66*, 182–194.
6. Ginde, A.A.; Liu, M.C.; Camargo, C.A. Demographic differences and trends of vitamin D insufficiency in the U.S. population, 1988–2004. *Arch. Intern. Med.* **2009**, *169*, 626–632.
7. DeLuca, H.F. Overview of general physiologic features and functions of vitamin D. *Am. J. Clin. Nutr.* **2004**, *80*, 1689–1696.

8. Lappe, J.; Cullen, D.; Haynatzki, G.; Recker, R.; Ahlf, R.; Thompson, K. Calcium and vitamin D supplementation decreased incidence of stress fractures in female navy recruits. *J. Bone Miner. Res.* **2008**, *23*, 741–749.

9. Valimaki, V.V.; Alfthan, H.; Lehmuskallio, E.; Loyttyniemi, E.; Sahi, T.; Stenman, U.H.; Suominen, H.; Valimaki, M.J. Vitamin D status as a determinant of peak bone mass in young Finnish men. *J. Clin. Endocr. Metab.* **2004**, *89*, 76–80.

10. Heaney, R.P. Vitamin D in health and disease. *Clin. J. Am. Soc. Nephrol.* **2008**, *3*, 1535–1541.

11. Ceglia, L.; Harris, S.S. Vitamin D and its role in skeletal muscle. *Calcif. Tissue Int.* **2013**, *92*, 151–162.

12. Holick, M.F. The vitamin D epidemic and its health consequences. *J. Nutr.* **2005**, *135*, 2739S–2748S.

13. Bischoff-Ferrari, H.A. Relevance of vitamin D in muscle health. *Rev. Endocr. Metab. Disord.* **2012**, *13*, 71–77.

14. Girgis, C.M.; Clifton-Bligh, R.J.; Hamrick, M.W.; Holick, M.F.; Gunton, J.E. The roles of vitamin D in skeletal muscle: Form, function, and metabolism. *Endocr. Rev.* **2013**, *34*, 33–83.

15. Hamilton, B. Vitamin D and athletic performance: The potential role of muscle. *Asian J. Sports Med.* **2011**, *2*, 211–219.

16. Marantes, I.; Achenbach, S.J.; Atkinson, E.J.; Khosla, S.; Melton, L.J., III; Amin, S. Is vitamin D a determinant of muscle mass and strength? *J. Bone Miner. Res.* **2011**, *26*, 2860–2871.

17. Foo, L.H.; Zhang, Q.; Zhu, K.; Ma, G.; Hu, X.; Greenfield, H.; Fraser, D.R. Low vitamin D status has an adverse influence on bone mass, turnover, and muscle strength in adolescent female girls. *J. Nutr.* **2009**, *139*, 1002–1007.

18. Wacker, M.; Holick, M.F. Vitamin D—Effects on skeletal and extraskeletal health and the need for supplementation. *Nutrients* **2013**, *5*, 111–148.

19. Wang, Y.; DeLuca, H.F. Is the vitamin D receptor found in muscle? *Endocrinology* **2011**, *152*, 354–363.

20. Cannell, J.J.; Hollis, B.W.; Sorenson, M.B.; Taft, T.N.; Anderson, J.J.B. Athletic performance and vitamin D. *Med. Sci. Sport Exerc.* **2009**, *41*, 1102–1110.

21. Bischoff-Ferrari, H.A.; Dietrich, T.; Orav, E.J.; Hu, F.B.; Zhang, Y.; Karison, E.W.; Dawson-Hughes, B. Higher 25-hydroxyvitamin D concentrations are associated with better lower-extremity function in both active and inactive persons aged > or =60 y. *Am. J. Clin. Nutr.* **2004**, *80*, 752–758.

22. Chan, R.; Chan, D.; Woo, J.; Ohlsson, C.; Mellstrom, D.; Kwok, T.; Leung, P.C. Not all elderly people benefit from vitamin D supplementation with respect to physical function: Results from the osteoporotic fractures in men study, Hong Kong. *J. Ame. Geriatr. Soc.* **2012**, *60*, 290–295.

23. Ward, K.A.; Das, G.; Berry, J.L.; Roberts, S.A.; Rawer, R.; Adams, J.E.; Mughal, Z. Vitamin D status and muscle function in postmenarchal adolescent girls. *J. Clin. Endocrinol. Metab.* **2004**, *94*, 559–563.

24. Chen, T.C.; Chimeh, F.; Zhiren, L.; Mathieu, J.; Person, K.S.; Zhang, A.; Holick, M.F. Factors that influence the cutaneous synthesis and dietary sources of vitamin D. *Arch. Biochem. Biophys.* **2007**, *460*, 213–217.

25. Mahan, L.K.; Escott-Stump, S. In *Krause's Food, Nutrition and Diet Therapy*, 11st ed.; Gallagher, M.G., Ed.; Elsevier: Philadelphia, PA, USA, 2004; pp. 83–88.

26. Moyad, M.A. Vitamin D: A rapid review. *Dermatol. Nurs.* **2009**, *21*, 25–30, 55.

27. Holick, M.F. Vitamin D and health: Evolution, biologic functions, and recommended dietary intakes for vitamin D. *Clin. Rev. Bone Min. Metab.* **2009**, *7*, 2–19.

28. Cannell, J.J.; Hollis, B.W. Use of vitamin D in clinical practice. *Altern. Med. Rev.* **2008**, *13*, 6–20.

29. Institute of Medicine of the National Academies. *Dietary Reference Intakes for Calcium and Vitamin D*; Catharine Ross, A., Taylor, C.L., Yaktine, A.L., Eds.; The National Academy of Sciences: Washington, DC, USA, 2011.

30. Holick, M.F.; Binkley, N.C.; Bischoff-Ferrari, H.A.; Gordon, C.M.; Hanley, D.A.; Heaney, R.P.; Murad, M.H.; Weaver, C.M. Evaluation, treatment, and prevention of vitamin D deficiency: An endocrine society clinical practice guideline. *J. Clin. Endocrinol. Metab.* **2011**, *96*, 1911–1930.

31. Bischoff-Ferrari, H.A.; Giovannucci, E.; Willett, W.C.; Dietrich, T.; Dawson-Hughes, B. Estimation of optimal serum concentrations of 25-hydroxyvitamin D for multiple health outcomes. *Am. J. Clin. Nutr.* **2006**, *84*, 18–28.

32. Willis, K.S.; Peterson, N.J.; Larson-Meyer, D.E. Should we be concerned about the vitamin D status of athletes? *Int. J. Sport Nutr. Exerc. Metab.* **2008**, *18*, 204–224.

33. Hamilton, B.; Grantham, J.; Racinais, S.; Hakim, C. Vitamin D deficiency is endemic in Middle Eastern sportsman. *Public Health Nutr.* **2009**, *10*, 1528–1534.

34. Tseng, M.; Giri, V.; Bruner, D.W.; Giovannucci, E. Prevalence and correlates of vitamin D status in African American men. *BMC Public Health* **2009**, *9*, 191–198.

35. Contantini, N.W.; Arieli, R.; Chodick, G.; Dubnov-Raz, G. High prevalence of vitamin D insufficiency in athletes and dancers. *Clin. J. Sport Med.* **2010**, *20*, 368–371.

36. Lovell, G. Vitamin D status of females in an elite gymnastics program. *Clin. J. Sport Med.* **2008**, *18*, 159–161.

37. Halliday, T.M.; Peterson, N.J.; Thomas, J.J.; Kleppinger, K.; Hollis, B.W.; Larson-Meyer, D.E. Vitamin D status relative to diet, lifestyle, injury and illness in college athletes. *Med. Sci. Sport Exerc.* **2010**, *42*, 335–343.

38. Storlie, D.M.; Pritchett, K.; Pritchett, R.; Cashman, L. 12-Week vitamin D supplementation trial does not significantly influence seasonal 25(OH)D status in male collegiate athletes. *Int. J. Health Nutr.* **2011**, *2*, 8–13.

39. Close, G.L.; Leckey, J.; Patterson, M.; Bradley, W.; Owens, D.J.; Fraser, W.D.; Morton, J.P. The effects of vitamin D3 supplementation on serum total 25(OH)D concentration and physical performance: A randomised dose-response study. *Br. J. Sports Med.* 2013, in press.

40. Close, G.L.; Russel, J.; Cobley, J.N.; Owens, D.J.; Wilson, G.; Gregson, W.; Fraser, W.D.; Morton, J.P. Assessment of vitamin D concentration in non-supplemented professional athlettes and healthy adults during the winter months in the UK: Implications for skeletal muscle function. *J. Sports Sci.* **2013**, *31*, 344–353.

41. Forney, L. Vitamin D status, adiposity and athletic performance measures in college-aged students. M.S. Thesis, Louisiana State University, Baton Rouge, LA, USA, June 2012.

42. Razavi, M.Z.; Nazarali, P.; Hanachi, P. The effect of an exercise programme and consumption of vitamin D on performance and respiratory indicators in patients with asthma. *Sport Sci. Health* **2011**, *6*, 89–92.

11

Vitamin D and Psoriasis Pathology in the Mediterranean Region, Valencia (Spain)

Maria Morales Suárez-Varela [1,2,3,*], Paloma Reguera-Leal [1,†], William B. Grant [4,†], Nuria Rubio-López [1,2,3,†] and Agustín Llopis-González [1,2,3,†]

[1] Unit of Public Health, Hygiene and Environmental Health, Department of Preventive Medicine and Public Health, Food Science, Toxicology and Legal Medicine, University of Valencia, 46100 Valencia, Spain; E-Mails: palomaregueraleal@hotmail.com (P.R.-L); nrubiolopez@hotmail.com (N.R.-L.); agustin.llopis@uv.es (A.L.-G.)

[2] CIBER Epidemiología y Salud Pública (CIBERESP), 28029 Madrid, Spain

[3] Center for Advanced Research in Public Health (CSISP-FISABIO), 46010 Valencia, Spain

[4] Sunlight, Nutrition and Health Research Center, P.O. Box 641603, San Francisco, CA 94164, USA; E-Mail: wbgrant@infionline.net

[†] These authors contributed equally to this work.

[*] Author to whom correspondence should be addressed; E-Mail: maria.m.morales@uv.es;

Abstract: Vitamin D has important immunomodulatory effects on psoriasis in the Mediterranean region. To measure vitamin D intake in subjects with and without psoriasis, and to find an association with relevant clinical features, a case-control study was performed using cases (n = 50, 50% participation rate) clinically diagnosed with psoriasis and 200 healthy subjects (39.5% participation rate), leaving a final sample of 104 people. A survey was conducted using a food frequency questionnaire and clinical histories. Cases and controls were compared using univariate and multivariate analyses. We observed insufficient intake of cholecalciferol (vitamin D3) or ergocalciferol (vitamin D2) for both cases and controls. Patients with psoriasis were at greater risk of associated pathologies: dyslipidaemia (OR: 3.6, 95% CI: 0.8–15.2); metabolic syndrome (OR: 3.3, 95% CI: 0.2–53.9);

hypertension (OR: 1.7, 95% CI: 0.4–7.2). Insufficient vitamin D intake in both psoriasis patients and controls in the Mediterranean population, and cardiovascular comorbility is more frequent in patients with psoriasis.

Keywords: vitamin D; psoriasis; Mediterranean region; diet

---

1. Introduction

Psoriasis is a common inflammatory skin disorder with variable morphology, distribution, severity and course [1]. Although the cause of psoriasis remains unknown, increasing evidence suggests that psoriasis is a complex disorder caused by the interaction of multiple genes, the immune system [2] and environmental factors [3]. Although psoriasis occurs worldwide [1,4,5], its prevalence varies between 0.6–4.8% [6]. While the genetic influence on psoriasis is well-established, the role of environmental factors is less well-defined. Overweight and obesity have also been identified as risk factors for psoriasis and/or a flare-up of the disease [7].

There has been much debate as to defining vitamin D insufficiency. Optimal concentration of vitamin D [25(OH)D] for maximum effects should be 30–50 ng/mL (75–125 nmol/L) [8]. It is generally agreed that a serum level of vitamin D [25(OH)D] below 20 ng/mL (or 50 nmol/L) is an indication of vitamin D deficiency [8,9], which has long since been recognised as a pathological condition characterised by muscle weakness, rickets or osteomalacia [9,10]. Vitamin D insufficiency, distinguished as a serum level of 25(OH)D ranging from 10 to 30 ng/mL (25–75 nmol/L) with no overt clinical symptoms, has recently become an important concern [11]. Vitamin D insufficiency is extremely common in Europe and the USA, where its prevalence in the general population is estimated to be as high as 50% [12].

Health authorities have used different cut-offs for their definitions of sufficient and optimal statuses, and defining a level of serum 25(OH)D as low or insufficient depends on the level that is defined as normal [13]. Substantial evidence suggests that vitamin D plays a pivotal role in modulating dendritic cell function and in regulating keratinocytes and T-cell proliferation [9,14,15,16]. Epidemiological data have also confirmed that vitamin D deficiency may be a risk for developing autoimmune disease, [10,14,17] including systemic lupus erythematosus [17], Crohn's disease [18], autoimmune thyroid disease [10], primary biliary cirrhosis [10] and rheumatoid arthritis [14,19].

In vitamin D (cholecalciferol and ergocalciferol), as 25(OH)D, acts via the Vitamin D Receptor (VDR) present in many tissues, skin being one, keratinocytes present VDR [20]. 25(OH)D displays marked growth inhibitory action and favours keratinocyte maturity. Given this activity, insufficient 25(OH)D could prove to be a risk factor in psoriasis whose fundamental pathogenic mechanism affects the cellular immune system (T lymphocytes), as well as the hyperproliferation and differentiation of keratinocytes and angiogenesis [9,15,16].

When psoriasis appears, it may involve a vicious circle where skin, aggravated by the disease, is less capable of synthesising 25(OH)D which, as is well-known, is synthesised by the action of ultraviolet radiation, leaving increasingly less 25(OH)D in the organism. Therefore, it is advisable to eat foods [20] which provide vitamin D to achieve suitable plasma levels because we have previously seen how 25(OH)D plays a key role in the modulation of dentritic cells, the regulation of keratinocytes and the proliferation of T-cells [15,16], which are altered as is case of autoimmune diseases [9,20].

This study estimates the prevalence of vitamin D deficiency intake in patients with chronic psoriasis and analyses the association of vitamin D intake with clinical features by paying special attention to the role of obesity.

2. Methods

2.1. Cases and Controls

The cases studied were persons who stated that they have been clinically diagnosed with psoriasis in the previous 12 months. For each case, four control subjects, matched for age (±1 year) and gender, were randomly selected from among the individuals of the sample who did not state that they had psoriasis, as confirmed by a dermatologist and/or general practitioner. Information was collected by revising clinical histories, face-to-face interviews and conducting an intake questionnaire. Information on smoking and drinking habits, body mass index (BMI) and drug intake was used.

Fifty adults with psoriasis and 200 subjects without psoriasis were recruited. Of these, 25 patients with psoriasis accepted to participate in the study, and 79 controls accepted (39.5% participation rate). All the participants were asked to complete the specific food frequency questionnaire on 3 days, validated by the Universidad Complutense de Madrid. [21] Of the participants, 79 did not present psoriasis (controls) and 25 were patients whose psoriasis was moderate to severe. Psoriasis plaques were diagnosed and evaluated by a specialised medical team. BMI was calculated by weight in kg divided by the square of height in m. A BMI of 18–25 kg/m^2 indicated normal weight, 25–29.9 overweight, ≥30.0 was obesity and ≥35.0 was morbid obesity [7].

The second part of the study involved studying and comparing the intake of nutrients between cases and controls to consider which diet type is capable of altering psoriasis by focusing on vitamin D intake. Cases and controls were recruited at the population level. The inclusion criterion for both cases and controls was if they wished to participate in the study. The exclusion criteria for both groups were if they did not wish to participate in the study and if they were on a special diet. All the subjects received a written informed consent before the study commenced. They were all seen by a dermatologist and a nutritionist, who collected the demographic, biometrics and health status data, and any other relevant details. The obtained data included age, gender, weight, height, BMI, psoriasis duration, concomitant diseases and medication. Cases were age- and gender-matched for comparison. After the data collection, diet was assessed with version 2.16 of the DIAL programme (January 2012) [22], which converts food into nutrients.

2.2. Statistical Analysis

Cases and controls were first compared using univariate analysis. All the continuous variables were revised with normal distribution using the Kolmogorov-Smirnov test. The Mann-Whitney U test was used to compare the quantitative variables, while the X2 and Fisher's exact tests were utilised to compare the qualitative variables. Odds ratios with 95% confidence intervals (95% CI) were estimated separately for each variable using standard case control methods with unconditional logistic regression models forcing the matching variable into all the models. The variables with $p > 0.15$ in the univariate analysis were considered for the multivariate analysis. The variables included in the final multivariate models were first selected using 2×2 analyses by assessing the first-order interaction and by confounding multiplicative models. Finally, a backward step-by-step regression was conducted.

Data are presented as the mean ($\pm$ 1SD) or number (and percentage), where appropriate. All the tests were 2-tailed. A p value of <0.05 was considered statistically significant. Data were analysed using the SPSS 14.0 for Windows (SPSS Inc, Chicago, IL, USA).

3. Results

Participation in this study was offered to fifty psoriasis patients. Of these, 20 (40%) did not completely answer the food questionnaire and 5 (10%) did not wish to participate. Thus, the final number of participants was 25 (50% participation rate). Of the 200 healthy subjects who were offered to participate, 121 did not wish to. Therefore, 79 healthy controls (39.5% participation rate) participated, leaving a final sample of 104 people (Figure 1).

Figure 1. Organizational chart of patients with psoriasis and without psoriasis.

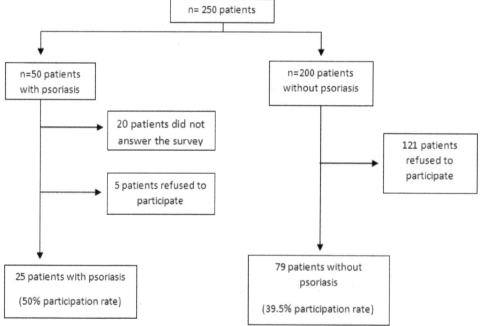

Table 1 provides the baseline characteristics and comorbidity of the psoriasis patients (cases) and of the subjects without psoriasis (controls). No statistically significant differences were found between cases and controls as far as age and gender are concerned. However, the weight of the cases with psoriasis was statistically heavier (78 $\pm$ 26 kg *vs.* 64 $\pm$ 20 kg) ($p = 0.01$). When evaluating BMI, a greater interval for overweight and obesity was maintained among the psoriasis cases (overweight 40%; obesity 36%), implying a risk of 3.39 of being overweight (95% CI: 1.1–10.8) and of 6.3 of being obese (95% CI: 1.8–21.3) among cases. For comorbidity, there were more pathologies found among the cases, of which dyslipidaemia (16%), hypertension (12%) and bone disease (8%) stand out.

Table 1. Baseline characteristics and comorbidity of subjects with and without psoriasis.

Baseline Characteristics and Comorbidity	Cases (n = 25) Fr (%)/Mean (SD)	Controls (n = 79) Fr (%)/Mean (SD)	p Value	Odds Ratio (95% CI)
Male gender	11 (44)	32 (40)	0.700	
Mean age ± SD, years	38 ± 15	42 ± 16	0.200	
Mean weight ± SD, kg	78 ± 26	64 ± 2	0.010	
Mean BMI ± SD	27 ± 8	23 ± 8	0.010	
Normal weight	6 (24)	46 (58)	-	1
Overweight	10 (40)	22 (28)	0.004	3.5 [1.1–10.8]
Obesity	9 (36)	11 (14)	0.003	6.3 [1.8–21.3]
Hypertension	3 (12)	6 (8)	0.004	1.6 [0.4–7.2]
Dyslipidaemia	4 (16)	4 (5)	0.001	3.6 [0.8–15.5]
Diabetes	1 (4)	3 (4)	0.700	1.1 [0.10–10.6]
Metabolic syndrome	1 (4)	1 (1)	0.001	3.2 [0.2–53.9]
Bone pathology	2 (8)	2 (2)	0.001	1.6 [0.3–9.5]

Notes: Fr: Frequency; SD: Standard Deviation; BMI: Body Mass Index; p value <0.05: was considered statistically significant, 95% CI, Confidence Interval.

Table 2 shows that no significant differences in either total macronutrients intake or level of carbohydrates, lipids, proteins and water was found between cases and controls. No bone diseases of genetic origin were taken into account. There were no differences in intake between both groups. The total energy intake was 1930 ± 704 kcal, carbohydrates 190 ± 72 g, lipids 84 ± 33 g, protein 84 ± 33 g and water 2055 ± 807 mL.

Table 2. Macronutrient intake in subjects with and without psoriasis.

Macronutrient	Cases (n = 25) Mean ± SD	Controls (n = 79) Mean ± SD	Total (n = 104) Mean ± SD	p Value
Energy (kilocalories)	1900 ± 1000	1940 ± 570	1930 ± 704	0.700
Carbohydrates (grams)	190 ± 100	190 ± 27	190 ± 72	0.800
Lipids (grams)	78 ± 41	85 ± 30	84 ± 33	0.300
Proteins (grams)	78 ± 41	86 ± 27	84 ± 33	0.400
Water (mL)	190 ± 1200	2100 ± 645	2055 ± 807	0.400

Notes: SD: Standard Deviation; p value < 0.05: was considered statistically significant.

Nevertheless, Table 3 reveals that both study groups consumed less vitamin D than the recommended amount. Psoriasis cases' vitamin D intake is 230 ± 190 UI/day (p = 0.03) and the recommended one is 620 ± 330 UI/day. The controls' vitamin D intake is 290 ± 280 UI/day (p = 0.001) and the recommended one 290 ± 280 UI/day.

Table 3. Vitamin D intake in subjects with and without psoriasis.

Intake	Cases	R_Cases	p Value	Controls	R_Controls	p Value
Vitamin D (UI/day)	230 ± 190	620 ± 330	0.030	290 ± 280	540 ± 220	0.001

Notes: R: recommended intake calculated by the DIAL programme; p value < 0.05: was considered statistically significant.

4. Discussion

In this study intake vitamin D were significantly lower in both groups regarding the recommendation, being higher in patients with psoriasis, which might account for the greater comorbidity relating to these patients' insufficient vitamin D intake.

The main vitamin D source is cutaneous synthesis via skin through UV radiation. There is some controversy as to exposure doses to UV radiation for skin cancer to appear. Therefore, additional vitamin D intake is necessary, preferably in the form of certain foods, or otherwise as diet supplements [23]. Since sun exposure is necessary for vitamin D synthesis, the benefit/risk ratio that this implies has to be taken into account since today's lifestyle tends to involve minimum yet habitual sun exposure, which intensifies during the holiday period, and implies a risk of developing skin cancer [16,24]. Thus moderate sun exposure all year round, along with a varied, healthy diet, should be a recommended practice to achieve adequate 25(OH)D levels in the blood. Unfortunately, very few foods contain 25(OH)D and many of them are not eaten regularly [24], which is one of the main reasons why the study population does not consume adequate quantities of vitamin D.

The relation between 25(OH)D and psoriasis has been studied since the 1930s. In 1985, Morimoto et al. [25] made a chance discovery; vitamin D3 administration improved psoriasis in isolated cases. The attempts made to employ oral 25(OH)D have been limited by its capacity to alter the calcium metabolism. Analogues of 25(OH)D present poorer hypercalcaemic activity to, for instance, Calcipotriol and tacalcitol and their biological actions, which include regulation of epidermal cell proliferation and differentiation, inhibition of angiogenesis and modulation of cytokines production [26]. Morimoto et al. [27] detected less circulating vitamin D3 in subjects with severe psoriasis, this relationship can be partially explained by the liposolubility of vitamin D and its reduced bioavailability in bodies with a high fat content [28]. This may be the reason why our psoriasis patients present more comorbidity as a higher prevalence of overweight or dyslipidaemia. Some research groups have centered their studies on vitamin D receptors. Okita et al. [29] studied the polymorphisms of VDR in psoriasis patients, they discovered a significant relation between genotype AA and liver failure in some patients. This finding suggests that 25(OH)D acts as regulator of the metabolic syndrome expression and dyslipidaemia, which accompanies psoriasis, as observed in the present study.

The type 1 diabetes mellitus is a frequent comorbidity in psoriasis patients. Seasonal variations have been found in the peaks of diabetes mellitus (DM) incidence, which have been associated with periodic oscillations in vitamin D levels [24]. In a large multicentre prospective 4-year study conducted in 51 regions worldwide, an inverse relation between UV radiation (UV-B) in all 51 regions and the incidence of type 1 DM has been verified [30]. Some studies found that vitamin D administration during infancy (2000 UI/day of 25(OH)D) with a follow-up lasting up to 30 years has been reported to significantly reduce the development of type 1 DM [31,32].

Arterial hypertension is another of the pathologies found more frequently among psoriasis patients and is regulated by 25(OH)D through Renin-Angiotensin System inhibition [33]. This relation has been supported by experimental studies, like that of Li et al. [34], who verified how administering 1,25-hydroxy vitamin D [1,25(OH)2D] inhibits the gene expression of renin in knockout mice for the expression of the 25(OH)D receptor. Likewise hypertension, which these mice generate spontaneously, can be reverted with both captopril and [1,25(OH)2D] [24,33] and UVA irradiation of human skin caused a significant drop in blood pressure even at moderate UVA doses [35].

The role that 25(OH)D plays in bone pathologies by regulating calcium in the blood to avoid hypocalcaemia and to stimulate mineralisationis well-known. 25(OH)D is able to stimulate the proteins involved in calcium absorption in the intestine, yet when calcium food intake is lacking, the mobilisation of its reserves from bone mass is favoured, which stimulates osteoclastogenesis. Furthermore, 25(OH)D acts with the parathyroid hormone to stimulate calcium re-absorption at the kidney tubules level [24].

Other studies also report the association with obesity found in the present study [7]. Nonetheless, these studies do not report a significant difference in calorie intake, but in BMI, which is greater in psoriasis patients. This led us to consider that there may be differences in their metabolism. Obesity is associated with basic systemic inflammation, characterised by an increase in pro-inflammatory markers such as TNF-α and IL-6 [36]. Adipokines are also dysregulated, which might be the basis of vascular diseases [37], and of insulin resistance and subsequent DM.

It is necessary to bear in mind that not only there is necessary the ingestion of rich food in vitamin D, but also the development of the vitamin D with the solar exposition exposure, as shown by the studies of the Dead Sea [38] with the normal incidence solar UVB radiation [39]. The quantity of 25(OH)D is very important for general population and psoriasis population, because this group display an altered metabolism [8]. Metabolic syndrome [10,40] (diabetes, hypertension, dyslipidemia, being overweight and obesity) is related with 25(OH)D. Thus evaluating its optimum levels in blood could prevent less comorbidities from appearing.

In short, there is recommended an increase of the vitamin D intake in general in the Mediterranean population and exposure to UV radiation, especially in the patients with psoriasis [8], with food rich in vitamin D such as blue fish (tuna, mackerel, salmon), fish liver, egg yolks and cheese [20]; also enriched food such as milk fortified with vitamin D or the use of vitamin D supplements. In addition new studies that determine both the intake and blood levels of 25(OH)D in psoriasis patients are required.

5. Conclusions

Although more research is need, the considerably low intake of vitamin D in both psoriasis patients and control group indicate the need for proper evaluation of vitamin D status in the Mediterranean population. Further, we identify more cardiovascular comorbililty in psoriasis patients.

Acknowledgments

The authors acknowledge the contribution made by the psoriasis patients and control that volunteered to participate in this study. The authors declare no conflict of interest.

Author Contributions

María Morales Suárez-Varela, Paloma Reguera-Leal and Agustín Llopis-González had the original idea for the study and, with all co-authors carried out the design. Paloma Reguera-Leal and Maria

Morales Suárez-Varela were responsible for recruitment and follow-up of study participants. William B. Grant, Nuria Rubio-López and María Morales Suárez-Varela was responsible for data cleaning and Paloma Reguera-Leal, María Morales Suárez-Varela and Nuria Rubio-López carried out the analyses. Agustín Llopis-González, Paloma Reguera-Leal, William B. Grant, Nuria Rubio-López and María Morales Suárez-Varela drafted the manuscript, which was revised by all authors.

Conflicts of Interest

The authors declare no conflict of interest.

References

1. Langley, R.G.; Krueger, G.G.; Griffiths, C.E. Psoriasis: Epidemiology, clinical features, and quality of life. *Ann. Rheum. Dis.* **2005**, *64*, ii18–ii23.

2. Gottlieb, S.L.; Gilleaudeau, P.; Johnson, R.; Estes, L.; Woodworth, T.G.; Gottlieb, A.B.; Krueger, J.G. Response of psoriasis to a lymphocyte-selective toxin (DAB389IL-2) suggests a primary immune, but not keratinocyte, pathogenic basis. *Nat. Med.* **1995**, *1*, 442–447.

3. Krueger, G.; Ellis, C.N. Psoriasis-recent advances in understanding its pathogenesis and treatment. *J. Am. Acad. Dermatol.* **2005**, *53*, S94–S100.

4. Nevitt, G.J.; Hutchinson, P.E. Psoriasis in the community: Prevalence, severity and patients beliefs and titudes towards the disease. *Br. J. Dermatol.* **1996**, *135*, 533–537.

5. Gelfand, J.M.; Weinstein, R.; Porter, S.B.; Neimann, A.L.; Berlin, J.A.; Margolis, D.J. Prevalence and treatment of psoriasis in the United Kingdom: A population-based study. *Arch. Dermatol.* **2005**, *141*, 1537–1541.

6. Koo, J. Population-based epidemiologic study of psoriasis with emphasis on quality of life assessment. *Dermatol. Clin.* **1996**, *14*, 485–496.

7. Naldi, L.; Chatenoud, L.; Linder, D.; Belloni Fortina, A.; Peserico, A.; Virgili, A.R.; Bruni, P.L.; Ingordo, V.; Lo Scocco, G.; Solaroli, C.; *et al.* Cigarette smoking, body mass index, and stress full if events as risk factors for psoriasis: Results from an Italian case control study. *J. Invest. Dermatol.* **2005**, *125*, 61–67.

8. Płudowski, P.; Karczmarewicz, E.; Bayer, M.; Carter, G.; Chlebna-Sokół, D.; Czech-Kowalska, J.; Dębski, R.; Decsi, T.; Dobrzańska, A.; Franek, E.; *et al.* Practical guidelines for the supplementation of vitamin D and the treatment of deficits in Central Europe—Recommended vitamin D intakes in the general population and groups at risk of vitamin D deficiency. *Endokrvnol. Pol.* **2013**, *64*, 319–327.

9. Pludowski, P.; Holick, M.F.; Pilz, S.; Wagner, C.L.; Hollis, B.W.; Grant, W.B.; Shoenfeld, Y.; Lerchbaum, E.; Llewellyn, D.J.; Kienreich, K.; *et al.* Vitamin D effects on musculoskeletal health, immunity, autoimmunity, cardiovascular disease, cancer, fertility, pregnancy, dementia and mortality-a review of recent evidence. *Autoimmun. Rev.* **2013**, *12*, 976–989.

10. Agmon-Levin, N.; Theodor, E.; Segal, R.M.; Shoenfeld, Y. Vitamin D in systemic and organ-specific autoimmune diseases. *Clin. Rev. Allergy Immunol.* **2013**, *45*, 256–266.

11. Giovannucci, E.; Liu, Y.; Hollis, B.W.; Rimm, E.B. 25-hydroxyvitamin D and risk of myocardial infarction in men: A rospective study. *Arch. Intern. Med.* **2008**, *168*, 1174–1180.

12. Ginde, A.A.; Liu, M.C.; Camargo, C.A., Jr. Demographic differences and trends of vitamin D insufficiency in the US population, 1988–2004. *Arch. Intern. Med.* **2009**, *169*, 626–632.

13. Mortimer, E.A.; Monson, R.R.; MacMahon, B. Reduction in mortality from coronary heart disease in men residing at high altitude. *N. Engl. J. Med.* **1977**, *296*, 581–585.

14. Ishikawa, L.L.; Shoenfeld, Y.; Sartori, A. Immunomodulation in human and experimental arthritis: including vitamin D, helminths and heat-shock proteins. *Lupus* **2014**, *23*, 577–587.

15. LoPiccolo, M.C.; Lim, H.W. Vitamin D in health disease. *Photodermatol. Photoinmunol. Photomed.* **2010**, *26*, 224–229.

16. Gniadecki, R.; Gajkowska, B.; Hansen, M. 1,25-dihydroxyvitamin D3 Stimulates the assembly of adherensjinctions in keratinocytes: Involvement of protein kinase C. *Endocrinology* **1997**, *138*, 2241–2248.

17. Yang, C.Y.; Leung, P.S.; Adamopoulos, I.E.; Gershwin, M.E. The Implication of Vitamin D and autoimmunity: A comprehensive review. *Clin. Rev. Allergy Immunol.* **2013**, *45*, 217–226.

18. Ananthakrishnan, A.N.; Khalili, H.; Higuchi, L.M.; Bao, Y.; Korzenik, J.R.; Giovannucci, E.L.; Richter, J.M.; Fuchs, C.S.; Chan, A.T. Higher predicted vitamin D status is associated with reduced risk of Crohn's disease. *Gastroenterology* **2012**, *142*, 482–489.

19. Haga, H.J.; Schmedes, A.; Naderi, Y.; Moreno, A.M.; Peen, E. Severe deficiency of 25-Hydroxyvitamin D(3) (25-OH-D (3)) is associated with high disease activity of rheumatoid arthritis. *Clin. Rheumatol.* **2013**, *32*, 629–633.

20. Borella, E.; Nesher, G.; Israeli, E.; Shoenfeld, Y. Vitamin D: A new anti-infective agent? *Ann. N Y Acad. Sci.* **2014**, *1317*, 76–83.

21. Ortega, R.M.; Requejo, A.M.; López-Sobaler, A.M. Modelos de cuestionarios para realización de estudios dietéticos en la valoración del estado nutricional. In *Manual de Nutrición Clínica en Atención Primaria*; Requejo, A.M., Ortega, R.M., Eds; Nutriguia: Madrid, Spain, 2006; pp. 456–459.

22. Ortega, R.M.; Lopez, A.M.; Andrés, P.; Requejo, A.M.; Aparicio, A.; Molinero, L.M. *DIAL programa para la* evaluación *de dietas y gestión de datos de alimentación*, Versión 2.16; Alce ingeniería: Madrid, Spain, 2012.

23. Biesalski, H.K.; Aggett, P.J.; Anton, R.; Bernstein, P.S.; Blumberg, J.; Heaney, R.P.; Henry, J.; Nolan, J.M.; Richardson, D.P.; van Ommen, B.; *et al.* 26th Hohenheim Consensus Conference, September 11, 2010 Scientific substantiation of health claims: Evidence-based nutrition. *Nutrition* **2011**, *27*, S1–S20.

24. Gilaberte, Y.; Aguilera, J.; Carrascosa, J.M.; Figueroa, F.L.; Romaní de Gabriel, J.; Nagore, E. Vitamin D: Evidence and controversies. *Actas Dermosifiliogr.* **2011**, *102*, 572–588.

25. Morimoto, S.; Kumahara, Y. A patient with psoriasis cured by 1 alpha-hydroxyvitamin D3. *Med. J. Osaka Univ.* **1985**, *35*, 51–54.

26. Wu-wong, J.R.; Tian, J.; Golzman, D. Vitamin D analogs as therapeutic agents: A clinical study update. *Curr. Opin. Investing Drugs* **2004**, *5*, 320–326.

27. Morimoto, S.; Yoshikawa, K.; Fukuo, K.; Shiraishi, T.; Koh, E.; Imanaka, S.; Kitano, S.; Ogihara, T. Inverse relation between severity of psoriasis and serum 1,25-dihydroxy-vitamin D level. *J. Dermatol. Sci.* **1990**, *1*, 277–282.

28. Orgaz-Molina, J.; Magro-Checa, C.; Arrabal-Polo, M.A.; Raya-Álvarez, E.; Naranjo, R.; Buendía-Eisman, A.; Arias-Santiago, S. Association of 25-hydroxyvitamin D with metabolic syndrome in patients with psoriasis: A case-control study. *Acta Derm. Venereol.* **2014**, *94*, 142–145.

29. Okita, H.; Ohtsuka, T.; Yamakage, A.; Yamazaki, S. Polymorphism of the vitamin D(3) receptor in patients with psoriasis. *Arch. Dermatol. Res.* **2002**, *294*, 159–162.

30. Svensson, J.; Lyngaae-Jørgensen, A.; Carstensen, B.; Simonsen, L.B.; Mortensen, H.B.; Danish Childhood Diabetes Registry. Long-term trends in the incidence of type 1 diabetes in Denmark: The seasonal variation changes over time. *Pediatr. Diabetes* **2009**, *10*, 248–254.

31. Mohr, S.B.; Garland, C.F.; Gorham, E.D.; Garland, F.C. The association between ultraviolet B irradiance, vitamin D status and incidence rates of type 1 diabetes in 51 regions worldwide. *Diabetologia* **2008**, *51*, 1391–1398.

32. Gorham, E.D.; Garland, C.F.; Burgi, A.A.; Mohr, S.B.; Zeng, K.; Hofflich, H.; Kimm, J.J.; Ricordi, C. Lower prediagnostic serum 25-hydroxyvitamin D concentration is associated with higher risk of insulin-requiring diabetes: A nested case-control study. *Diabetologia* **2012**, *55*, 3224–3227.

33. Yamshchikov, A.; Desai, N.S.; Blumberg, H.M.; Ziegler, T.R.; Tangpricha, V. Vitamin D for the treatment and prevention of infectious diseases: A systematic review of randomized controlled trials. *Endocr. Pract.* **2009**, *15*, 438–449.

34. Li, Y.C. Vitamin D regulation of the renin-angiotensin system. *J. Cell. Biochem.* **2003**, *88*, 327–331.

35. Opländer, C.; Volkmar, C.M.; Paunel-Görgülü, A.; van Faassen, E.E.; Heiss, C.; Kelm, M.; Halmer, D.; Mürtz, M.; Pallua, N.; Suschek, C.V. Whole body UVA irradiation lowers systemic blood pressure by release of nitric oxide from intracutaneous photolabile nitric oxide derivates. *Circ. Res.* **2009**, *105*, 1031–1040.

36. Grimble, R.F.; Tappia, P.S. Modulation of pro-inflammatory cytokine biology by unsaturated fatty acids. *Z Ernahrungswiss.* **1998**, *37*, 57–65.

37. Gerdes, S.; Rostami-Yazdi, M.; Mrowietz, U. Adipokines and psoriasis. *Exp. Dermatol.* **2011**, *20*, 81–87.

38. Katz, U.; Shoenfeld, Y.; Zakin, V.; Sherer, Y.; Sukenik, S. Scientific evidence of the therapeutic effects of dead sea treatments: A systematic review. *Semin. Arthritis Rheum.* **2012**, *42*, 186–200.

39. Kudish, A.I.; Harari, M.; Evseev, E.G. The measurement and analysis of normal incidence solar UVB radiation and its application to the photoclimatherapy protocol for psoriasis at the Dead Sea, Israel. *Photochem. Photobiol.* **2011**, *87*, 215–222.

40. Love, T.J.; Qureshi, A.A.; Karlson, E.W.; Gelfand, J.M.; Choi, H.K. Prevalence of metabolic syndrome in psoriasis: Results from the national health and nutrition examination survey 2003–2006. *Arch. Dermatol.* **2011**, *147*, 419–424.

Does Sufficient Evidence Exist to Support a Causal Association between Vitamin D Status and Cardiovascular Disease Risk? An Assessment Using Hill's Criteria for Causality

Patricia G. Weyland [1,]*, **William B. Grant** [2] **and Jill Howie-Esquivel** [1]

[1] Department of Physiological Nursing, School of Nursing, University of California, San Francisco (UCSF), #2 Koret Way Box 0610, San Francisco, CA 94143, USA;
E-Mail: jill.howie-esquivel@nursing.ucsf.edu

[2] Sunlight, Nutrition, and Health Research Center, P.O. Box 641603, San Francisco, CA 94164-1603, USA; E-Mail: wbgrant@infionline.net

* Author to whom correspondence should be addressed; E-Mail: patricia.weyland@ucsf.edu;

Abstract: Serum 25-hydroxyvitamin D (25(OH)D) levels have been found to be inversely associated with both prevalent and incident cardiovascular disease (CVD) risk factors; dyslipidemia, hypertension and diabetes mellitus. This review looks for evidence of a causal association between low 25(OH)D levels and increased CVD risk. We evaluated journal articles in light of Hill's criteria for causality in a biological system. The results of our assessment are as follows. Strength of association: many randomized controlled trials (RCTs), prospective and cross-sectional studies found statistically significant inverse associations between 25(OH)D levels and CVD risk factors. Consistency of observed association: most studies found statistically significant inverse associations between 25(OH)D levels and CVD risk factors in various populations, locations and circumstances. Temporality of association: many RCTs and prospective studies found statistically significant inverse associations between 25(OH)D levels and CVD risk factors. Biological gradient (dose-response curve): most studies assessing 25(OH)D levels and CVD risk found an inverse association exhibiting a linear biological gradient. Plausibility of biology: several plausible cellular-level causative mechanisms and biological pathways may lead from a low 25(OH)D level to increased risk for CVD with mediators, such as dyslipidemia, hypertension and diabetes mellitus. Experimental evidence: some well-designed RCTs found increased CVD risk factors with decreasing 25(OH)D levels. Analogy: the association between serum 25(OH)D levels and CVD risk is analogous to that between 25(OH)D levels and the risk of overall cancer, periodontal disease, multiple sclerosis and breast cancer. Conclusion: all relevant Hill criteria for a causal association in a biological system are satisfied to indicate a low 25(OH)D level as a CVD risk factor.

Keywords: association; cardiovascular disease; causation; Hill criteria; vitamin D

---

1. Introduction

Cardiovascular disease (CVD) is the leading cause of death in the United States and has been since the early 1900s [1]. CVD incidence peaked in the 1960s and then gradually declined over the next 50 years. From 1980 to 2000, the death rate for coronary heart disease (CHD) for men, adjusted for age, decreased from 543 to 267 per 100,000, and for women, the death rate decreased from 263 to 134 per 100,000. Almost half of the decline can be attributed to decreasing CVD risk factors, including hypertension (HTN), smoking and dyslipidemia [2]. The CVD death rate has now plateaued, but, alarmingly, may be increasing [1], reducing life expectancy for the first time [3]. To decrease CVD morbidity and mortality, we must identify and effectively treat all risk factors and their causes.

Robert Scragg [4] first hypothesized that increasing ultra-violet (UV)-related vitamin D status affords protection against CVD. The serum 25-hydroxyvitamin D (25(OH)D) level is the most widely used measurement to assess overall vitamin D status [5]. Serum 25(OH)D levels are inversely associated with several CVDs, including myocardial infarction (MI) [6,7], coronary artery disease (CAD), heart failure, atrial fibrillation, ventricular tachycardia [8], peripheral vascular disease (PVD) [8–11], stroke [8,12], incident coronary artery calcium (CAC) [13–16], cardiac valve and vascular calcification [17] and all CVDs [18].

Study findings have inversely associated risk factors for CVD with serum 25(OH)D levels, including lower serum high-density lipoprotein cholesterol (HDL-C) levels, higher serum triglyceride (TG) levels [15], diabetes mellitus (DM) [8,19], increased blood pressure (BP) [15,20–25], dysfunctional changes in the characteristics of plasma lipids [26–28], inflammation [29] and increased serum parathyroid hormone (PTH) levels [30].

Isolating primary risk factors that cause CVD is challenging, because the human body responds to disrupted homeostasis by up- and down-regulating cellular function. Multiple pathways may exist between a low serum 25(OH)D level and increased CVD risk. Some pathways may be direct and not include any intermediate factors, whereas others may be indirect and include an intermediate factor(s). Moreover, CVD is not a single diagnosis, but rather, according to the National Center for Health Statistics, a group of diagnoses, including CAD, heart failure, essential HTN, hypertensive renal disease, cardiac dysrhythmias, rheumatic heart disease, cardiomyopathy, pulmonary heart disease and cerebrovascular disease [31].

The level of sufficiency for serum 25(OH)D is still being debated. Two schools of thought exist regarding what constitutes a sufficient level: 20 ng/mL [32,33] and 30 ng/mL [34–37]. Approximately 32% of the U.S. population has a deficient serum 25(OH)D level (defined as <20 ng/mL) [38]. The worldwide prevalence of deficient serum 25(OH)D levels is approximately one billion [39]. The primary causes of low serum 25(OH)D levels are strict sun protection and inadequate dietary or supplemental vitamin D intake [40]. Levels are easily elevated by oral vitamin D supplementation [41]. A daily intake of 10,000–20,000 IU of cholecalciferol (vitamin D_3) per day is unlikely to result in vitamin D toxicity [42]. Results from epidemiological studies suggest that if a low serum 25(OH)D level is a primary risk factor for CVD and then corrected, all-cause mortality could decrease significantly, both in the United States [43] and worldwide [44].

2. Approach and Rationale

The research studies used for this evaluation were located in the PubMed database by using the following search terms: Hill's criteria for causality, vitamin D, cardiovascular disease, randomized controlled trial, seasonality, hypertension, dyslipidemia, coronary artery calcium, parathyroid hormone, inflammation, diabetes mellitus and high-density lipoprotein cholesterol. Studies were also sought in the references of the preceding studies. We evaluated studies for relevance to this assessment and being representative of current research. We included them regardless of whether they supported criteria for a causal association between serum 25(OH)D levels and CVD risk.

We evaluated the likelihood of a causal association between a low serum 25(OH)D level and increased risk for CVD by applying Sir Austin Bradford Hill's criteria for causality in a biological system [45] (see Table 1). Causality is multifaceted, and certain conditions must be met to determine that a causal association is likely. Hill stated that the criteria are useful, as we most often depend on observed events to detect relationships between sickness and its antecedents. Waiting to take action until research results explain the entire chain of events that lead to disease may not be necessary when discovering a few links in the chain may suffice.

Table 1. Hill's criteria for causality in a biological system.

Criterion	Defining Question
Strength of the association	Is there a large difference in the outcome between exposed and non-exposed persons?
Consistency of the observed association	Has the outcome been observed by multiple researchers, in various circumstances, places and at different times?
Specificity of the association	Are there specific persons or geographic locations associated with specific outcomes?
Temporality (temporal relationship of the association)	Does the cause always precede the effect?
Biological gradient	Is there a dose-response curve?
Plausibility of the biology	Is the suspected causation consistent with current knowledge of biology?
Coherence	Are there any serious conflicts with the biology or natural history of the disease?
Experiment (experimental or quasi-experimental evidence)	Has an observed association led to a preventive action that has prevented the outcome?
Analogy	Is there an analogous exposure and outcome?

The criteria relevant to this evaluation include all, except specificity and coherence. This evaluation does not include specificity, because evidence supports low serum 25(OH)D levels and increased risk of several other disease processes [43]. This evaluation does not include coherence, because of its similarity to plausibility (see Table 2), and the information would be redundant. Hill's criteria have been used to assess a causal association between serum 25(OH)D levels and cancer risk [46], periodontal disease [37], multiple sclerosis (MS) [47], breast cancer risk [48] and the most prevalent cancers [49].

To arrive at the most accurate conclusions and to intervene with the most effective treatments, a thorough understanding of causality and of the limitations inherent in how we determine whether a causal association exists is essential. No single type of study, including randomized controlled trials (RCTs), can evaluate each of Hill's criteria. This evaluation used Hill's criteria, because it can consider the results of RCTs, prospective, cross-sectional and epidemiological studies.

Table 2. Studies used to evaluate causality between low vitamin D and increased risk of CVD. HTN, hypertension; DM, diabetes mellitus; PWV, pulse wave velocity.

Criterion	Proposed Mechanism	Reference	No Effect	Satisfied?
Strength of association		[6,8,12,50–53]		Yes
Consistency		[7,15,54–56]		Yes
Temporality		[8,18,55,57,58]		Yes
Biological Gradient		[8,55,59,60]		Yes
Plausibility	Blunts renin-angiotensin system	[61,62]		Yes
	Arterial stiffness (HTN)	[15,62–66]		
	Reduced risk of DM	[19]		
	Insulin resistance	[67]		
	Glucose regulation	[58,67,68]		
	Seasonal variations in serum 25(OH)D	[4]		
	Lipids	[69,70]		
	Metabolic syndrome	[71–75]		
	DM type 2 and its progression	[19,57,76]		
Experiment	RCTs	[77]	[78]	Yes
	Blood pressure reduction	[79]		
	Blunts renin-angiotensin system	[61]		
	Arterial stiffness (PWV)	[25]		
	Insulin resistance	[80,81]		
	Glucose	[80,81]		
	Lipids		[82–84]	
	Metabolic syndrome	[85,86]		

Table 2. *Cont.*

Criterion	Proposed Mechanism	Reference	No Effect	Satisfied?
Analogy	Cancer	[46,87]		Yes
	DM type 2	[19]		
Confounding Factors	Nitric oxide liberated by solar UV	[88–90]		
	Calcium supplementation	[91]		
	Reverse causation	[91]		
	CVD risk factors affect 25(OH)D levels (obesity)	[91]		Yes
	Physical activity	[92]		
	Statins	[75,93]		
	Seasonal variations in temperature	[94,95]		
Concerns				
Excess vitamin D		[96]		
Hypercalcemia		[97]		
DM	Limited effect of vitamin D	[98–101]		

3. Findings: Evaluation Using Hill's Criteria for Causality

The studies included in this criteria section and all of the studies in the subsequent criteria sections are ordered by design; first are the meta-analyses, then prospective, retrospective, cross-sectional, case-control and lastly ecological studies. They are then ordered from the highest to the lowest relative risk ration (RR), hazards ratio (HR) or odds ratio (OR) when available.

3.1. Strength of the Association

The stronger the positive or negative association between two variables, the more likely the association is causal. However, this may not always be true. One must consider all that is known about the two variables before concluding that an association is causal. For example, a very strong association may exist between an exposure and a disease, but another unknown variable may mediate the two. Alternatively, an exposure may directly cause a disease, but only under certain, sometimes very limited, circumstances; therefore, the association between the exposure and the disease would be weak. Therefore, a strong association is neither necessary nor sufficient to determine the likelihood of a causal association.

Satisfying the strength of association criterion requires a thorough evaluation of the correlation between vitamin D status and CVD risk. To come as close as possible to determining the true strength of an association, one must determine and then consistently use the most accurate and precise measures of the exposure and the disease [102]. Most researchers agree that the serum 25(OH)D level is the most accurate measure of overall vitamin D status. Several investigators have found statistically significant associations between serum 25(OH)D levels and CVD risk factors or CVDs.

Correia and colleagues [51] performed a prospective study in which they examined the association between serum 25(OH)D levels and the incidence of CVD-related mortalities during hospitalization. Ten percent of their 206 participants were severely deficient, defined as serum 25(OH)D levels ≤10 ng/mL. Incident CVD-related mortality was much higher at 24% for the group of patients with severe serum 25(OH)D deficiency *versus* 4.9% in the group of patients with levels >10 ng/mL

(RR 4.3, 95% CI, 1.8, 10, $p = 0.001$). These results are impressive, but the authors acknowledge that the CIs were very wide. Anderson and colleagues [8] completed a study with both cross-sectional and prospective data, which offered support for an association between serum 25(OH)D levels and CVD risk. The researchers examined 41,504 electronic health records and concluded from the cross-sectional data that there is an inverse association between prevalence of CVD risk factors and serum 25(OH)D levels. A significant increase in the prevalence of HTN (30% relative increase RI), DM (90% RI), PVD (53% RI) and hyperlipidemia (9% RI) was present in the group with serum 25(OH)D levels ≤15 ng/mL compared with the group with levels >30 ng/mL ($p < 0.0001$ for all, significant after Bonferroni correction for multiple comparisons). The authors acknowledge that selection bias may have been present, because only individuals who had serum 25(OH)D levels in their record were included in the study.

Researchers outside North America have also found inverse associations between serum 25(OH)D levels and risk factors for CVD, although sun exposure and diet may differ. Jang and colleagues [50] performed a cross-sectional study with 320 Korean girls whose average age was 13 years, 63.8% of whom had serum 25(OH)D levels <20 ng/mL. After adjusting for physical activity and BMI Z-score, the researchers found that serum 25(OH)D levels were negatively associated with fasting blood glucose levels ($r = -0.1748$, $p = 0.0033$) and insulin resistance ($r = -0.1441$, $p = 0.0154$), both risk factors for metabolic disorders.

The 2013 study by Deleskog and colleagues [53] had mixed results. The researchers performed a cross-sectional study with 3430 participants, 8% of whom had deficient serum 25(OH)D levels defined as <51 nmol/L (<20 ng/mL), 82% had insufficient levels defined as 51–75 nmol/L (20–30 ng/mL) and 10% had sufficient levels defined as >75 nmol/L (>30 ng/mL). No independent association emerged between serum 25(OH)D level insufficiency and carotid intima media thickness. However, those with deficient levels were more likely to have CVD risk factors, including higher BP, blood glucose, TG levels and lower serum HDL-C levels. Additionally, they were more likely to have DM.

Sun and colleagues [12] performed a case-control study in which they examined the association between ischemic stroke risk and serum 25(OH)D levels in 464 females with ischemic stroke and 464 female matched controls. The researchers compared participants in the lowest *versus* highest tertiles of serum 25(OH)D levels after adjusting for dietary and lifestyle covariates. Lower serum 25(OH)D levels were associated with an increased risk for ischemic stroke (OR 1.49, 95% CI, 1.01, 2.18, $p < 0.04$).

Scragg and colleagues [6] were one of the first research teams to examine the association between serum 25(OH)D levels and CVD. The researchers performed a case-control study with 179 MI cases with controls matched for age, sex and date of blood collection. They found an RR for MI of 0.43 (95% CI, 0.27, 0.69) for participants with serum 25(OH)D levels at or above their study median value of 32 nmol/L (12.8 ng/mL) *versus* below the median.

Deleskog and colleagues [52] included 774 participants in a case-control study to evaluate the association between serum 25(OH)D levels and premature MI (younger than 60 years). Serum 25(OH)D levels were analyzed twice as a categorical variable; insufficiency was defined as <50 nmol/L (20 ng/mL) and was compared with levels ≥50 nmol/L; a separate analysis defined insufficiency as <75 nmol/L (30 ng/mL), which was compared with levels ≥75 nmol/L. Neither of the definitions of serum 25(OH)D level insufficiency were independently associated with premature

MI. Therefore, the results do not support the criterion. The researchers concluded that the serum 25(OH)D level insufficiency may promote risk factors that are already established and known to promote atherothrombosis.

The criterion strength of the association has thus been met for 25(OH)D levels and CVD or CVD risk factors, including MI, CVD-related mortality, ischemic stroke risk, HTN, DM, PVD, hyperlipidemia, elevated blood glucose and increased insulin resistance.

3.2. Consistency of the Association

An association is consistent if it is observed under different circumstances, at different times, in various places and by various researchers [45]. Consistency is also confirmed if the results of a study can be replicated with a different sample of participants with the same study design and analytic methods. Inconsistent study results may occur when differences exist in study design, lab assays, definitions of serum 25(OH)D level deficiency, insufficiency *versus* sufficiency and statistical methods. Confidence in the results of meta-analyses depends on an assessment of the comparability of all studies included in the analysis [103].

Parker and colleagues [54] carried out the study with the strongest support for the criterion of consistency. In their meta-analysis, they systematically reviewed 28 studies with a total of 99,745 participants. The researchers reported important variations among studies included in their review, including categories of serum 25(OH)D levels, study design and analyses. Despite these differences, 29 of 33 ORs from the 28 studies showed an inverse association between serum 25(OH)D levels and the prevalence of cardio-metabolic disorders. One study demonstrated no effect, and three studies showed a positive association. Parker and colleagues [54] found a 43% reduction in cardio-metabolic disorders with the highest levels of serum 25(OH)D (OR 0.57, 95% CI, 0.48, 0.68).

The meta-analysis by Wang and colleagues [55] offers additional strong support. They included 19 prospective studies with a total of 65,994 participants, of whom 6123 developed CVD. The 19 studies included CVD, CVD mortality, CHD and stroke as outcomes. Wang and colleagues found an inverse linear association between serum 25(OH)D in the range 20–60 nmol/L (8–24 ng/mL) and the risk of CVD (RR, 1.03, 95% CI, 1.00, 1.06).

Giovannucci and colleagues [7] found results consistent with the previous studies. This prospective, nested, case-control study included 454 male participants who were CHD cases and 900 male controls matched for age, HTN, aspirin use, physical activity, serum TG and low-density lipoprotein cholesterol (LDL-C) levels, as well as alcohol use. The median values for each of the four categories of serum 25(OH)D levels were entered as continuous variables in a regression model. The researchers found a two-fold increase in risk for MI if the serum 25(OH)D level was less than 16 ng/mL compared with those with a level of at least 30 ng/mL (RR, 2.42, 95% CI, 1.53, 3.84; $p < 0.001$). They also found a 2.1% decreased risk of MI for every 1 ng/mL increase in serum 25(OH)D levels. Only including males in the study prevents the generalizability of the results to females.

Support for the consistency criterion is also evident in the prospective study by de Boer and colleagues [15] ($N = 1370$). At baseline, 723 (53%) had CAC. Over a three-year period, 135 participants developed CAC. The researchers adjusted for gender, age, ethnicity/race, location, season, activity level, smoking status, body mass index (BMI), DM, BP and serum lipid and C-reactive protein (CRP) levels. They found that serum 25(OH)D levels were inversely associated with incident, but not prevalent, CAC; for every 10 ng/mL decrease in the serum 25(OH)D level, the risk of developing CAC increased by 23% (RR, 1.23, 95% CI, 1.00, 1.52, $p = 0.049$).

Finally, a cross-sectional study by Kendrick and colleagues [56] found similar supporting results by using data from 16,603 participants of the Third National Health and Nutrition Examination Survey (NHANES III). Serum 25(OH)D level deficiency, defined as <20 ng/mL, was associated with a 57% increased odds for prevalent CVD. After adjusting for gender, age, ethnicity/race, season, activity level, smoking status, HTN, DM, BMI, dyslipidemia, chronic kidney disease and vitamin D use, the odds decreased to 20% (OR, 1.20, 95% CI, 1.01, 1.36, $p = 0.03$).

A study-participant characteristic that should be included in the evaluation of the consistency criterion is ethnicity. A prospective study by Michos and colleagues [82] found that serum 25(OH)D levels less than 15 ng/mL were not associated with fatal stroke in blacks, but were associated with fatal stroke in whites. One limitation of this study is that because the median time to fatal stroke was 14.1 years and the serum 25(OH)D levels were only drawn once at baseline, there could have been undetected significant changes in serum 25(OH)D levels during the study. Differences in CHD events, including angina, MI, cardiac arrest or CHD death, by ethnicity were found in a prospective study by Robinson-Cohen and colleagues [66]. The researchers found an association between lower serum 25(OH)D levels and incident CHD events for white or Chinese, but not black or Hispanic participants. The same limitation is present in this study; only a baseline serum 25(OH)D level was drawn, and there was a median follow-up period of 8.5 years.

An unexplained difference by ethnicity was found by Gupta and colleagues [104], who performed a cross-sectional study. The researchers found significant associations between both pre-diabetes and pre-hypertension and gender, age and BMI in Mexican-Americans. However, they did not find an association between either pre-diabetes or pre-hypertension and serum 25(OH)D levels, as has been found for both non-Hispanic whites and non-Hispanic blacks. The authors stated that the reason for these results was unclear.

Results from a study performed by Rezai and colleagues [14] found that there was an association between serum 25(OH)D levels and left ventricular end-diastolic volumes for men of all ethnicities. The results of this cross-sectional study add support to the criterion of consistency, because low 25(OH)D levels showed the same association with poorer CV status for all ethnicities. This may mean that disparities in the prevalence of low vitamin D status among ethnicities may cause the disparities among ethnicities in the prevalence of CVD. Webb and colleagues [12] found that the pulse wave velocity (PWV) was higher in British South Asians of Indian descent than in white Europeans (9.32 m/s *vs.* 8.68 m/s, $p = 0.001$) using a cross-sectional design. They also found that the serum 25(OH)D level was independently associated with PWV, when adjusted for age, mean arterial pressure, sex, glucose, heart rate, vasoactive medications and South Asian ethnicity ($R^2 = 0.73$, $p = 0.004$). The researchers concluded that vitamin D insufficiency may mediate an increase in aortic stiffness without a difference in the risk profile, including vascular disease.

The preceding studies have shown mixed results, and the reasons for the differences are multifaceted. One reason for the disparity in serum 25(OH)D levels among different ethnic groups is that vitamin D production is inversely proportional to skin pigmentation [105]. Skin pigmentation varies among members of the same ethnic group, and designing a study in which skin pigmentation is objectively quantified and included as a variable may help to clarify differences between individuals *versus* groups. Studies that use ethnicity self-reporting or that have the investigator determine the ethnicity of the participants can also decrease the validity of the findings.

The consistency of the association criterion has thus been met due to the research results regarding the systematic review by Parker and colleagues and the smaller described supporting studies. The studies regarding ethnicity have mixed results. Parker and colleagues in their meta-analysis found overall associations between serum 25(OH)D levels and MI, stroke, ischemic heart disease, PVD, DM and metabolic syndrome.

3.3. Temporality

Temporality refers to the direction of influence in a sequence of events. An event or phenomenon cannot cause another event or phenomenon if the presumed cause does not precede the presumed effect. Determining whether a potential risk factor precedes a disease process is particularly difficult when the disease is chronic and progresses slowly [45]. Determining the temporal direction of influence of low serum 25(OH)D levels in relation to CVD risk by examining the results of prospective studies or meta-analyses that have included only prospective studies will help determine if the criterion of temporality has been met.

DM is a well-established risk factor for CVD, and the association between serum 25(OH)D levels and DM has been prospectively studied. Song and colleagues [57] included 21 prospective studies with 76,220 participants, 4996 incident type 2 DM cases and serum 25(OH)D in a meta-analysis. The researchers compared the highest to lowest serum 25(OH)D levels using categories and found that the summary RR for type 2 DM was 0.62 (95% CI, 0.54, 0.70). The statistical significance of the inverse association between DM risk and serum 25(OH)D levels remained after controlling for sex, criteria for DM diagnosis, follow-up time, sample size and 25(OH)D assay type. Each 10 nmol/mL (4 ng/mL) increase in the serum 25(OH)D level was associated with a 4% lower risk of type 2 DM (95% CI, 3, 6; p linear trend = 0.0001). Therefore, low 25(OH)D levels may be a risk factor for CVD with type 2 DM as the mediator.

Wang and colleagues [55] examined the association between CVD mortality along with CVD risk and serum 25(OH)D levels in a meta-analysis of 19 prospective studies. Collectively, these studies had 65,994 participants, of whom 6123 developed CVD. The researchers used the median serum 25(OH)D levels, or if unavailable, they compared the mean or the midpoint of the upper and lower bounds in each of the 25(OH)D categories from each of the 19 studies to the category of the risk of CVD. Being in the lowest category was associated with a higher risk for all CVDs (pooled RR 1.52, 95% CI, 1.30, 1.77), for CVD mortality (pooled RR 1.42, 95% CI, 1.19, 1.71), for CHD (pooled RR 1.38, 95% CI, 1.21, 1.57) and for stroke (pooled RR 1.64, 95% CI, 1.27, 2.10) than the highest category.

Although the study by Anderson and colleagues [8] was included in both the Song and colleagues and Wang and colleagues meta-analyses, it is a landmark study, and the results are important to cite. This study offers strong support for temporality. The prospective study using electronic health records monitored participants for an average of 1.3 years and a maximum of 9.3 years. The prevalence of serum 25(OH)D levels ≤30 ng/mL was 63.6%. Participants without risk factors for CVD with serum 25(OH)D levels ≤15 ng/mL had a higher risk of incident HTN, dyslipidemia and DM than those with levels >30 ng/mL. Adjusted relative rates for death increased by 20% for serum 25(OH)D levels of 16–30 ng/mL and increased by 77% for serum 25(OH)D levels ≤15 ng/mL. The researchers concluded that these data provide support for low serum 25(OH)D level as a primary risk factor for CVD. Schöttker and colleagues [18], in a prospective study with 9578 participants, found an increased risk of cardiovascular mortality associated with decreased serum 25(OH)D levels (hazards ratio (HR) 1.39, 95% CI, 1.02, 1.89).

Tsur and colleagues [58] conducted a prospective cohort study over a two-year period that assessed incident impaired fasting glucose (IFG) and DM type 2 in 117,960 participants. The researchers adjusted for several variables, including sex, age, BMI, serum LDL-C, HDL-C, TG levels, history of HTN, smoking status and CVD. Participants with a serum 25(OH)D level ≤25 nmol/L (10 ng/mL) had an OR for progression from normoglycemia to IFG of 1.13 (95% CI, 1.03, 1.24), from normoglycemia to DM of 1.77 (95% CI, 1.11, 2.83) and from IFG to DM of 1.43 (95% CI, 1.16, 1.76), compared with a serum 25(OH)D level >75 nmol/L (30 ng/mL). The researchers concluded that a low serum 25(OH)D level may be an independent risk factor for IFG and DM that can eventually lead to CVD.

The previously described meta-analyses of prospective studies and the additional prospective studies offer evidence that temporality is satisfied, because they all use serum 25(OH)D levels taken at the time of enrollment, which precedes the incident event or death. Furthermore, most reviewed individual prospective studies, and a meta-analysis of prospective studies showed an increased incidence of CVD or CVD risk factors with decreasing serum 25(OH)D. The CVDs or risk factors for CVD included CVD mortality, CHD, stroke, dyslipidemia, HTN, type 2 DM and IFG.

3.4. Biological Gradient (Dose-Response Relation)

In the context of this assessment, the biological gradient, or dose-response relation, refers to the change in the prevalence or incidence rate of CVD or risk factors for CVD as serum 25(OH)D levels change. The biological gradient criterion is satisfied when the value of the dependent variable (effect) can be predicted, with some degree of confidence, when the value of the independent variable (cause) is known. Hill [45] states that securing a satisfactory quantitative measure to use for this purpose is often difficult.

Wang and colleagues [55] showed a biological gradient effect in their 2012 meta-analysis. They found a linear (graded) and inverse association between serum 25(OH)D levels of 20–60 nmol/L (8–24 ng/mL) and the risk of CVD. They found a linear trend for the RR = 1.03 (95% CI, 1.00, 1.06) for every 25 nmol/L (10 ng/mL) decrease in 25(OH)D ([55]; Figure 3). Wang and colleagues had similar results in an earlier study [60]. They examined low serum 25(OH)D levels and incident CVD prospectively in 1739 participants from the Framingham Offspring Study. A serum 25(OH)D level <15 ng/mL was associated with a two-fold increase in an age and sex-adjusted five-year incident rate for CVD compared with those with a level of ≥15 ng/mL (multivariable-adjusted HR = 1.62, 95% CI, 1.11, 2.36; $p = 0.01$). The researchers also found a graded increase in CVD risk for serum 25(OH)D levels of 10–14 ng/mL (multivariable-adjusted HR = 1.53, 95% CI, 1.00, 2.36; $p = 0.01$) *versus* levels <10 ng/mL (multivariable-adjusted HR = 1.80, 95% CI, 1.05, 3.08; $p = 0.01$).

Anderson and colleagues [8] performed a prospective study, which was included in the Wang and colleagues meta-analysis. The researchers found statistically significant and biologically-graded inverse associations between serum 25(OH)D levels and the prevalence of CVD and CVD risk factors, including PVD, HTN, DM and hyperlipidemia (all $p < 0.0001$). The researchers categorized serum 25(OH)D levels; levels of serum 25(OH)D ≤15 ng/mL *versus* those >30 ng/mL were associated with increased prevalence of DM (90% relative and 14% absolute) and HTN (30% relative and 12% absolute) (p trend for both <0.0001).

Vacek and colleagues [59] performed a retrospective study ($n = 10,899$) for a 68-month period. Using univariate analysis, the researchers found statistically significant ORs for vitamin D deficiency, defined as <30 ng/mL, and CAD (OR, 1.16, 95% CI, 1.012, 1.334, $p = 0.03$), cardiomyopathy (OR, 1.29, 95% CI, 1.019, 1.633, $p = 0.03$) and HTN (OR, 1.40, 95% CI, 1.285, 1.536, $p \leq 0.0001$).

The criterion, biological gradient, or dose-response curve, has thus been met. Most reviewed studies used serum 25(OH)D levels as categorical or continuous variables and found strong evidence for a graded association between levels and CVD/CVD risk factors, including nonspecific CVD, PVD, HTN, DM, hyperlipidemia, elevated BMI, elevated serum LDL-C and TG levels and decreased serum HDL-C levels.

3.5. Plausibility

Biological plausibility can be confirmed when the suspected causation mechanism is consistent with the current knowledge of biology. The actual physiological pathway of the hypothesized causal association between low serum 25(OH)D levels and increased risk for CVD may include mediators that are known CVD risk factors or other unknown factors. Specific cellular-level causative mechanisms that explain the increase in CVD associated with low vitamin D status need to be identified in order to definitively state that the criterion, biological plausibility, has been met.

Several cellular-level causative mechanisms have been proposed. It should be taken into consideration that, in contrast to the causative agent of an infectious disease, these proposed causative mechanisms do not necessarily compete with one another and are not mutually exclusive. Some or all of the proposed mechanisms may be accurate. This is because CVD is a broad category of diseases, and each of the diseases has multiple causes.

An *in vitro* study by Oh and colleagues [17] found an inhibition of foam cell formation when macrophages from persons with type 2 DM exposed to modified LDL were cultured in the bio-active form of vitamin D; $1\alpha,25$-dihydroxyvitamin D_3 ($1\alpha,25(OH)_2D_3$). They also found accelerated foam cell formation when the vitamin D receptors (VDRs) were deleted from the macrophages. A reduction in the formation of atherosclerotic lesions in mice with the administration of the vitamin D analog, calcitriol ($1\alpha,25(OH)_2D_3$), was seen by Takeda and colleagues [32]. They hypothesize that calcitriol modulates the systemic and intestinal immune systems by inducing immunologically-tolerant dendritic cells and T-cells, both of which are anti-atherogenic.

Additionally, an *in vitro* study by Riek and colleagues [106] was performed in order to determine if vitamin D plays a role in monocyte migration and adhesion. The researchers examined monocytes from study participants ($n = 12$) with type 2 DM and obesity who were vitamin D deficient. The researchers found a 20% reduction in monocyte migration in monocytes incubated with $25(OH)D_3$ compared to vitamin D-deficient conditions ($p < 0.005$). They also found that, compared to monocytes maintained in vitamin D-deficient conditions, incubation with $25(OH)D_3$ also significantly decreased adhesion ($p < 0.05$). The researchers concluded that hydroxylation of 25(OH)D$_3$ to 1,25(OH)$_2$D$_3$ at the cellular level may play a role in vitamin D anti-atherogenic effects.

VDRs were also found in human coronary artery smooth muscle cells (CASMC) by Wu-Wong and colleagues [107]. When CASMC were treated with the vitamin D analogs, calcitriol or paricalcitol (19-nor-1α,25(OH)$_2$D$_2$) there was an upregulation of 24-hydroxylase and also an upregulation of thrombomodulin (TM) mRNA. Downregulation of TM mRNA has been associated with atherosclerosis and thrombosis. Finding that upregulation occurred led the researchers to hypothesize that this is the mechanism that leads to a decrease in morbidity and mortality with vitamin D analog use in persons with chronic kidney disease.

Many studies have shown inverse associations between established CVD risk factors, such as dyslipidemia, HTN and DM [108] and serum 25(OH)D levels (see Table 2). The following research studies further assist in evaluating the plausibility of a causal association.

3.5.1. Dyslipidemia

A proposed causal mechanism for the association between low serum 25(OH)D levels and increased risk for CVD involves dysfunctional changes in the characteristics of plasma lipids, including metabolism or transport [26], the ability to promote macrophage efflux, [27] and changes in serum levels of total cholesterol (total-C), HDL-C, LDL-C and TGs [15,28].

Skaaby and colleagues [70] investigated the association between serum 25(OH)D levels at baseline and incident dyslipidemia over five years in a prospective study with 4330 participants. A serum 25(OH)D level of 10 nmol/L (4 ng/mL) higher at baseline was associated with decreased serum TG levels (β = −0.52, 95% CI, −0.99, −0.05, $p = 0.03$) and decreased serum very-low-density lipoprotein cholesterol (VLDL-C) levels (β = −0.66, 95% CI, −1.1, −0.2, $p = 0.005$). With the same higher serum 25(OH)D level at baseline, the OR for incident hypercholesterolemia was 0.94 (95% CI, 0.90, 0.99, $p = 0.01$). The researchers concluded that higher serum 25(OH)D levels may favorably change lipid profiles and therefore positively influence cardiovascular health.

Karhapää and colleagues [109] performed a cross-sectional study in which they examined the relationship between serum 25(OH)D levels and total-C, LDL-C, HDL-C and TG levels in a study that included 909 male participants. The researchers found a significant inverse association between serum 25(OH)D levels and total-C, LDL-C and TG levels (β = −0.15, −0.13 and −0.17, respectively; $p < 0.001$), which supports lower serum 25(OH)D levels leading to a less favorable lipid profile. However, they found no association between serum 25(OH)D and HDL-C levels, which does not support an association between lower serum 25(OH)D levels and a more favorable lipid profile.

Jorde and colleagues [28] also examined the association between serum 25(OH)D levels and serum lipid levels by using both cross-sectional and longitudinal data collected over 14 years. The cross-sectional study included 10,105 participants, and the researchers found that with increasing quartiles of serum 25(OH)D levels, serum HDL-C and LDL-C levels increased and serum TG levels decreased. In the longitudinal study with 2159 participants, the researchers found that increasing quartiles of serum 25(OH)D levels were associated with decreased serum TG levels. These results, except for the increase in serum LDL-C levels, support associating higher serum 25(OH)D levels with a more favorable lipid profile.

Researchers have also conducted genomic and cytochrome P450 enzyme studies to determine mechanisms that cause low serum 25(OH)D levels to lead to dysfunctional changes in lipids. Shirts and colleagues [69], in a cross-sectional study with 1060 participants, investigated the influence of single-nucleotide polymorphisms on serum HDL-C, LDL-C and TG levels for gene-25(OH)D interactions. Participants with deficient levels of serum 25(OH)D were more likely to also have lower serum HDL-C levels ($p = 0.0003$). Chow and colleagues [110] incubated human hepatocytes with $1,25(OH)_2D_3$ and found a reduction in cholesterol production due to an increase in cytochrome P450 enzyme 7A1 activation of the VDR.

Guasch and colleagues [29] found an association between low plasma 25(OH)D levels and atherogenic dyslipidemia after adjusting for BMI in a cross-sectional study with 316 participants. When the researchers introduced serum-ultrasensitive CRP levels as a covariable, an association was no longer present. They suggested that inflammation may mediate the effect of serum 25(OH)D levels on lipid profiles.

3.5.2. Hypertension

The cause of HTN is usually unknown. Researchers have investigated the association between serum 25(OH)D levels and both prevalent and incident idiopathic HTN and pre-HTN [20,22–25]. Carrara and colleagues [61] conducted a prospective interventional trial in which they administered 25,000 IU of oral cholecalciferol (vitamin D_3) weekly over two months to 15 participants with essential HTN. There was neither randomization to different interventions or a placebo group. Because the researchers found reduced aldosterone ($p < 0.05$) and renin plasma levels ($p < 0.05$) after supplementation, they concluded that for persons with essential HTN and a low serum 25(OH)D level, vitamin D supplementation may help decrease BP.

Forman and colleagues [21] performed a prospective study with 1811 participants with measured plasma 25(OH)D levels. The researchers found that incident HTN was greater for participants with a plasma 25(OH)D level of <15 ng/mL compared to those with a level ≥30 ng/mL (RR 3.18, 95% CI, 1.39, 7.29). For men only ($n = 613$), the RR for the same comparison was much greater (RR 6.13, 95% CI, 1.0, 37.8) compared to women only ($n = 1198$) (RR 2.67, 95% CI, 1.05, 6.79). Forman and colleagues [62] also conducted a prospective study that included only women participants aged 32–52 years. The researchers found that incident HTN increased for the lowest quartile (6.2–21.0 ng/mL) *versus* the highest quartile (32.3–89.5 ng/mL) for 25(OH)D levels (OR, 1.66, 95% CI, 1.11, 2.48, $p = 0.01$).

Increased arterial stiffness may be an effect of low serum 25(OH)D level. Giallauria and colleagues [63], in a cross-sectional study with 1228 participants, found a statistically significant inverse association between serum 25(OH)D levels and arterial stiffness, measured with PWV (adjusted $R^2 = 0.27$, $\beta = -0.43$; $p = 0.001$). Furthermore, measuring PWV, Mayer and colleagues [64] performed a cross-sectional study and found a negative association with serum 25(OH)D level quartiles. The lowest serum 25(OH)D level quartile (<20 ng/mL) had the highest PWV score compared with the second, third or fourth quartile ($p = 0.0001$).

Three studies with only female participants had similar results. Pirro and colleagues conducted a cross-sectional study with 150 postmenopausal and serum 25(OH)D-insufficient (<30 ng/mL) participants [65]. The researchers found a significant association between arterial stiffness, measured with PWV and serum 25(OH)D levels, but not after controlling for logarithmically-transformed serum PTH levels. Serum PTH levels were associated with arterial stiffness ($\beta = 0.23$, $p = 0.007$). Reynolds and colleagues [66] in a cross-sectional study found a similar association between serum 25(OH)D levels and aortic stiffness (PWV scores) ($\beta = -0.0217$, 95% CI, -0.038, -0.005, $p = 0.010$) for 75 female participants with systemic lupus erythematosus. The authors did not state that serum PTH levels were measured and controlled for, and therefore, PTH levels may have mediated the association.

3.5.3. Diabetes Mellitus

DM is an important risk factor for CVD. Several studies have associated serum 25(OH)D levels and both prevalent and incident DM. Afzal and colleagues [19], in a prospective study with 9841 white participants, found an increased risk of type 2 DM for study participants with plasma 25(OH)D levels <5 ng/mL $versus$ ≥20 ng/mL (HR, 1.22, 95% CI, 0.85, 1.74). The researchers also performed a meta-analysis of 13 studies and found a greater prevalence of type 2 DM for those in the lowest $versus$ highest quartile for the serum 25(OH)D level (cut-points for the quartiles varied among the 13 studies) (OR, 1.39, 95% CI, 1.21, 1.58). Anderson and colleagues [8], found an adjusted RI in incident DM of 89% for very low (≤15 ng/mL) $versus$ sufficient (>30 ng/mL) categories of serum 25(OH)D levels (HR, 1.89, 95% CI, 1.54, 2.33, $p < 0.0001$). Forouhi and colleagues [67] found in a prospective study with 524 participants that baseline 25(OH)D levels were inversely associated with the 10-year risk of hyperglycemia (fasting glucose: $\beta = -0.002$, $p = 0.02$) and insulin resistance (fasting insulin $\beta = -0.15$, $p = 0.01$).

3.5.4. Metabolic Syndrome

Studies have been conducted to assess the association between both incident and prevalent metabolic syndrome and serum 25(OH)D levels. A prospective study by Gagnon and colleagues [74] found that 12.7% of 4164 participants developed metabolic syndrome over a five-year follow-up period. A higher risk of metabolic syndrome was present for those with serum 25(OH)D levels in the first quintile (<18 ng/mL) (OR = 1.41, 95% CI, 1.02, 1.95) and second quintile (18–23 ng/mL) (OR = 1.74, 95% CI, 1.28, 2.37) compared with the highest quintile (≥34 ng/mL). Serum 25(OH)D levels were inversely associated with fasting glucose ($p < 0.01$), homeostasis model assessment for insulin resistance ($p < 0.001$), TG ($p < 0.01$) and waist circumference ($p < 0.001$). No association with two-hour plasma glucose ($p = 0.29$), HDL-C ($p = 0.70$) or BP ($p = 0.46$) was evident at the five-year follow-up.

Another cross-sectional study conducted by Brenner and colleagues [72] with 1818 participants found an 8.9% prevalence of metabolic syndrome. The researchers found an inverse association between plasma 25(OH)D levels and the number of components for metabolic syndrome ($\beta = -0.1$, $p < 0.0001$). Components of metabolic syndrome included serum HDL-C level <40 mg/dL (males) or <50 mg/dL (females), serum TG level >1.7 mmol/L, fasting plasma glucose >110 mg/dL, BP > 130/85 mmHg and waist circumference >102 cm (males) or >88 cm (females). A lower OR (0.50, 95% CI, 0.24, 1.06) for metabolic syndrome was evident for study participants whose plasma 25(OH)D level was in the highest $versus$ lowest quartile. After adjusting for age, sex, ethnicity, smoking status, physical activity and month of interview, researchers found that a 10-nmol/mL

(4 ng/mL) increase in the plasma 25(OH)D level was inversely associated with the homeostasis model assessment for insulin resistance score (β = -0.08, p = 0.006). Another cross-sectional study by Reis and colleagues [71] that included 1654 participants with DM assessed the prevalence of metabolic syndrome. The researchers divided serum 25(OH)D levels into quintiles and found an OR of 0.27 (CI, 0.15, 0.46; p trend <0.001) for metabolic syndrome for the highest quintile (median = 88 nmol/L (35 ng/mL)) *versus* the lowest quintile (median = 26.8 nmol/L (10.7 ng/mL)).

In a case-control study by Makariou and colleagues, 52 participants with metabolic syndrome had lower serum 25(OH)D levels (mean = 11.8 ng/mL, range = 0.6–48.3 ng/mL) than 58 controls (mean = 17.2 ng/mL, range = 4.8–62.4 ng/mL; p = 0.027) [75]. Serum 25(OH)D levels were inversely associated with serum TG levels (r = -0.42, p = 0.003) and small dense LDL-C (r = -0.31, p = 0.004).

The criterion for plausibility has thus been satisfied. There are several proposed biologically-plausible cellular-level mechanisms for the increase in CVD associated with low vitamin D status. Studies involving the assessment of an association between serum 25(OH)D levels and dyslipidemia, HTN, DM and metabolic syndrome have also been evaluated. Dyslipidemia, HTN, DM and metabolic syndrome are all plausible mediators between low serum 25(OH)D levels and increased risk of CVD. Specifically, the studies support increased serum LDL-C, VLDL-C and TG levels, decreased serum HDL-C levels, increased arterial stiffness, increased insulin resistance, hyperglycemia and increased incident metabolic syndrome as potentially plausible mediators.

3.6. Experiment

Researchers have conducted RCTs to assess the effect of serum 25(OH)D levels on CVD risk factors. However, vitamin D RCTs conducted to date have mixed results. The main reason is that vitamin D RCTs have been designed largely on the model used for pharmaceutical drugs, which assumes that the agent used in the trial is the only source of the agent and that a linear dose-response relation exists. Neither assumption is valid for vitamin D.

Another consideration is that chronic disease is caused by more than one risk factor and may occur only after long-term *versus* short-term vitamin deficiency. Vitamin supplementation studies are usually designed to assess the decrease in risk due to increasing vitamin intake to meet the minimum sufficiency level. Additional information would be gained from studies that also test the effects of supplementation on levels beyond those previously established for disease risk [111].

Robert Heaney [112] recently outlined the steps to design and conduct vitamin D RCTs: (1) start with the 25(OH)D level-health outcome relation; (2) measure the 25(OH)D levels of prospective participants; (3) enroll only those with low 25(OH)D levels; (4) supplement with enough vitamin D_3 to increase 25(OH)D levels to the upper end of the quasi-linear region of the 25(OH)D level-health outcome relation; and (5) re-measure 25(OH)D levels after supplementation. For CVD, these recommendations would translate to enrolling people with 25(OH)D levels below about 15 ng/mL and then supplementing with 2000–4000 IU of vitamin D_3 per day to raise 25(OH)D levels to >30–40 ng/mL.

The effect of vitamin D supplementation on CVD risk factors for women with polycystic ovarian syndrome was investigated by Rahimi-Ardabili and colleagues [113]. The study participants taking the vitamin D supplement had a statistically significant increase in serum vitamin D level and statistically significant decreases in serum total-C, TGs and VLDL-C levels (all $p < 0.05$). They did not have any changes in serum levels of HDL-C, LDL-C, apolipoprotein-A1 (Apo-A1) or high-sensitivity C-reactive protein (hs-CRP). The placebo group had no changes.

Schnatz and colleagues [77] supplemented participants ($n = 600$) with 1000 mg of elemental calcium and 400 IU of vitamin D per day. The researchers found a 1.28 mg/dL decrease in LDL-C ($p = 0.04$) with a 38% increase in the 25(OH)D level. The researchers also found an increase in HDL-C and a decrease in TGs.

Breslavsky and colleagues [68] conducted an RCT, including 47 participants with type 2 DM, who were randomized into two groups. One group received cholecalciferol (vitamin D_3) at 1000 IU per day for 12 months, whereas the other group received a placebo. After being similar at baseline, the group receiving cholecalciferol had significantly decreased hemoglobin A1c levels ($p < 0.0001$), but no change occurred in the placebo group.

Grimnes and colleagues [114] performed an RCT with 94 participants with low serum 25(OH)D levels. The participants were randomly assigned to receive a 20,000 IU supplement of oral D_3 or a placebo twice weekly for six months. The supplement did not improve the lipid profile, which included total-C, LDL-C, HDL-C and TGs.

Ponda and colleagues [82] conducted a randomized, placebo-controlled, double-blinded trial. They randomized 151 vitamin D-deficient participants to receive oral D_3 at 50,000 IU weekly for eight weeks or placebo and then examined the effect on serum cholesterol levels. In the supplemented group, serum 25(OH)D levels increased, serum PTH levels decreased and serum calcium levels increased. When participants were stratified by the change in serum 25(OH)D level and the serum calcium level, those whose response was greater than the median response had an increase in serum LDL-C of 15.4 mg/dL compared with those who had lower than the median response. The analysis of the group receiving placebo did not show this relationship. Table 3 shows results from RCTs in order of serum 25(OH)D level at time of enrollment. This RCT does not support a beneficial effect on lipid status.

In a manuscript under preparation, it was found that for vitamin D RCTs related to CVD risk factors, the median baseline serum 25(OH)D level for the RCT with significant beneficial effects was 15 ng/mL, while the median baseline serum 25(OH)D for those without beneficial effects was 19 ng/mL (Grant, in preparation). This finding underscores the importance of having a low baseline serum 25(OH)D level when designing and conducting vitamin D RCTs to evaluate the findings of observational studies, as proposed by Heaney [112].

The criterion for experiment has thus been met. We reviewed RCTs that supplemented participants with vitamin D and found that most well-designed RCTs supported a causal association between serum 25(OH)D levels and CVD risk.

Does Sufficient Evidence Exist to Support a Causal Association between Vitamin D Status and Cardiovascular...   189

Table 3. Results of studies on vitamin D supplementation and CVD risk factors (ordered by mean serum 25(OH)D (ng/mL)).

Mean Serum 25(OH)D (ng/mL)	Vitamin D₃ Dose (IU/day)	Increase in 25(OH)D (ng/mL)	Mean Age (year)	Health Outcome of Interest	Findings	Reference
8.4	4000	19.6	42	Insulin sensitivity	5.9 *vs.* −5.9 (*p* = 0.003)	[115]
8.4	4000	19.6	42	Fasting serum glucose	−3.6 *vs.* 1.1 (*p* = 0.02)	[115]
13	400 or 1000	13	64	HDL-C, LDL-C, TG, ApoA1, ApoB100, HOMA-IR, hs-CRP, sICAM-1, IL-6	Not significant	[83]
<20	2000 *			Total cholesterol, HDL-C, LDL-C, TGs	Not significant	[82]
14.7	1000	15	38	Total cholesterol, LDL-C, ApoA1, ApoA1:ApoB-100	Significant to *p* < 0.01	[108]
14.7	1000	15	38	HDL-C, LDL-C:ApoB-100	Significant to *p* < 0.04	[108]
14.7	1000	15	38	ApoB-100, lipoprotein(a)	Not significant	[108]
16.1	2857 *	40	52	Insulin sensitivity	Not significant	[114]
16.3	0		51	Systolic BP	+1.7 mm	[79]
16.3	1000		51		−0.66 mm	[79]
14.5	2000		51		−3.4 mm	[79]
15.6	4000		51		−4.0 mm	[79]
19.6	4000	19.5	14.1	Insulin sensitivity	−1.36 *vs.* +0.27 (*p* = 0.03)	[116]
				Fasting insulin	−6.5 *vs.* +1.2 (*p* = 0.03)	[116]
19.6	2857 * or 5714 *	40	52	HDL-C, LDL-C, TGs, ApoA1, ApoB, hs-CRP	Not significant	[84]
22.9	2857 * or 5714 *	22.8	50	TNF-α, IL-6, HOMA-IR, QUICKI	Not significant	[117]
23	1000	21	61	Systolic BP	−1.5 mm *vs.* +0.4 mm (*p* = 0.26)	[25]
30.3	2500	16	64	Glucose, CRP, FMD, diastolic BP, systolic BP, PWV	Not significant	[118]

* Average daily oral intake from a bolus dose; FMD, flow-mediated dilation; QUICKI, qualitative insulin sensitivity check index; hs-CRP, high-sensitivity C-reactive protein; TNF-α, tissue necrosis factorα; IL-6, interleukin 6; ApoA1, apolipoprotein A1; ApoB, apolipoprotein B.

3.7. Analogy

The likelihood of a causal association between low vitamin D status and several diseases has been evaluated using Hill's criteria for causality in a biological system. Hill's criteria were met when Grant [46] evaluated overall cancer risk, when breast cancer risk was evaluated by Mohr and colleagues [48], when Grant and Boucher [37] evaluated periodontal disease and when Hanwell and Banwell [47] evaluated multiple sclerosis. Hanwell and Banwell found that all of the criteria were satisfied, except the criterion for disease prevention by intervention (experiment). The researchers state that fulfilling this criterion will be difficult because multiple sclerosis has a low incidence, the age of onset is highly variable and there is a lack of consensus regarding optimal vitamin D dose and the timing of treatment.

The criterion, analogy, has thus been met. Several assessments with various diseases have shown an analogous association to low serum 25(OH)D levels and CVD risk.

3.8. Confounding Factors

Potischman and colleagues [119] discussed the inadequacies of traditional causal criteria for assessing nutrients, but they acknowledged that they are necessary for public health recommendations. The authors stated that additional important considerations exist, such as confounding, errors in measurement and dose-response curves for nutrients.

Opländer and colleagues [88] discovered a potentially confounding factor for the association between production of vitamin D in the skin and a decrease in BP. UVB irradiation is responsible for vitamin D production and is associated with a decrease in BP, but UVA irradiation was found to also decrease BP. The effect was attributed to UVA irradiation-induced release of nitric oxide.

Beveridge and colleagues identified other confounders [91]. Associations in vitamin D studies may be confounded by the effects of other CVD risk factors in addition to those being studied, and confounding related to the possibility of reverse causality may also occur. Liberopoulos and colleagues [93] found that statins have different effects on the increase of serum 25(OH)D levels. Woodhouse and colleagues [94] found a seasonal variation in serum total-C, HDL-C and TG levels. These confounders can be controlled for with the use of appropriate statistical analyses, just as age, gender, ethnicity, BMI and smoking status are often controlled for in research studies.

Essential to the credibility of study results is the measurement and reporting of adherence to the intervention. The evaluation of adherence to oral vitamin D supplements given in a study may be either absent or inadequate. Furthermore, an inquiry about concurrent use of personal oral vitamin D supplementation may differ across studies. Negative study results may simply be attributed to a lack of adherence to the intervention, because it leads to bias and a decrease in the statistical power.

4. Conclusions

Despite the identification and treatment of currently recognized CVD risks, CVD remains the leading cause of death. The focus of vitamin D research has recently expanded to include the effects of vitamin D status on CVD and CVD risk factors. Low serum 25(OH)D levels are associated with increased incidence [8], prevalence [56] and risk factors for CVD [15]. This assessment demonstrates that Hill's criteria were satisfied.

Potential benefits of decreasing the impact of a risk factor for CVD should outweigh potential risks. Repletion of vitamin D stores with a supplemental dose of 10,000 IU per day or less is unlikely to lead to toxic effects [39]. Repletion can be accomplished by a sensible increase in sun exposure [37] or by consuming vitamin D-rich foods, but this goal is most easily accomplished with oral supplementation. Furthermore, more severe deficiencies in serum 25(OH)D levels show a more rapid increase than less severe deficiencies [103]. Treatment for some CVD risk factors is expensive and may be difficult to access, but oral vitamin D supplements are readily accessible and reasonably priced. Other considerations for individualized treatment should include attention to skin melanin content, latitude and altitude of residence, dietary habits and amount of sun exposure.

The physiological mechanisms hypothesized to cause low vitamin D status to increase CVD risk have not yet been confirmed. Nearly all research studies regarding low vitamin D status and increased risk of CVD use observational study designs. More RCTs are needed that incorporate the complex pharmacokinetic and pharmacodynamic properties of vitamin D in the study design: dose-response curve, half-life, avoidance of toxicity and use of the most accurate and precise serum assays.

Exposure to sunlight or vitamin D supplementation may be used in an RCT, although having a control group with a zero serum 25(OH)D level would not be possible. This approach is possible only in drug studies [120]. Nutrients are more appropriately studied in the context of proving negative causation: the absence of an antecedent caused the consequence. This study design would be consistent with research involving preventive healthcare strategies.

Current scientific evidence supports a causal association between serum 25(OH)D levels and increased risk for CVD on the basis of Hill's criteria for causality in a biological system. Only RCTs starting with low serum 25(OH)D levels found significant beneficial effects of vitamin D supplementation in reducing risk factors associated with CVD. However, evidence to date suggests that raising serum 25(OH)D levels to at least 30 ng/mL will reduce the risk of CVD.

Whether it is ethical to design a study in which a group of people is deprived of a known essential nutrient to measure an endpoint should be carefully determined. Furthermore, waiting for completion of long-term RCTs to change treatment recommendations, especially when risks are minimal, may adversely affect the health of countless individuals. According to Hill [45]: "All scientific work is incomplete—whether it be observational or experimental. All scientific work is liable to be upset or modified by advancing knowledge. That does not confer upon us a freedom to ignore the knowledge we already have, or to postpone the action that it appears to demand at a given time."

Acknowledgements

The authors would like to acknowledge and thank Steven M. Paul, Principal Statistician, School of Nursing, UCSF, for his expert assistance with the interpretation of statistical analyses in the research studies we included in this review.

Author Contributions

All of the authors contributed to the conception and design of this review as well as the analyses performed in order to determine if the criteria had been met. Patricia G. Weyland drafted the review with considerable assistance with the review of literature, organization and editing from Jill Howie-Esquivel and William B. Grant. All of the authors have approved all of the manuscript revisions as well as the final version prior to submission for publication.

Conflicts of Interest

The authors declare no conflicts of interest. Patricia G. Weyland receives funding from Bio-Tech Pharmacal (Fayetteville, AR, USA) and the Sunlight Research Forum (Veldhoven, The Netherlands).

References

1. Jones, D.S.; Podolsky, S.H.; Greene, J.A. The burden of disease and the changing task of medicine. *N. Engl. J. Med.* **2012**, *366*, 2333–2338.
2. Ford, E.S.; Ajani, U.A.; Croft, J.B.; Critchley, J.A.; Labarthe, D.R.; Kottke, T.E.; Giles, W.H.; Capewell, S. Explaining the decrease in U.S. deaths from coronary disease, 1980–2000. *N. Engl. J. Med.* **2007**, *356*, 2388–2398.
3. Olshansky, S.J.; Passaro, D.J.; Hershow, R.C.; Layden, J.; Carnes, B.A.; Brody, J.; Hayflick, L.; Butler, R.N.; Allison, D.B.; Ludwig, D.S. A potential decline in life expectancy in the United States in the 21st century. *N. Engl. J. Med.* **2005**, *352*, 1138–1145.
4. Scragg, R. Seasonality of cardiovascular disease mortality and the possible protective effect of ultra-violet radiation. *Int. J. Epidemiol.* **1981**, *10*, 337–341.
5. DeLuca, H.F. Overview of general physiologic features and functions of vitamin D. *Am. J. Clin. Nutr.* **2004**, *80*, 1689S–1696S.
6. Pludowski, P.; Grant, W.B.; Bhattoa, H.P.; Bayer, M.; Povoroznyuk, V.; Rudenka, E.; Ramanau, H.; Varbiro, S.; Rudenka, A.; Karczmarewicz, E.; *et al.* Vitamin D status in Central Europe. *Int. J. Endocrinol.* **2014**, *2014*, 589587, doi:10.1155/2014/589587.
7. Giovannucci, E.; Liu, Y.; Hollis, B.W.; Rimm, E.B. 25-Hydroxyvitamin D and risk of myocardial infarction in men: A prospective study. *Arch. Intern. Med.* **2008**, *168*, 1174–1180.
8. Anderson, J.L.; May, H.T.; Horne, B.D.; Bair, T.L.; Hall, N.L.; Carlquist, J.F.; Lappe, D.L.; Muhlestein, J.B. Relation of vitamin D deficiency to cardiovascular risk factors, disease status, and incident events in a general healthcare population. *Am. J. Cardiol.* **2010**, *106*, 963–968.
9. Zagura, M.; Serg, M.; Kampus, P.; Zilmer, M.; Eha, J.; Unt, E.; Lieberg, J.; Cockcroft, J.R.; Kals, J. Aortic stiffness and vitamin D are independent markers of aortic calcification in patients with peripheral arterial disease and in healthy subjects. *Eur. J. Vasc. Endovasc. Surg.* **2011**, *42*, 689–695.
10. Gaddipati, V.C.; Bailey, B.A.; Kuriacose, R.; Copeland, R.J.; Manning, T.; Peiris, A.N. The relationship of vitamin D status to cardiovascular risk factors and amputation risk in veterans with peripheral arterial disease. *J. Am. Med. Dir. Assoc.* **2011**, *12*, 58–61.

11. Van de Luijtgaarden, K.M.; Voute, M.T.; Hoeks, S.E.; Bakker, E.J.; Chonchol, M.; Stolker, R.J.; Rouwet, E.V.; Verhagen, H.J. Vitamin D deficiency may be an independent risk factor for arterial disease. *Eur. J. Vasc. Endovasc. Surg.* **2012**, *44*, 301–306.

12. Webb, D.R.; Khunti, K.; Lacy, P.; Gray, L.J.; Mostafa, S.; Talbot, D.; Williams, B.; Davies, M.J. Conduit vessel stiffness in British South Asians of Indian descent relates to 25-hydroxyvitamin D status. *J. Hypertens.* **2012**, *30*, 1588–1596.

13. Pletcher, M.J.; Tice, J.A.; Pignone, M.; Browner, W.S. Using the coronary artery calcium score to predict coronary heart disease events: A systematic review and meta-analysis. *Arch. Intern. Med.* **2004**, *164*, 1285–1292.

14. Rezai, M.R.; Balakrishnan Nair, S.; Cowan, B.; Young, A.; Sattar, N.; Finn, J.D.; Wu, F.C.; Cruickshank, J.K. Low vitamin D levels are related to left ventricular concentric remodelling in men of different ethnic groups with varying cardiovascular risk. *Int. J. Cardiol.* **2012**, *158*, 444–447.

15. De Boer, I.H.; Kestenbaum, B.; Shoben, A.B.; Michos, E.D.; Sarnak, M.J.; Siscovick, D.S. 25-Hydroxyvitamin D levels inversely associate with risk for developing coronary artery calcification. *J. Am. Soc. Nephrol.* **2009**, *20*, 1805–1812.

16. Taylor, A.J.; Fiorilli, P.N.; Wu, H.; Bauer, K.; Bindeman, J.; Byrd, C.; Feuerstein, I.M.; O'Malley, P.G. Relation between the Framingham risk score, coronary calcium, and incident coronary heart disease among low-risk men. *Am. J. Cardiol.* **2010**, *106*, 47–50.

17. Oh, J.; Weng, S.; Felton, S.K.; Bhandare, S.; Riek, A.; Butler, B.; Proctor, B.M.; Petty, M.; Chen, Z.; Schechtman, K.B.; *et al.* 1,25(OH)2 vitamin D inhibits foam cell formation and suppresses macrophage cholesterol uptake in patients with type 2 diabetes mellitus. *Circulation* **2009**, *120*, 687–698.

18. Grant, W.B.; Mascitelli, L.; Goldstein, M.R. Comment on Ryan; *et al.* An investigation of association between chronic musculoskeletal pain and cardiovascular disease in the Health Survey for England (2008). *Eur. J. Pain* **2014**, *18*, 893–894.

19. Afzal, S.; Bojesen, S.E.; Nordestgaard, B.G. Low plasma 25-hydroxyvitamin D and risk of tobacco-related cancer. *Clin. Chem.* **2013**, *59*, 771–780.

20. Krause, R.; Buhring, M.; Hopfenmuller, W.; Holick, M.F.; Sharma, A.M. Ultraviolet B and blood pressure. *Lancet* **1998**, *352*, 709–710.

21. Forman, J.P.; Giovannucci, E.; Holmes, M.D.; Bischoff-Ferrari, H.A.; Tworoger, S.S.; Willett, W.C.; Curhan, G.C. Plasma 25-hydroxyvitamin D levels and risk of incident hypertension. *Hypertension* **2007**, *49*, 1063–1069.

22. Zhao, G.; Ford, E.S.; Li, C.; Kris-Etherton, P.M.; Etherton, T.D.; Balluz, L.S. Independent associations of serum concentrations of 25-hydroxyvitamin D and parathyroid hormone with blood pressure among US adults. *J. Hypertens.* **2010**, *28*, 1821–1828.

23. Goel, R.K.; Lal, H. Role of vitamin D supplementation in hypertension. *Indian J. Clin. Biochem.* **2011**, *26*, 88–90.

24. Gupta, A.K.; Brashear, M.M.; Johnson, W.D. Prediabetes and prehypertension in healthy adults are associated with low vitamin D levels. *Diabetes Care* **2011**, *34*, 658–660.

25. Larsen, T.; Mose, F.H.; Bech, J.N.; Hansen, A.B.; Pedersen, E.B. Effect of cholecalciferol supplementation during winter months in patients with hypertension: A randomized, placebo-controlled trial. *Am. J. Hypertens.* **2012**, *25*, 1215–1222.

26. Schwartz, J.B. Effects of vitamin D supplementation in atorvastatin-treated patients: A new drug interaction with an unexpected consequence. *Clin. Pharmacol. Ther.* **2009**, *85*, 198–203.

27. De la Llera-Moya, M.; Drazul-Schrader, D.; Asztalos, B.F.; Cuchel, M.; Rader, D.J.; Rothblat, G.H. The ability to promote efflux via ABCA1 determines the capacity of serum specimens with similar high-density lipoprotein cholesterol to remove cholesterol from macrophages. *Arterioscler. Thromb. Vasc. Biol.* **2010**, *30*, 796–801.

28. Jorde, R.; Figenschau, Y.; Hutchinson, M.; Emaus, N.; Grimnes, G. High serum 25-hydroxyvitamin D concentrations are associated with a favorable serum lipid profile. *Eur. J. Clin. Nutr.* **2010**, *64*, 1457–1464.

29. Guasch, A.; Bullo, M.; Rabassa, A.; Bonada, A.; del Castillo, D.; Sabench, F.; Salas-Salvado, J. Plasma vitamin D and parathormone are associated with obesity and atherogenic dyslipidemia: A cross-sectional study. *Cardiovasc. Diabetol.* **2012**, *11*, 149.

30. Van Ballegooijen, A.J.; Snijder, M.B.; Visser, M.; van den Hurk, K.; Kamp, O.; Dekker, J.M.; Nijpels, G.; Stehouwer, C.D.; Henry, R.M.; Paulus, W.J.; *et al.* Vitamin D in relation to myocardial structure and function after eight years of follow-up: The Hoorn Study. *Ann. Nutr. Metab.* **2012**, *60*, 69–77.

31. Minino, A. Mortality among teenagers aged 12–19 years: United States, 1999–2006. *NCHS Data Brief* **2010**, *37*, 1–8.

32. Takeda, M.; Yamashita, T.; Sasaki, N.; Nakajima, K.; Kita, T.; Shinohara, M.; Ishida, T.; Hirata, K. Oral administration of an active form of vitamin D_3 (calcitriol) decreases atherosclerosis in mice by inducing regulatory T cells and immature dendritic cells with tolerogenic functions. *Arterioscler. Thromb. Vasc. Biol.* **2010**, *30*, 2495–2503.

33. Bouillon, R.; van Schoor, N.M.; Gielen, E.; Boonen, S.; Mathieu, C.; Vanderschueren, D.; Lips, P. Optimal vitamin D status: A critical analysis on the basis of evidence-based medicine. *J. Clin. Endocrinol. Metab.* **2013**, *98*, E1283–E1304.

34. Grant, W.B. Using findings from observational studies to guide vitamin D randomized controlled trials. *J. Intern. Med.* **2014**, *59*, 1–4.

35. Holick, M.F.; Binkley, N.C.; Bischoff-Ferrari, H.A.; Gordon, C.M.; Hanley, D.A.; Heaney, R.P.; Murad, M.H.; Weaver, C.M. Evaluation, treatment, and prevention of vitamin D deficiency: An endocrine society clinical practice guideline. *J. Clin. Endocrinol. Metab.* **2011**, *96*, 1911–1930.

36. Holick, M.F.; Binkley, N.C.; Bischoff-Ferrari, H.A.; Gordon, C.M.; Hanley, D.A.; Heaney, R.P.; Murad, M.H.; Weaver, C.M. Guidelines for preventing and treating vitamin D deficiency and insufficiency revisited. *J. Clin. Endocrinol. Metab.* **2012**, *97*, 1153–1158.

37. Grant, W.B.; Boucher, B.J. Are Hill's criteria for causality satisfied for vitamin D and periodontal disease? *Derm. Endocrinol.* **2010**, *2*, 30–36.

38. Looker, A.C.; Johnson, C.L.; Lacher, D.A.; Pfeiffer, C.M.; Schleicher, R.L.; Sempos, C.T. Vitamin D status: United States, 2001–2006. *NCHS Data Brief* **2011**, *59*, 1–8.

39. Holick, M.F. Vitamin D deficiency. *N. Engl. J. Med.* **2007**, *357*, 266–281.

40. Vieth, R. What is the optimal vitamin D status for health? *Prog. Biophys. Mol. Biol.* **2006**, *92*, 26–32.

41. Heaney, R.P.; Recker, R.R.; Grote, J.; Horst, R.L.; Armas, L.A. Vitamin D_3 is more potent than vitamin D_2 in humans. *J. Clin. Endocrinol. Metab.* **2011**, *96*, E447–E452.

42. Garland, C.F.; French, C.B.; Baggerly, L.L.; Heaney, R.P. Vitamin D supplement doses and serum 25-hydroxyvitamin D in the range associated with cancer prevention. *Anticancer Res.* **2011**, *31*, 607–611.

43. Grant, W.B. In defense of the sun: An estimate of changes in mortality rates in the United States if mean serum 25-hydroxyvitamin D levels were raised to 45 ng/mL by solar ultraviolet-B irradiance. *Derm. Endocrinol.* **2009**, *1*, 207–214.

44. Grant, W.B. An estimate of the global reduction in mortality rates through doubling vitamin D levels. *Eur. J. Clin. Nutr.* **2011**, *65*, 1016–1026.

45. Hill, A.B. The environment and disease: Association or causation? *Proc. R. Soc. Med.* **1965**, *58*, 295–300.

46. Grant, W.B. How strong is the evidence that solar ultraviolet B and vitamin D reduce the risk of cancer? An examination using Hill's criteria for causality. *Derm. Endocrinol.* **2009**, *1*, 14–21.

47. Hanwell, H.E.; Banwell, B. Assessment of evidence for a protective role of vitamin D in multiple sclerosis. *Biochim. Biophys. Acta* **2011**, *1812*, 202–212.

48. Mohr, S.B.; Gorham, E.D.; Alcaraz, J.E.; Kane, C.I.; Macera, C.A.; Parsons, J.K.; Wingard, D.L.; Garland, C.F. Does the evidence for an inverse relationship between serum vitamin D status and breast cancer risk satisfy the Hill criteria? *Derm. Endocrinol.* **2012**, *4*, 152–157.

49. Robsahm, T.E.; Schwartz, G.G.; Tretli, S. The inverse relationship between 25-hydroxyvitamin D and cancer survival: Discussion of causation. *Cancers* **2013**, *5*, 1439–1455.

50. Jang, H.B.; Lee, H.J.; Park, J.Y.; Kang, J.H.; Song, J. Association between serum vitamin D and metabolic risk factors in Korean schoolgirls. *Osong Public Health Res. Perspect.* **2013**, *4*, 179–186.

51. Correia, L.C.; Sodre, F.; Garcia, G.; Sabino, M.; Brito, M.; Kalil, F.; Barreto, B.; Lima, J.C.; Noya-Rabelo, M.M. Relation of severe deficiency of vitamin D to cardiovascular mortality during acute coronary syndromes. *Am. J. Cardiol.* **2013**, *111*, 324–327.

52. Deleskog, A.; Piksasova, O.; Silveira, A.; Samnegard, A.; Tornvall, P.; Eriksson, P.; Gustafsson, S.; Ostenson, C.G.; Ohrvik, J.; Hamsten, A. Serum 25-hydroxyvitamin D concentration, established and emerging cardiovascular risk factors and risk of myocardial infarction before the age of 60 years. *Atherosclerosis* **2012**, *223*, 223–229.

53. Deleskog, A.; Piksasova, O.; Silveira, A.; Gertow, K.; Baldassarre, D.; Veglia, F.; Sennblad, B.; Strawbridge, R.J.; Larsson, M.; Leander, K.; *et al.* Serum 25-hydroxyvitamin D concentration in subclinical carotid atherosclerosis. *Arterioscler. Thromb. Vasc. Biol.* **2013**, *33*, 2633–2638.

54. Parker, J.; Hashmi, O.; Dutton, D.; Mavrodaris, A.; Stranges, S.; Kandala, N.B.; Clarke, A.; Franco, O.H. Levels of vitamin D and cardiometabolic disorders: Systematic review and meta-analysis. *Maturitas* **2010**, *65*, 225–236.

55. Wang, L.; Song, Y.; Manson, J.E.; Pilz, S.; Marz, W.; Michaelsson, K.; Lundqvist, A.; Jassal, S.K.; Barrett-Connor, E.; Zhang, C.; *et al.* Circulating 25-hydroxy-vitamin D and risk of

cardiovascular disease: A meta-analysis of prospective studies. *Circ. Cardiovasc. Qual. Outcomes* **2012**, *5*, 819–829.

56. Kendrick, J.; Targher, G.; Smits, G.; Chonchol, M. 25-Hydroxyvitamin D deficiency is independently associated with cardiovascular disease in the Third National Health and Nutrition Examination Survey. *Atherosclerosis* **2009**, *205*, 255–260.

57. Song, Y.; Wang, L.; Pittas, A.G.; del Gobbo, L.C.; Zhang, C.; Manson, J.E.; Hu, F.B. Blood 25-hydroxy vitamin D levels and incident type 2 diabetes: A meta-analysis of prospective studies. *Diabetes Care* **2013**, *36*, 1422–1428.

58. Tsur, A.; Feldman, B.S.; Feldhammer, I.; Hoshen, M.B.; Leibowitz, G.; Balicer, R.D. Decreased serum concentrations of 25-hydroxycholecalciferol are associated with increased risk of progression to impaired fasting glucose and diabetes. *Diabetes Care* **2013**, *36*, 1361–1367.

59. Vacek, J.L.; Vanga, S.R.; Good, M.; Lai, S.M.; Lakkireddy, D.; Howard, P.A. Vitamin D deficiency and supplementation and relation to cardiovascular health. *Am. J. Cardiol.* **2012**, *109*, 359–363.

60. Wang, T.J.; Pencina, M.J.; Booth, S.L.; Jacques, P.F.; Ingelsson, E.; Lanier, K.; Benjamin, E.J.; D'Agostino, R.B.; Wolf, M.; Vasan, R.S. Vitamin D deficiency and risk of cardiovascular disease. *Circulation* **2008**, *117*, 503–511.

61. Carrara, D.; Bernini, M.; Bacca, A.; Rugani, I.; Duranti, E.; Virdis, A.; Ghiadoni, L.; Taddei, S.; Bernini, G. Cholecalciferol administration blunts the systemic renin-angiotensin system in essential hypertensives with hypovitaminosis D. *J. Renin Angiotensin Aldosterone Syst.* **2014**, *15*, 82–87.

62. Forman, J.P.; Curhan, G.C.; Taylor, E.N. Plasma 25-hydroxyvitamin D levels and risk of incident hypertension among young women. *Hypertension* **2008**, *52*, 828–832.

63. Giallauria, F.; Milaneschi, Y.; Tanaka, T.; Maggio, M.; Canepa, M.; Elango, P.; Vigorito, C.; Lakatta, E.G.; Ferrucci, L.; Strait, J. Arterial stiffness and vitamin D levels: The Baltimore Longitudinal Study of Aging. *J. Clin. Endocrinol. Metab.* **2012**, *97*, 3717–3723.

64. Mayer, O., Jr.; Filipovsky, J.; Seidlerova, J.; Vanek, J.; Dolejsova, M.; Vrzalova, J.; Cifkova, R. The association between low 25-hydroxyvitamin D and increased aortic stiffness. *J. Hum. Hypertens.* **2012**, *26*, 650–655.

65. Pirro, M.; Manfredelli, M.R.; Helou, R.S.; Scarponi, A.M.; Schillaci, G.; Bagaglia, F.; Melis, F.; Mannarino, E. Association of parathyroid hormone and 25-OH-vitamin D levels with arterial stiffness in postmenopausal women with vitamin D insufficiency. *J. Atheroscler. Thromb.* **2012**, *19*, 924–931.

66. Robinson-Cohen, C.; Hoofnagle, A.N.; Ix, J.H.; Sachs, M.C.; Tracy, R.P.; Siscovick, D.S.; Kestenbaum, B.R.; de Boer, I.H. Racial differences in the association of serum 25-hydroxyvitamin D concentration with coronary heart disease events. *JAMA* **2013**, *310*, 179–188.

67. Forouhi, N.G.; Luan, J.; Cooper, A.; Boucher, B.J.; Wareham, N.J. Baseline serum 25-hydroxyvitamin D is predictive of future glycemic status and insulin resistance: The Medical Research Council Ely Prospective Study 1990–2000. *Diabetes* **2008**, *57*, 2619–2625.

68. Breslavsky, A.; Frand, J.; Matas, Z.; Boaz, M.; Barnea, Z.; Shargorodsky, M. Effect of high doses of vitamin D on arterial properties, adiponectin, leptin and glucose homeostasis in type 2 diabetic patients. *Clin. Nutr.* **2013**, *32*, 970–975.

69. Grant, W.B.; Garland, C.F. Vitamin D has a greater impact on cancer mortality rates than on cancer incidence rates. *Br. Med. J.* **2014**, *348*, g2862, doi:http://dx.doi.org/10.1136/bmj.g2862.

70. Grant, W.B. Primary malignancy in patients with nonmelanoma skin cancer-letter. *Cancer Epidemiol. Biomark. Prev.* **2014**, *23*, 1438, doi:10.1158/1055-9965.

71. Savic, L.; Mrdovic, I.; Perunicic, J.; Asanin, M.; Lasica, R.; Marinkovic, J.; Vasiljevic, Z.; Ostojic, M. Impact of the combined left ventricular systolic and renal dysfunction on one-year outcomes after primary percutaneous coronary intervention. *J. Interv. Cardiol.* **2012**, *25*, 132–139.

72. Brenner, D.R.; Arora, P.; Garcia-Bailo, B.; Wolever, T.M.; Morrison, H.; El-Sohemy, A.; Karmali, M.; Badawi, A. Plasma vitamin D levels and risk of metabolic syndrome in Canadians. *Clin. Investig. Med.* **2011**, *34*, E377.

73. Boucher, B.J. Is vitamin D status relevant to metabolic syndrome? *Derm. Endocrinol.* **2012**, *4*, 212–224.

74. Gagnon, C.; Lu, Z.X.; Magliano, D.J.; Dunstan, D.W.; Shaw, J.E.; Zimmet, P.Z.; Sikaris, K.; Ebeling, P.R.; Daly, R.M. Low serum 25-hydroxyvitamin D is associated with increased risk of the development of the metabolic syndrome at five years: Results from a national, population-based prospective study (The Australian Diabetes, Obesity and Lifestyle Study: Ausdiab). *J. Clin. Endocrinol. Metab.* **2012**, *97*, 1953–1961.

75. Makariou, S.; Liberopoulos, E.; Florentin, M.; Lagos, K.; Gazi, I.; Challa, A.; Elisaf, M. The relationship of vitamin D with non-traditional risk factors for cardiovascular disease in subjects with metabolic syndrome. *Arch. Med. Sci.* **2012**, *8*, 437–443.

76. De Boer, I.H.; Katz, R.; Chonchol, M.; Ix, J.H.; Sarnak, M.J.; Shlipak, M.G.; Siscovick, D.S.; Kestenbaum, B. Serum 25-hydroxyvitamin D and change in estimated glomerular filtration rate. *Clin. J. Am. Soc. Nephrol.* **2011**, *6*, 2141–2149.

77. Schnatz, P.F.; Jiang, X.; Vila-Wright, S.; Aragaki, A.K.; Nudy, M.; O'Sullivan, D.M.; Jackson, R.; Leblanc, E.; Robinson, J.G.; Shikany, J.M.; *et al.* Calcium/vitamin D supplementation, serum 25-hydroxyvitamin D concentrations, and cholesterol profiles in the Women's Health Initiative calcium/vitamin D randomized trial. *Menopause* **2014**, *8*, 823–833.

78. Bolland, M.J.; Grey, A.; Gamble, G.D.; Reid, I.R. The effect of vitamin D supplementation on skeletal, vascular, or cancer outcomes: A trial sequential meta-analysis. *Lancet Diabetes Endocrinol.* **2014**, *2*, 307–320.

79. Forman, J.P.; Scott, J.B.; Ng, K.; Drake, B.F.; Suarez, E.G.; Hayden, D.L.; Bennett, G.G.; Chandler, P.D.; Hollis, B.W.; Emmons, K.M.; *et al.* Effect of vitamin D supplementation on blood pressure in blacks. *Hypertension* **2013**, *61*, 779–785.

80. George, P.S.; Pearson, E.R.; Witham, M.D. Effect of vitamin D supplementation on glycaemic control and insulin resistance: A systematic review and meta-analysis. *Diabet. Med.* **2012**, *29*, e142–e150.

81. Talaei, A.; Mohamadi, M.; Adgi, Z. The effect of vitamin D on insulin resistance in patients with type 2 diabetes. *Diabetol. Metab. Syndr.* **2013**, *5*, 8, doi:10.1186/1758-5996-5-8.

82. Michos, E.D.; Reis, J.P.; Post, W.S.; Lutsey, P.L.; Gottesman, R.F.; Mosley, T.H.; Sharrett, A.R.; Melamed, M.L. 25-Hydroxyvitamin D deficiency is associated with fatal stroke among whites but not blacks: The NHANES-III linked mortality files. *Nutrition* **2012**, *28*, 367–371.

83. Wood, A.D.; Secombes, K.R.; Thies, F.; Aucott, L.; Black, A.J.; Mavroeidi, A.; Simpson, W.G.; Fraser, W.D.; Reid, D.M.; Macdonald, H.M. Vitamin D$_3$ supplementation has no effect on conventional cardiovascular risk factors: A parallel-group, double-blind, placebo-controlled RCT. *J. Clin. Endocrinol. Metab.* **2012**, *97*, 3557–3568.

84. Jorde, R.; Strand Hutchinson, M.; Kjaergaard, M.; Sneve, M.; Grimnes, G. Supplementation with high doses of vitamin D to subjects without vitamin D deficiency may have negative effects: Pooled data from four intervention trials in Tromsø. *ISRN Endocrinol.* **2013**, *2013*, 348705, doi:10.1155/2013/348705.

85. Liu, S.; Song, Y.; Ford, E.S.; Manson, J.E.; Buring, J.E.; Ridker, P.M. Dietary calcium, vitamin D, and the prevalence of metabolic syndrome in middle-aged and older U.S. women. *Diabetes Care* **2005**, *28*, 2926–2932.

86. Fung, G.J.; Steffen, L.M.; Zhou, X.; Harnack, L.; Tang, W.; Lutsey, P.L.; Loria, C.M.; Reis, J.P.; van Horn, L.V. Vitamin D intake is inversely related to risk of developing metabolic syndrome in African American and white men and women over 20 y: The Coronary Artery Risk Development in Young Adults study. *Am. J. Clin. Nutr.* **2012**, *96*, 24–29.

87. Moukayed, M.; Grant, W.B. Molecular link between vitamin D and cancer prevention. *Nutrients* **2013**, *5*, 3993–4021.

88. Oplander, C.; Volkmar, C.M.; Paunel-Gorgulu, A.; van Faassen, E.E.; Heiss, C.; Kelm, M.; Halmer, D.; Murtz, M.; Pallua, N.; Suschek, C.V. Whole body UVA irradiation lowers systemic blood pressure by release of nitric oxide from intracutaneous photolabile nitric oxide derivates. *Circ. Res.* **2009**, *105*, 1031–1040.

89. Andrukhova, O.; Slavic, S.; Zeitz, U.; Riesen, S.C.; Heppelmann, M.S.; Ambrisko, T.D.; Markovic, M.; Kuebler, W.M.; Erben, R.G. Vitamin D is a regulator of endothelial nitric oxide synthase and arterial stiffness in mice. *Mol. Endocrinol.* **2014**, *28*, 53–64.

90. Jamaluddin, S.; Liang, Z.; Lu, J.M.; Yao, Q.; Chen, C. Roles of cardiovascular risk factors in endothelial nitric oxide synthase regulation: An update. *Curr. Pharm. Des.* **2013**, *22*, 3563–3578.

91. Beveridge, L.A.; Witham, M.D. Vitamin D and the cardiovascular system. *Osteoporos. Int.* **2013**, *24*, 2167–2180.

92. Zittermann, A.; Iodice, S.; Pilz, S.; Grant, W.B.; Bagnardi, V.; Gandini, S. Vitamin D deficiency and mortality risk in the general population: A meta-analysis of prospective cohort studies. *Am. J. Clin. Nutr.* **2012**, *95*, 91–100.

93. Liberopoulos, E.N.; Makariou, S.E.; Moutzouri, E.; Kostapanos, M.S.; Challa, A.; Elisaf, M. Effect of simvastatin/ezetimibe 10/10 mg *versus* simvastatin 40 mg on serum vitamin D levels. *J. Cardiovasc. Pharmacol. Ther.* **2013**, *18*, 229–233.

94. Woodhouse, P.R.; Khaw, K.T.; Plummer, M. Seasonal variation of blood pressure and its relationship to ambient temperature in an elderly population. *J. Hypertens.* **1993**, *11*, 1267–1274.

95. Burkart, K.; Schneider, A.; Breitner, S.; Khan, M.H.; Kramer, A.; Endlicher, W. The effect of atmospheric thermal conditions and urban thermal pollution on all-cause and cardiovascular mortality in Bangladesh. *Environ. Pollut.* **2011**, *159*, 2035–2043.

96. Brandenburg, V.M.; Vervloet, M.G.; Marx, N. The role of vitamin D in cardiovascular disease: From present evidence to future perspectives. *Atherosclerosis* **2012**, *225*, 253–263.

97. Hathcock, J.N.; Shao, A.; Vieth, R.; Heaney, R. Risk assessment for vitamin D. *Am. J. Clin. Nutr.* **2007**, *85*, 6–18.

98. Gradinaru, D.; Borsa, C.; Ionescu, C.; Margina, D.; Prada, G.I.; Jansen, E. Vitamin D status and oxidative stress markers in the elderly with impaired fasting glucose and type 2 diabetes mellitus. *Aging Clin. Exp. Res.* **2012**, *24*, 595–602.

99. Alkharfy, K.M.; Al-Daghri, N.M.; Sabico, S.B.; Al-Othman, A.; Moharram, O.; Alokail, M.S.; Al-Saleh, Y.; Kumar, S.; Chrousos, G.P. Vitamin D supplementation in patients with diabetes mellitus type 2 on different therapeutic regimens: A one-year prospective study. *Cardiovasc. Diabetol.* **2013**, *12*, 113, doi:10.1186/1475-2840-12-113.

100. Wilmot, E.G.; Edwardson, C.L.; Biddle, S.J.; Gorely, T.; Henson, J.; Khunti, K.; Nimmo, M.A.; Yates, T.; Davies, M.J. Prevalence of diabetes and impaired glucose metabolism in younger "at risk" UK adults: Insights from the STAND programme of research. *Diabet. Med.* **2013**, *30*, 671–675.

101. Yiu, Y.F.; Yiu, K.H.; Siu, C.W.; Chan, Y.H.; Li, S.W.; Wong, L.Y.; Lee, S.W.; Tam, S.; Wong, E.W.; Lau, C.P.; *et al.* Randomized controlled trial of vitamin D supplement on endothelial function in patients with type 2 diabetes. *Atherosclerosis* **2013**, *227*, 140–146.

102. DeKeyser, F.G.; Pugh, L.C. Assessment of the reliability and validity of biochemical measures. *Nurs. Res.* **1990**, *39*, 314–317.

103. Lappe, J.M.; Heaney, R.P. Why randomized controlled trials of calcium and vitamin D sometimes fail. *Derm. Endocrinol.* **2012**, *4*, 95–100.

104. Gupta, A.K.; Brashear, M.M.; Johnson, W.D. Predisease conditions and serum vitamin D levels in healthy Mexican American adults. *Postgrad. Med.* **2012**, *124*, 136–142.

105. Harris, S.S. Vitamin D and African Americans. *J. Nutr.* **2006**, *136*, 1126–1129.

106. Riek, A.E.; Oh, J.; Darwech, I.; Moynihan, C.E.; Bruchas, R.R.; Bernal-Mizrachi, C. 25(OH) vitamin D suppresses macrophage adhesion and migration by downregulation of ER stress and scavenger receptor A1 in type 2 diabetes. *J. Steroid Biochem. Mol. Biol.* **2013**, *144*, 172–179, doi:10.1016/j.jsbmb.2013.10.016.

107. Wu-Wong, J.R.; Nakane, M.; Ma, J.; Ruan, X.; Kroeger, P.E. VDR-mediated gene expression patterns in resting human coronary artery smooth muscle cells. *J. Cell. Biochem.* **2007**, *100*, 1395–1405.

108. Yusuf, S.; Hawken, S.; Ounpuu, S.; Dans, T.; Avezum, A.; Lanas, F.; McQueen, M.; Budaj, A.; Pais, P.; Varigos, J.; *et al.* Effect of potentially modifiable risk factors associated with myocardial infarction in 52 countries (the INTERHEART study): Case-control study. *Lancet* **2004**, *364*, 937–952.

109. Karhapaa, P.; Pihlajamaki, J.; Porsti, I.; Kastarinen, M.; Mustonen, J.; Niemela, O.; Kuusisto, J. Diverse associations of 25-hydroxyvitamin D and 1,25-dihydroxy-vitamin D with dyslipidaemias. *J. Intern. Med.* **2010**, *268*, 604–610.

110. Chow, E.C.; Magomedova, L.; Quach, H.P.; Patel, R.; Durk, M.R.; Fan, J.; Maeng, H.J.; Irondi, K.; Anakk, S.; Moore, D.D.; *et al.* Vitamin D receptor activation down-regulates the

small heterodimer partner and increases CYP7A1 to lower cholesterol. *Gastroenterology* **2014**, *146*, 1048–1059.

111. Moser, U. Vitamins—Wrong approaches. *Int. J. Vitam. Nutr. Res.* **2012**, *82*, 327–332.

112. Heaney, R.P. Guidelines for optimizing design and analysis of clinical studies of nutrient effects. *Nutr. Rev.* **2014**, *72*, 48–54.

113. Rahimi-Ardabili, H.; Pourghassem Gargari, B.; Farzadi, L. Effects of vitamin D on cardiovascular disease risk factors in polycystic ovary syndrome women with vitamin D deficiency. *J. Endocrinol. Investig.* **2013**, *36*, 28–32.

114. Grimnes, G.; Figenschau, Y.; Almas, B.; Jorde, R. Vitamin D, insulin secretion, sensitivity, and lipids: Results from a case-control study and a randomized controlled trial using hyperglycemic clamp technique. *Diabetes* **2011**, *60*, 2748–2757.

115. Von Hurst, P.R.; Stonehouse, W.; Coad, J. Vitamin D supplementation reduces insulin resistance in South Asian women living in New Zealand who are insulin resistant and vitamin D deficient—A randomised, placebo-controlled trial. *Br. J. Nutr.* **2010**, *103*, 549–555.

116. Belenchia, A.M.; Tosh, A.K.; Hillman, L.S.; Peterson, C.A. Correcting vitamin D insufficiency improves insulin sensitivity in obese adolescents: A randomized controlled trial. *Am. J. Clin. Nutr.* **2013**, *97*, 774–781.

117. Beilfuss, J.; Berg, V.; Sneve, M.; Jorde, R.; Kamycheva, E. Effects of a 1-year supplementation with cholecalciferol on interleukin-6, tumor necrosis factor-alpha and insulin resistance in overweight and obese subjects. *Cytokine* **2012**, *60*, 870–874.

118. Gepner, A.D.; Ramamurthy, R.; Krueger, D.C.; Korcarz, C.E.; Binkley, N.; Stein, J.H. A prospective randomized controlled trial of the effects of vitamin D supplementation on cardiovascular disease risk. *PLoS One* **2012**, *7*, e36617, doi:10.1371/journal.pone.0036617.

119. Potischman, N.; Weed, D.L. Causal criteria in nutritional epidemiology. *Am. J. Clin. Nutr.* **1999**, *69*, 1309S–1314S.

120. Biesalski, H.K.; Aggett, P.J.; Anton, R.; Bernstein, P.S.; Blumberg, J.; Heaney, R.P.; Henry, J.; Nolan, J.M.; Richardson, D.P.; van Ommen, B.; *et al.* 26th Hohenheim Consensus Conference, September 11, 2010 Scientific substantiation of health claims: Evidence-based nutrition. *Nutrition* **2011**, *27*, S1–S20.

13

The ABC of Vitamin D: A Qualitative Study of the Knowledge and Attitudes Regarding Vitamin D Deficiency amongst Selected Population Groups

Billie Bonevski [1],*, Jamie Bryant [2], Sylvie Lambert [3], Irena Brozek [4] and Vanessa Rock [4]

[1] Priority Research Centre for Translational Neuroscience and Mental Health, Level 5 McAuley Building, Mater Hospital, Cnr Edith & Platt Streets, Waratah, NSW, 2298, Australia
[2] Priority Research Centre in Health Behaviour, School of Medicine and Public Health, University of Newcastle, Hunter Medical Research Institute, Newcastle, 2305, Australia;
     E-Mail: Jamie.Bryant@newcastle.edu.au
[3] Translational Cancer Research Unit, Ingham Institute for Applied Medical Research, South Western Sydney Clinical School, UNSW Medicine, The University of New South Wales, Sydney, 2170, Australia; E-Mail: s.lambert@unsw.edu.au
[4] Cancer Council NSW, PO Box 572 Kings Cross, NSW, 1340, Australia;
     E-Mails: irenab@nswcc.org.au (I.B.); vanessar@nswcc.org.au (V.R.)

*   Author to whom correspondence should be addressed; E-Mail: Billie.bonevski@newcastle.edu.au;

Abstract: Objective: In Australia, vitamin D supply in food is limited, and sun exposure is the main source of vitamin D. However skin cancer risk is high, and the need to gain some sun exposure for adequate vitamin D is challenging public health messages to use protection in the sun. The complex vitamin D public health message may be confusing the public and, in particular, those at highest risk for vitamin D deficiency. This study explored vitamin D and sun exposure attitudes, knowledge and practices of some groups considered at risk of vitamin D deficiency and those delivering healthy sun exposure messages to children. Method: 52 adults participated in six focus groups. Results: Results corroborated with previous research showing low levels of vitamin D knowledge. Individual and environmental barriers to receiving adequate sun exposure were also identified. Conclusions and Implications: The message advocating balanced sun exposure to produce adequate vitamin D needs to be made clearer and be more effectively communicated.

Findings provide insights to aid development of appropriate public health messages for safe sun exposure and vitamin D, especially for vulnerable groups.

Keywords: vitamin D; focus groups; knowledge and attitudes

1. Introduction

While there continues to be uncertainty about recent claims of vitamin D's preventive role with some types of cancers [1,2], autoimmune disorders (such as multiple sclerosis) and possibly cardiovascular diseases [2] and diabetes [3], its essential benefits in the normal development and maintenance of bone health [2,4] have been long known.

In Australia, vitamin D content in food is almost non-existent, and it is predominantly gained from exposure to ultraviolet (UV) sun exposure. Because of its relationship to UV exposure, vitamin D status is associated with geography. There is greater insufficiency of vitamin D at high latitudes, like northern European countries [5–7], but it is also found at low latitudes, like Australia, where UV levels are generally high and rates of skin cancer are amongst the highest in the world [8,9]. This co-occurrence of vitamin D insufficiency and skin cancer is puzzling and has led to the development of guidelines for a balanced approach to sun exposure for both the public [10,11] and health professionals [12]. The balance message suggests some sunlight exposure each day for adequate vitamin D production, but not so much that would lead to increased skin cancer risk.

Population groups at higher risk of vitamin D deficiency include the elderly living in residential care (22%–86% [13,14]), dark skinned and veiled pregnant women (80% [15]), individuals with hip fracture (63% deficiency [16]) and those who cover their skin for religious reasons [17].

Findings from Australian surveys suggest that there is a limited awareness and understanding about vitamin D in the general community [18]. For example, 80% of participants in a community survey were unable to name a health benefit of adequate vitamin D and 15% were unable to give an estimate of the amount of sun exposure needed for vitamin D maintenance [18].

Successful communication of a health message has been associated with changes in people's beliefs about and attitudes toward a risky behaviour and, in turn, changes in that behaviour [19] and the need for messages to be consistent has been highlighted [20,21]. The current vitamin D and sun "balance" message, however, is complex requiring an up-to-date understanding of factors, such as personal skin type, amount of sun exposure, time of day and UV rating, season, latitude and clothing worn [10–12]. While broad community surveys provide valuable prevalence data on the attitudes, knowledge and actions of populations, they often fail to capture more subtle influential factors. For example, is uncertainty regarding amount of sun exposure required for adequate vitamin D [18], due to the sometimes contradictory vitamin D and sun "balance" messages or other factors? Qualitative methods can address these types of issues in the development of public health messages providing a deeper understanding behind reasons for low knowledge or misperceptions. Specifically, focus groups provide an understanding of a target group's motivations, environments, belief systems and health practices [22–24]. To date, no qualitative research exploring these constructs with people with increased risk of vitamin D deficiency or individuals responsible for delivering healthy sun exposure messages to children (teachers) has been published. This study aimed to explore vitamin D and sun exposure attitudes, knowledge and practices of the selected populations using focus groups.

2. Methods

2.1. Study Design

Qualitative focus groups ($n = 6$) were conducted in November 2010, in Sydney, Australia. The Consolidated Criteria for Reporting Qualitative Research framework was used to guide the reporting of the findings [25].

Two health behaviour theories—*Social Cognitive Theory* [26] and *The Health Belief Model* [27]—informed sampling, development of the interview guide and analysis. Social Cognitive Theory suggests that behaviour is influenced by social and physical environments, along with the features of the behaviour [26]. The Health Belief Model specifies that individuals adopt a health protective behaviour (e.g., sun protection for skin cancer or sun exposure for vitamin D), to the extent that they perceive themselves to be susceptible to a health threat (*i.e.*, skin cancer or deficiency), perceive the threat to be severe, perceive the benefits of the proposed health action for mitigating the threat and can overcome perceived barriers to the health behaviour.

2.2. Sample & Recruitment

Participants were English-speaking adults aged over 18 years, living in Sydney, Australia. Purposive sampling ensured participants were recruited from the three groups of interest: (1) teachers (two groups—primary and secondary); (2) office workers (two groups); and (3) elderly (two groups—community dwelling and those in residential aged care facilities).

Recruitment of participants was conducted by an accredited recruitment agency—Stable Research. Participants were recruited from pre-existing registers and supplemented by additional methods (e.g., contacting local aged care facilities). Equal numbers of males and females were targeted across groups. Four focus groups were held in a location with a high migrant population to increase the cultural mix of the sample. "Office workers" were defined as those working in an indoor office at least four days a week. "Community living elderly" were persons aged 65 years living independently and "Elderly living in aged care" were persons aged 65 years and over living in an aged care facility or assisted retirement village.

2.3. Procedure

An independent social market research organisation (IPSOS-Eureka) with experience in qualitative research was engaged to conduct the focus groups. Groups were conducted in four locations across Sydney. Following initial telephone contact by the recruitment agency to determine interest in participating, each participant was mailed an information statement and consent form prior to attending the group discussions. All focus groups were recorded. One of the authors was an observer in the focus groups (IB). All participants were offered $80 reimbursement for time and travel expenses. Ethics approval was granted by the University of Newcastle Human Ethics Research Committee.

2.4. Discussion Guide Content

Each focus group was led by an experienced moderator who used a discussion guide to focus the discussion. Informed by theoretical models outlined above, the discussion guide included items within the broad domains of: knowledge of vitamin D; awareness of vitamin D message; barriers to receiving adequate sun exposure; and communicating the vitamin D message.

2.5. Data Coding and Analysis

Audio recordings were transcribed verbatim. Transcripts were coded by two independent coders (JB & SL) using NVivo version 8 [28]. Each transcript was reviewed line-by-line, and through inductive reasoning, words, statements and paragraphs related to the broad domains of the interview guide were extracted. Through this in-depth analysis, similar excerpts were identified using the same label or code [29]. Codes were either single words (e.g., "*food*", "*sun*") or short phrases (e.g., "*balance between sun exposure and protection*") that captured the essence of the excerpts. Codes were grouped under broad domains of the discussion guide and theoretical constructs (e.g., personal susceptibility to health effects of vitamin D deficiency). Where appropriate, sub-categories were developed to further describe the categories. Three of the six focus groups were analysed by two coders (JB and SL), with discrepancies in coding discussed until a kappa of >0.6 was achieved across 75% of central nodes. The remaining transcripts ($n = 3$) were coded independently by one coder (JB or SL).

3. Results

Fifty-two participants (23 males, 29 females) took part in six focus groups. Groups contained seven to nine participants and ranged from 1 to 1.5 h in duration. Whilst we aimed to include approximately equal numbers of males and females in each group, the group with primary school teachers included only one male participant (see Table 1).

Table 1. Focus group schedule.

	Participants	Male N	Female N
Group 1	Office workers	4	5
Group 2	Independent living adults (65 years+)	5	4
Group 3	Office workers	4	5
Group 4	Community aged home residents (65 years+)	4	5
Group 5	Primary School teachers	1	6
Group 6	Secondary School teachers	5	4

3.1. Knowledge

3.1.1. General Vitamin D Knowledge

Most participants felt they knew less about the benefits or role of Vitamin D in comparison to other vitamins. This was mainly attributed to comparatively limited media attention given to vitamin D compared to other vitamins, such as vitamin C or B. Many participants presumed vitamin D had to be essential and offer some health benefits, but few could name what these were.

3.1.2. Sources of Information about Vitamin D

Several participants could not recall a specific source of information for their knowledge of vitamin D. Sources of information on vitamin D mentioned by participants included (in descending order):

- *Media:* articles in newspapers, magazines and current affairs programs;
- *Doctors*: some participants (primarily with a deficiency in vitamin D) had learnt about vitamin D from their doctor, although often information they had received was limited;
- *Family members/friends:* few participants mentioned that they had heard about vitamin D through family members, friends or significant others;
- *School and further education:* a small number of participants said they had learnt what they know from school or further education.

3.1.3. Vitamin D Testing and Education

Most participants did not know whether their vitamin D level had ever been tested or assumed it had been tested as part of a blood test for a range of things.

> *"... I have a cholesterol test usually at least once a year, but I have got no idea whether there is a vitamin D component in that."* (Independent aged)

Most participants tested and found to be low in vitamin D did not recall being told by their doctor why it was important, the consequences of inadequate vitamin D or how much sun was needed each day to ensure adequate vitamin D. Rather, it was common for participants to report that they had simply been told they *"need to get out in the sun more"* or advised to take a supplement.

> *"No, he [doctor] didn't [explain why Vitamin D was important], he just recommended [...] I take Caltrac with vitamin D. That was it."* (Office worker)

3.2. Awareness

3.2.1. Knowledge of Times and Seasons for Sun Protection

Many participants identified mid-day or the hottest time of the day as the critical period when sun protection is needed.

Early morning (e.g., before 10:00) or late afternoon (e.g., after 15:00) was perceived as the ideal time to spend time in the sun, because *"you still get the sunshine, but you are not getting it as intense."* (Primary school teacher).

3.2.2. Knowledge about Amount of Sun Exposure Required for Adequate Vitamin D

Many participants admitted they were unsure of how long was needed to be in the sun for adequate vitamin D. There was a tendency however to overestimate the time required in summer, with 15–20 min being the most common response. Participants identified that time needed in the sun to get enough vitamin D might vary according to age, skin colour/type and nutrition. Discussion about the amount of sun exposure raised many questions regarding the impact of clothing and sunscreen.

"How much exposure, too, I mean, I was out in the sun yesterday with arms exposed. I mean, is that the same as, do I need 20 min of that, whereas I can stay outside in the nude for three minutes?" (Primary school teacher)

3.2.3. Knowledge about Groups at Higher Risk of Vitamin D Deficiency

Participants identified groups that may be at increased risk of vitamin D deficiency in Australia, including; the elderly or individuals who might have difficulty getting outside (e.g., immobile due to disability), workers confined to an office during the day, shift workers and those who cover their skin for religious reasons.

3.3. Personal Behaviours and Perceived Risk

Personal UV Exposure for Adequate Vitamin D

Current guidelines for vitamin D were communicated to participants (see Table 2), and most felt they were getting adequate sunlight in the summer months on most days of the week. Most school teachers and office workers thought they would easily meet the recommendations on most days in summer, spring and autumn, largely through incidental exposure. While most adults over 65 also thought they would meet recommendations on most days, this was often dependent on the weather. Several participants were surprised at the length of exposure needed in winter, and most reported that they would not meet recommendations in winter.

"No. I don't think in winter I would in a day. Especially when you have a week, like days of rain and ... I don't think in winter." (Primary school teacher)

Table 2. Summary of key Australian guidelines for sun exposure for vitamin D sufficiency for the general population (moderate fair skin) and people at high risk of vitamin D deficiency.

	General Population
a	Fair skinned people can achieve adequate vitamin D levels (>50 nmol/L) in summer by exposing the face, arms and hands or the equivalent area of skin to a few minutes of sunlight on either side of peak UV periods on most days of the week. In winter, in the southern regions of Australia, where UV radiation levels are less intense, maintenance of vitamin D levels may require 2–3 h of sunlight exposure to the face, arms and hands or equivalent area of skin over a week.
b	In Sydney, in December to January (Australian summer), 6 to 8 min at 10 am or 2 pm. In Sydney, in July to August (Australian winter), 26 to 28 min at 10 am or 2 pm or 16 min at 12 noon.
	People at high risk of vitamin D deficiency
a	Naturally dark skinned people (Fitzpatrick skin type 5 and 6) are relatively protected from skin cancer by the pigment in their skin; they could safely increase their sun exposure. Other people at high risk of vitamin D deficiency should discuss their vitamin D status with their medical practitioner, as some might benefit from dietary supplementation with vitamin D.
b	Vitamin D supplementation is likely to be required for this population group.

[a] The Risks and Benefits of Sun Exposure Position Statement. Approved by the Australian and New Zealand Bone and Mineral Society, Osteoporosis Australia, The Australasian College of Dermatologists and the Cancer Council Australia; updated 2007; [b] Calcium, Vitamin D and Osteoporosis [12].

Communication of the guidelines prompted questions from participants seeking more detail about the type of exposure needed. Participants were unsure how sunscreen and protective clothing affected the absorption of vitamin D and whether it is possible to "store" vitamin D by having longer period of sun exposure, but on fewer days per week. Several participants also wondered whether it would be equally acceptable to spend a shorter period of time in the more 'intense' sunlight during the middle of the day to get a *"boost [...] of vitamin D"* (Independent aged).

3.4. Barriers

3.4.1. Barriers to Receiving Sun Exposure for Adequate Vitamin D

A number of barriers to receiving adequate sun exposure were identified: lack of information and knowledge about the effects of vitamin D deficiency, concern about skin cancer and sun burn, ability to go outside, the weather and work. Overall, participants were much more aware of the "SunSmart" message than the "vitamin D" message and almost unanimously more concerned about preventing skin cancer than about ensuring they get enough vitamin D. Two reasons seemed to underpin these findings. Promotion of the "SunSmart" message, as well as an awareness of the dangers of skin cancer has led to participants purposefully limiting their sun exposure. In comparison, vitamin D deficiency seemed inconsequential and not serious enough to warrant any specific action.

> *"The consequences I think are greater. It's [skin cancer] deadly, and you die a lot quicker*
> *from cancer than you can from vitamin D deficiency..."* (Secondary school teacher)

Several participants highlighted that the "SunSmart" and "vitamin D" messages seem contradictory—on the one hand, the recommendation is to cover up and on the other hand, the recommendation is to expose skin. A few participants also mentioned that in addition to skin cancer, they were concerned about sunburn and, consequently, limited their exposure. Extremes of weather, including the summer heat and wet weather, being unable to go outside due to medical conditions and physical ability were identified as barriers to sun exposure.

3.4.2. Ways to Address the Barriers to Increase Sun Exposure

The majority of participants' suggestions to help them meet recommendations for sun exposure centred around increasing incidental exposure, such as by parking the car further away from their destination, a brief walk at lunchtime and eating meals outdoors. Only one office worker and a secondary school teacher identified fortifying food with vitamin D or taking a supplement as a way of receiving adequate vitamin D.

3.4.3. Communicating the Vitamin D Message

Overall, participants felt the vitamin D message had not been effectively communicated. Participants made recommendations as to how to communicate the vitamin D message (communication medium) and what needs to be communicated (type of message).

Communication medium: Television advertising was considered the communication medium of choice, followed by newspapers, magazines and radio. New media, including the internet, Facebook and "pop-up" ads on websites, such as Google, were identified as potentially effective ways of communicating the message, particularly to adolescents and young adults.

Doctors and pharmacists were considered a good source of information about vitamin D, especially for the elderly.

Type of message: Participants suggested that messages relating to vitamin D should focus on providing education, but stressed that "It's got to be a simple message. If it's too complicated, your eyes just glaze over and you think about something else." (Independent aged).

While number of participants suggested combining recommendations for acquiring adequate vitamin D with related messages, such as the *Slip! Slop! Slap!* Message, an equal number of participants were concerned this could cause confusion and be counter-productive. There was particular concern that mixed messages could be used as an excuse by children and adolescents to be out in the sun without sun protection. One participant suggested that the message should only be targeted at those who are at-risk.

4. Discussion

This study used qualitative methods to explore understanding and awareness of the vitamin D message and opportunities and barriers to UV exposure. Focus groups were conducted with individuals at risk for vitamin D deficiency, including people who have limited access to outdoor sunlight through the day, including indoor office workers and elderly people in aged care facilities. The study provides new and unique knowledge in this emerging area, with implications for the development of the "balance" message.

4.1. Low Knowledge and Awareness about Balancing the Benefits and Risks of Sun Exposure

The almost complete lack of awareness of the balance message and low levels of knowledge about vitamin D were not surprising. Previous quantitative community surveys conducted in Australia, although mostly in Queensland, have found similar results [18,30]. Furthermore, some research suggests that people who intentionally tan claim to do so for their vitamin D status. Thus, the misunderstanding about vitamin D may be placing people at risk of skin cancer. Our participants were unable to name the health benefits of vitamin D with certainty, had little awareness of UV times of the day for adequate vitamin D exposure and most were unaware of the amount of time in the sun they required. Most participants had not had previous exposure to the current guidelines for sun exposure, and when the message was communicated, it prompted several questions. These results and previous quantitative studies suggest that current communication of the "balance" message is not reaching most of the community. Unlike previous studies that have found that the vitamin D message is being misinterpreted, particularly by people who intentionally suntan putting themselves at risk of skin cancer [30], the current study found people continued to heed the sun protection message, even during winter and outside of peak UV times. These results suggest that even those at risk of deficiency are not aware of the need to increase their vitamin D intake.

One factor, which may be contributing to the low levels of knowledge and difficulty in communicating the "balance" sun exposure message, is the lack of conclusive research evidence regarding how much time the public needs in direct UV exposure in order to assist their vitamin D status. Currently, the message is complex and different according to location, season and individual characteristics. Broad recommendations for the amount of skin an individual needs to expose to the sun and the amount of time to be exposed are based on incomplete data. As further research evidence is gathered, the messages will be made clearer and communicated more confidently.

4.2. High Levels of SunSmart Awareness and Sun Avoidance Behaviours

Slogans, such as *Slip! Slop! Slap!* and SunSmart, have very high public recognition, and there has been considerable policy and practice in place in Australia since the early 1980s that reinforces sun protective behaviour [31]. Two related themes emerged in the discussions that reflect this situation. Firstly, the SunSmart message has been effectively communicated and adopted by study participants. Use of sun protection amongst this group was largely "normalised", and most participants reported frequently using sun protection measures. Secondly, the message that skin cancer is a high risk concern had been effectively communicated and taken up by participants. Participants stated they were more concerned about skin cancer than vitamin D deficiency.

One consequence of the success of the SunSmart messages is that some participants reported the need to use sun protection at all times, with some participants feeling that there was no safe time to be exposed, especially in summer. Encouragingly, most participants identified the middle of the day as unsuitable, and some believed that early morning or late afternoon were suitable for safe sun exposure. No participants offered "outside of peak UV times" as appropriate times to be in the sun. Instead, generic "early" and "late" in the day times were offered. This suggests that the UV Alert, which may be an appropriate tool for displaying safe and unsafe sun exposure times of the day, requires further promotion and education for people to understand and use the ratings.

4.3. Barriers to Sun Exposure for Vitamin D

Incidental exposure during the day was the most common type of sun exposure reported, with more time spent outside on weekends than weekdays. This type of sun exposure may not be sufficient for vitamin D, given that the recommendation of up to 10 min outside of peak UV time is based on estimates from ideal conditions of sun exposure (clear, open sky and an unshaded, horizontal surface) and may not correspond to typical outdoor behaviours [32]. This is the first study to explore barriers to sun exposure for vitamin D. Types of barriers participants in all groups reported included lack of knowledge about the need for vitamin D, concerns about sunburn, the need to use sun protection when outdoors and environmental barriers, including the weather (wet, hot and cold weather), work hours indoors (indoor workers group) and physical inabilities to go outside (aged care group). Development of vitamin D public health education and campaigns need to address these barriers.

4.4. Strategies to Overcome the Barriers

Increasing incidental sun exposure through routine, daily, outdoor activities was the main strategy identified by participants for increasing sun exposure for vitamin D. Examples included parking the car ten minutes away from work and walking the distance and eating lunch outside the workplace. Improving education about the need for sun exposure and vitamin D was also suggested. Channels for communicating the vitamin D message included the mass media and internet, schools, doctors and pharmacists. While the mass media has been informally used to date, it's reporting of health news is less than optimal [33] and has been accused of misrepresenting the vitamin D issue and confusing the message further [34,35]. Alternatively, doctors and pharmacists may be better placed as providers of information, where the benefits and risks can be communicated in a balanced manner and various factors considered in calculating risk and need (including latitude, skin type, season and time of day). Doctors, in particular, frequently need to manage the communication of uncertainties, risks and benefits of medical therapies [36]. However, the results of this study suggest that participants' doctors were not informing their patients about their vitamin D status. Other research suggests this may be due to low levels of knowledge about vitamin D amongst doctors [37]. Clearly, further efforts into educating both the media and health professionals about vitamin D is needed.

There was a division of opinion regarding whether the vitamin D message should be linked to the *Slip! Slop! Slap! Seek and Slide* message. Whilst some participants felt it was a natural way to communicate the balance message, others believed this strategy would confuse the messages and cause negative consequences, including increased tanning. Others have suggested that the vitamin D message can complement SunSmart messages in Australia [31], particularly if the UV Alert is effectively incorporated. Some research has started to suggest that younger tanners are using the need for vitamin D as a reason for their sun tanning behaviours [38]. This highlights the need to carefully explore all the factors that may affect the interpretation and use of a balance message among a variety of target groups and identify methods for communicating the message. A tailored approach with messages designed for different groups may be the most effective and safe. The need for a consistent and simple message was reinforced.

4.5. Study Strengths and Weaknesses

This study is one of the first qualitative studies of the knowledge and attitudes of groups at risk of vitamin D deficiency. The use of the theoretical models proved instrumental to shaping aspects of the study. The focus groups found that social and physical environments, as proposed in the Social Cognitive Model, played a role in lack of UV exposure, both for office workers and elderly persons. As predicted by the Health Belief Model, perceived susceptibility to skin cancer and sunburn was greater than risk of vitamin D deficiency, and perceptions of the severity of the skin cancer and sunburn threats were greater than the threat of vitamin D deficiency. An examination of the barriers to the desired health behaviour revealed suggestions for overcoming the barriers. As a result, the study provides valuable insight into peoples' understanding of the vitamin D and sun exposure message. Other strengths of this formative research are its inclusion of groups at higher risk for vitamin D deficiency and a high number of participants. The use of multiple researchers to collect and analyse the qualitative data also reduced the potential for investigator bias in interpreting the findings. The generalizability of study results is limited, due to two main reasons. First, only select groups were included in the study. Secondly, detailed demographic or skin cancer history information about participants was not collected. Further research is required to generalise these findings to other types of community groups or individuals, including those with darker skin types or those who wear veiled clothing.

Conflict of Interest

The authors declare no conflict of interest.

Author Contributions

BB and VR conceived of the study and developed the study protocol. BB and JB developed study materials. IB was an observer during focus groups. JB and SL conducted coding and analysis. All authors contributed to paper writing.

References

1. Garland, C.F.; Garland, F.C.; Gorham, E.D.; Lipkin, M.; Newmark, H.; Mohr, S.B.; Holick, M. The role of vitamin D in cancer prevention. *Am. J. Public Health* **2005**, *96*, 252–261.
2. Holick, M.F. Sunlight and vitamin D for bone health and the prevention of autoimmune diseases, cancers and cardiovasular disease. *Am. J. Clin. Nutr.* **2004**, *80*, 1678s–1688s.
3. Hypponen, E. Vitamin D and the Risk of Type 1 Diabetes. In *Vitamin D: Physiology, Molecular Biology, and Clinical Applications (Nutrition and Health)*; Hollick, M.F., Ed.; Humana Press: New York, NY, USA, 2010; pp. 867–879.
4. Holick, M.F. vitamin D and bone health. *J. Nutr.* **1996**, *126*, 11595–11645.
5. Moan, J.; Porojnicu, A.C.; Dahlback, A.; Setlow, R.B. Addressing the health benefits and risks, involving vitamin D or skin cancer, of increased sun exposure. *Proc. Natl. Acad. Sci. USA* **2008**, *105*, 668–673.
6. Vik, T.; Try, K.; Stromme, J.H. The vitamin D status of man at 70 degrees north. *Scand. J. Clin. Lab. Invest.* **1980**, *40*, 227–232.
7. Brustad, M.; Alaser, E.; Engelsen, O.; Aksnes, L.; Lund, E. Vitamin D status of middle aged women at 65–71 degrees north in relation to dietary intake and exposure to ultraviolet radiation. *Public Health Nutr.* **2004**, *7*, 327–335.
8. McGrath, J.J.; Kimlin, M.G.; Saha, S.; Eyles, D.; Parisi, A. Vitamin D insufficiency in southeast queensland. *Med. J. Aust.* **2001**, *174*, 150–151.
9. Pasco, J.A.; Henry, M.J.; Nicholson, G.C.; Sanders, K.M.; Kotowicz, M.A. Vitamin D status of women in the geelong osteoporosis study: Association with diet and casual exposure to sunlight. *Med. J. Aust.* **2001**, *175*, 401–405.
10. Australian New Zealand Bone and Mineral Society; Osteoporosis Australia; The Australasian College of Dermatologists; and the Cancer Council Australia. Risks and benefits of sun exposure position statement, updated 2007. Available online: http://www.Dermcoll.Asn.Au/downloads/ccrisksandbenefitsmarch8.Pdf (accessed on 20 January 2011).
11. American Academy of Dermatology Updated position statement on vitamin D. Available online: http://www.aad.org/media/background/news/Releases/American_Academy_of_Dermatology_Issues_Updated_Pos/ (accessed on 20 January 2011).
12. Osteoporosis Australia. Calcium, vitamin D and osteoporosis. A guide for gps, 2nd ed.; 2008. Available online: http:/www.Osteoporosis.Org.Au/files/factsheets/oth-7665-eng.Pdf (accessed on 20 January 2011).

13. Flicker, L.; Mead, K.; Macinnis, R.J.; Nowson, C.; CScherer, S.; Stein, M.S.; Thomasx, J.; Hopper, J.L.; Wark, J.D. Serum vitamin D and falls in older women in residential care in australia. *J. Am. Geriatr. Soc.* **2003**, *51*, 1533–1538.

14. Sambrook, P.N.; Cameron, I.D.; Cumming, R.G.; Lord, S.R.; Schwarz, J.M.; Trube, A.; March, L.M. Vitamin D deficiency is common in frail institutionalised older people in northern sydney. *Med. J. Aust.* **2002**, *176*, 560.

15. Grover, S.R.; Morley, R. Vitamin D deficiency in veiled or dark skinned pregnant women. *Med. J. Aust.* **2001**, *175*, 251–252.

16. Diamond, T.; Smerdely, P.; Kormas, N.; Sekel, R.; Vu, T.; Day, P. Hip fracture in elderly men: The importance of subclinical vitamin D deficiency and hypogonadism. *Med. J. Aust.* **1998**, *169*, 138–141.

17. Hatun, S.; Islam, O.; Cizmecioglu, F.; Kara, B.; Babaoglu, K.; Berk, F.; Gökalp, A.S. Subclinical vitamin D deficiency is increased in adolescent girls who wear concealing clothing. *J. Nutr.* **2005**, *135*, 218–222.

18. Janda, M.; Youl, P.; Bolz, K.; Niland, C.; Kimlin, M. Knowledge about the health benefits of vitamin D in queensland australia. *Prev. Med.* **2010**, *50*, 215–216.

19. Rosenstock, I.M.; Strecher, V.J.; Becker, M.H. Social learning theory and the health belief model. *Health Educ. Q.* **1988**, *15*, 175–183.

20. McGuire, W.J. Public communication as a strategy for inducing health-promoting behavioural change. *Prev. Med.* **1984**, *13*, 299–319.

21. Rogers, E.M. *Diffusion of Innovations*; The Free Press: New York, NY, USA, 1993.

22. Kirby, S.; Baranowski, T.; Reynolds, K.D.; Taylor, G.; Binkley, D. Children's fruit and vegetable intake: Socioeconomic, adult-child, regional, and urban-rural influences. *J. Nutr. Educ.* **1995**, *27*, 261–271.

23. Green, L.W.; Kreuter, M. *Health Promotion Planning: An Educational and Environmental Approach*, 2nd ed.; Mayfield: Mountain View, CA, USA, 1991.

24. Glanz, K.; Lewis, F.M.; Rimer, B.K. *Health Behavior and Health Education: Theory, Research, and Practice*, 2nd ed.; Jossey-Bass: San Francisco, CA, USA, 1997.

25. Tong, A.; Sainsbury, P.; Craig, J. Consolidated criteria for reporting qualitative research (coreq): A 32-item checklist for interviews and focus groups. *Int. J. Qual. Health Care* **2007**, *19*, 349–357.

26. Bandura, A. *Social Foundations of Thought and Action: A Social Cognitive Theory*; Prentice-Hall: Englewood Cliffs, NJ, USA, 1986.

27. Strecher, V.J.; Rosenstock, I.M. *The Health Belief Model*, 2nd ed.; Jossey-Bass: San Francisco, CA, USA, 1997.

28. *NVivo Qualitative Data Analysis Software*, version 8; QSR International Pty Ltd.: Doncaster, Australia, 2008.

29. Holloway, I.; Wheeler, S. *Qualitative Research in Nursing*, 2nd ed.; Blackwell Publishing: Melbourne, Australia, 2002.

30. Youl, P.; Janda, M.; Kimlin, M.G. vitamin D and sun protection: The impact of mixed messages in australia. *Int. J. Cancer* **2008**, *124*, 1963–1970.

31. Sinclair, C. Risks and benefits of sun exposure: Implications for public health practice based on the australian experience. *Prog. Biophys. Mol. Biol.* **2006**, *92*, 173–178.

32. Diffey, B.L. Is casual exposure to summer sunlight effective at maintaining adequate vitamin D status? *Photodermatol. Photoimmunol. Photomed.* **2010**, *26*, 172–176.

33. Wilson, A.; Bonevski, B.; Jones, A.; Henry, D. Deconstructing cancer: What makes a good quality news story. *Med. J. Aust.* **2010**, *193*, 702–706.

34. Kemp, G.A.; Eagle, L.; Verne, J. Mass media barriers to social marketing interventions: The example of sun protection in the uk. *Health Promot. Int.* **2010**, *26*, 37–45.

35. Scully, M.; Wakefield, M.; Dixon, H. Trends in news coverage about skin cancer prevention, 1993-2006: Increasingly mixed messages for the public. *Aust. N. Z. J. Public Health* **2008**, *32*, 461–466.

36. Politi, M.C.; Han, P.K.J.; Col, N.F. Communicating the uncertainty of harms and benefits of medical interventions. *Med. Decis. Mak.* **2007**, *27*, 681.

37. Bonevski, B.; Girgis, A.; Magin, P.; Horton, G.; Brozek, I.; Armstrong, B. Prescribing sunshine: A survey of general practitioners' knowledge, attitudes and practices relating to the sun and vitamin D. *Int. J. Cancer* **2011**, *130*, 2138–2145.

38. Woo, D.K.; Eide, M.J. Tanning beds, skin cancer, and vitamin D: An examination of the scientific evidence and public health implications. *Dermatol. Ther.* **2010**, *23*, 61–71.

14

Increased Plasma Concentrations of Vitamin D Metabolites and Vitamin D Binding Protein in Women Using Hormonal Contraceptives

Ulla K. Møller [1,*], **Susanna við Streym** [1], **Lars T. Jensen** [2], **Leif Mosekilde** [1], **Inez Schoenmakers** [3], **Shailja Nigdikar** [3] and **Lars Rejnmark** [1]

[1] Department of Endocrinology and Internal Medicine, THG, Aarhus University Hospital, Tage Hansens Gade 2, DK, Aarhus 8000, Denmark;
E-Mails: susanna.vid.streym@gmail.com (S.S.); leif.mosekilde@gmail.com (L.M.); rejnmark@post6.tele.dk (L.R.)

[2] Department of Clinical Physiology, Glostrup University Hospital, Copenhagen DK-2900, Denmark;
E-Mail: lars.thorbjoern.jensen@regionh.dk

[3] MRC Human Nutrition Research, Cambridge CB1 9NL, UK;
E-Mails: inez.schoenmakers@mrc-hnr.cam.ac.uk (I.S.); shailja.nigdikar@mrc-hnr.cam.ac.uk (S.N.)

* Author to whom correspondence should be addressed; E-Mail: kristine.moller@ki.au.dk;

Abstract: Use of hormonal contraceptives (HC) may influence total plasma concentrations of vitamin D metabolites. A likely cause is an increased synthesis of vitamin D binding protein (VDBP). Discrepant results are reported on whether the use of HC affects free concentrations of vitamin D metabolites. *Aim*: In a cross-sectional study, plasma concentrations of vitamin D metabolites, VDBP, and the calculated free vitamin D index in users and non-users of HC were compared and markers of calcium and bone metabolism investigated. *Results:* 75 Caucasian women aged 25–35 years were included during winter season. Compared with non-users (n = 23), users of HC (n = 52) had significantly higher plasma concentrations of 25-hydroxyvitamin D (25OHD) (median 84 interquartile range: [67–111] *vs.* 70 [47–83] nmol/L, p = 0.01), 1,25-dihydroxyvitamin D (1,25(OH)$_2$D) (198 [163–241] *vs.* 158 [123–183] pmol/L, p = 0.01) and VDBP (358 [260–432] *vs.* 271 [179–302] µg/mL, p < 0.001). However, the calculated free indices (FI-25OHD and FI-1,25(OH)$_2$D) were not significantly different between groups (p > 0.10). There were no significant differences in indices of calcium homeostasis (plasma concentrations of calcium, parathyroid hormone, and calcitonin, $p > 0.21$) or bone metabolism (plasma bone specific alkaline phosphatase, osteocalcin, and urinary NTX/creatinine ratio) between groups. *In conclusion:* Use of HC is associated with 13%–25% higher concentrations of total vitamin D metabolites and VDBP. This however is not reflected in indices of calcium or bone metabolism. Use of HC should be considered in the interpretation of plasma concentrations vitamin D metabolites.

Keywords: hormonal contraceptives; 25hydroxyvitamin D; 1,25-dihydroxyvitamin D; vitamin D binding protein; parathyroid hormone; calcitonin; bone turnover; bone mineral density

---

1. Introduction

Vitamin D (calciferol) is obtained from endogenous synthesis in the skin in response to solar UV-B radiation and intake from the diet and supplements [1,2]. Once in the circulation, calciferol is converted to 25-hydroxyvitamin D (25OHD) in the liver and, subsequently, to its circulating biologically active form 1,25-dihydroxyvitamin D ($1,25(OH)_2D$) in the kidney [3]. This conversion may also occur in other tissues for auto- or paracrine actions [4]. It has been estimated that 85% to 90% of 25OHD and $1,25(OH)_2D$ is bound to vitamin D binding protein (VDBP) [5], 10% to 15% to albumin, whereas only a very small fraction (<0.1%) circulates in its free form [5,6]. VDBP binding protects vitamin D metabolites from hydroxylase-mediated catabolism, affects their cellular uptake, and modulates their biological activity [5,6].

Total plasma concentrations of 25OHD are considered an indicator of vitamin D status due to its long plasma half-life (approximately 15–35 days) and lack of hormonal control of the hepatic 25-hydroxylase [3].

Vitamin D is known to affect several health outcomes. Classically, low vitamin D concentrations are known to be associated with an increased risk of myopathy, rickets or osteomalacia, and low bone mineral density and fracture. In a number of recent studies, an impaired vitamin D status has also been associated with various adverse non-skeletal health outcomes such as an increased risk of malignancies or cardiovascular diseases [1].

Plasma 25OHD concentrations are influenced by many factors. In addition to variations in UVB-exposure and dietary intake, 25OHD concentrations are influenced by several host factors such as age, adiposity [2,7,8], ethnicity, and skin tone as well as certain genotypes [8,9], and plasma VDBP concentrations [5].

Pregnancy is known to be associated with an increase in VDBP through its oestrogen mediated increase in synthesis [10,11]. Plasma concentrations of 25OHD are reported to be unaltered and $1,25(OH)_2D$ to be elevated compared to non-pregnant women [12–14]. The use of hormonal contraceptives (HC) may also affect 25OHD concentrations and metabolism due to their oestrogenic components. The limited data on the effects of HC on 25OHD concentrations report no change or an increase in total 25OHD [9,12,15–17], whereas most studies consistently report an increase in levels of $1,25(OH)_2D$ and VDBP [10,15,18–20].

These data suggest that HC may cause differential effects on 25OHD and 1,25(OH)$_2$D; the free 25OHD index (the molar ratio of 25OHD- to VDBP-concentrations) may be decreased due to an absence of a parallel increase in VDBP and 25OHD, whereas the free index of 1,25(OH)$_2$D may remain unchanged.

In order to study the possible effects of HC, we compared plasma concentrations of 25OHD, 1,25(OH)$_2$D, VDBP, and the calculated free vitamin D index in users and non-users of HC. In addition, we assessed possible impacts of HC on calcium homeostasis and bone metabolism.

2. Subjects and Methods

This paper reports a secondary analysis of the effects of HC on vitamin D metabolism in a subset of women participating in a population based controlled cohort study, using cross-sectional data obtained at baseline. The design of the study has previously been reported in detail [12,21]. In brief, we included 153 healthy Caucasian women, aged 25–35 years, trying to conceive, and 75 age-matched women not planning a pregnancy for the next 21 months. All women were recruited by direct mailing of 11,175 randomly selected women from a population of 21,317 women aged 25–35 years living in the community of Aarhus, Denmark. We obtained names and addresses from the Danish Civil Registration System. A total of 561 wished to participate, from which 333 were excluded as based on predefined exclusion criteria (Pregnant or breastfeeding at the start of the study ($n = 85$), known infertility ($n = 46$), miscarriage within last 6 months ($n = 3$), withdrawal or moved residence ($n = 84$), age, illness, foreign origin ($n = 25$), or responded after closure of recruitment ($n = 90$)). Analyses reported in this paper only include data obtained in the group of women ($n = 75$) not planning a pregnancy, of which 52 were using hormonal contraception (including oral, subdermal contraceptive implant, or hormonal spiral methods). They were all included between October 2006 and April 2007. The study was performed according to The Helsinki Declaration II. The study was notified to the Danish Data Protection Agency (#2004-41-4737) and approved by the Regional Scientific Ethical Committee of Aarhus County (#20040186).

2.1. Measurements

Standing height and body weight were measured (Seca, Sa-med, Kvistgaard, Denmark) wearing indoor clothing. Incident diseases and the use of drugs were recorded. Participants were asked to fill in a questionnaire on medical conditions, smoking habits, and dietary intake of calcium as well as use of calcium and vitamin D containing supplements. Dietary intake of calcium was assessed as previously described [22] and total calcium intake was calculated as dietary intake plus intake from supplements.

2.2. Biochemistry

A non-fasting blood sample was drawn between 8 a.m. and 2 p.m. according to standardized procedures and centrifuged at 4 °C with a relative centrifugal force of 2500 g for 10 min. Plasma was separated and stored at −80 °C until analyzed. Urine and plasma samples were assessed in batches, *i.e.*, all samples from each participant were analyzed in the same run, except for analysis of calcium, creatinine, and phosphate, which were analyzed within two hours after collection. A second void morning urine sample was collected at home. Urine samples were collected under fasting conditions or before any consumption of calcium rich foods. Plasma 25-hydroxyvitamin D (25OHD) concentrations were measured by isotope dilution liquid chromatography–tandem mass spectrometry (LC-MS/MS) by a method adapted from Maunsell *et al.* [23,24]. The method separately quantifies $25OHD_2$ and total $25OHD_3$ (including the 3-epimer). The total 25OHD concentration was calculated and used for further analyses. Calibrators traceable to NIST SRM 972 (Chromsystems, DE) were used. The inter-assay CV was <10%, at plasma concentrations of 23.4 nmol/L ($25OHD_2$) and 24.8 nmol/L ($25OHD_3$). We determined plasma 1,25-dihydroxyvitamin D ($1,25(OH)_2D$) concentrations by a radioimmunoassay (Gamma-B 1,25-Dihydroxy Vitamin D, Immunodiagnostic Systems (IDS) Ltd., Boldon, England). The inter- and intra-assay CV was 9.0% and 8.0%, respectively, at 220 pmol/L.

Vitamin D binding protein concentration was determined by ELISA (R & D Systems, Abingdon, UK) with both an inter- and intra-assay CV < 6%. Assay performance was monitored using kit and in-house controls and under strict standardization according to ISO 9001:2000.

The free fraction of 25OHD and $1,25(OH)_2D$ were calculated as the free 25OHD index (FI-25OHD) and the free $1,25(OH)_2D$ index (FI-$1,25(OH)_2D$) using the molar ratio of 25OHD and $1,25(OH)_2D$ to VDBP [11].

We determined plasma and urinary concentrations of calcium and creatinine (Cr) by standard laboratory methods and calculated the albumin adjusted calcium concentration according to the formula: plasma calcium, adjusted [mmol/L] = plasma calcium, total [mmol/L] + 0.00086 × (650-plasma albumin μmol/L) [22].

Calcitonin was measured by a radioimmunoassay as described by Schifter [25]. The plasma concentrations of intact parathyroid hormone (PTH) and osteocalcin were measured with electro-chemiluminescence immunoassays using an automated instrument (Cobas 601e, Roche Diagnostics, GmbH, Mannheim, Germany). We measured plasma bone specific alkaline phosphatase concentrations by an immunoassay (METRA BAP EIA kit, Quidel Corporation, San Diego, CA, USA). The renal excretion of cross-linked *N*-terminal telopeptide of type 1 collagen (NTx) was quantified by ELISA using an automated instrument (Vitros ECI, Ortho Clinical Diagnostics, Amersham, UK). Results were expressed relative to creatinine (Cr) excretion (NTx/Cr), as nmol of bone collagen equivalents (nMmol BCE) per mmol of creatinine. The CV was 9.6% at 41.5 nmol BCE/mmol Cr.

We measured bone mineral density (BMD) of the whole body, the lumbar spine, and total hip. Total body fat and lean mass were measured. All DXA scans were performed using a Hologic Discovery scanner (Hologic, Waltham, MA, USA). We assessed long-term stability through daily scans of an anthropometrical phantom. Precision error for BMD was 1% at the lumbar spine and 2% at the total hip.

2.3. Statistics

The majority of the data were non-normally distributed, therefore descriptive statistics are reported as medians with the 25 and 75-percentile (p25; p75), unless stated otherwise. We explored the differences between groups using chi-square tests for categorical variables and a Mann-Whitney *U*-test for continuous variables. Spearman's rho correlation was used to calculate the magnitude and direction of the correlations between measured variables.

Vitamin D status was described according to plasma 25OHD concentrations categorized into three groups: 25OHD < 50 nmol/L; 25OHD between 50.1 and 75 nmol/L, 25OHD > 75.1 nmol/L [26].

All statistical analyses were performed using the Statistical Package for Social Sciences (SPSS 17, Chicago, IL, USA) for Windows. *P*-values below 0.05 were considered statistically significant.

3. Results

Table 1 shows characteristics of the 75 included women. Anthropometric-, diet-, and lifestyle-characteristics did not differ between women using hormonal contraceptives (HC) ($n = 52$) and non-users ($n = 23$), except that daily calcium intake was slightly higher in users- compared with non-users of HC ($p = 0.02$).

Table 1. Characteristic of the 75 studied women stratified by use of hormonal contraceptives. Median with interquartile (p25; p75) ranges unless otherwise indicated.

	All, *n* = 75	Users of hormonal contraceptive (*n* = 52)	Non-users of hormonal contraceptives (*n* = 23)	*p* value [1]
Age, mean	29 (27; 32)	29 (27; 32)	29 (26; 33)	0.81
Weight, kg	67 (60; 77)	69 (63; 77)	63 (57; 80)	0.12
Height, cm	168 (163; 172)	167 (162; 172)	169 (163; 172)	0.61
BMI	24 (22; 27)	25 (23; 27)	23 (20; 27)	0.12
Total calcium intake, mg/day	800 (660; 975)	850 (700; 1000)	700 (500; 853)	*0.02*
Use of vitamin D supplements, *n* (%)	24 (32)	17 (33)	7 (30)	1.00
Vitamin D intake from supplements (μg/day)	5 (5; 9)	5 (5; 10)	5 (5; 5)	
Smoking, *n* (%)	11 (15)	7 (14)	4 (17)	0.71

[1] Independent-Samples Mann-Whitney U Test.

Of the 52 HC users, 44 used oral HC, six used intrauterine hormonal device, one used sub-dermal contraceptive implant, and one used a vaginal ring. No differences in biochemical markers were seen between the 44 using oral HC and the six using intrauterine hormonal device (data not shown).

Physical activity, time spend outdoor, and the time of the day for blood sampling did not differ between the HC users and no-users of HC (data not shown). The number of women with a BMI above 25 was not different between users- and non-HC users. BMD at whole body, lumbar spine, and total hip, as well as fat and lean mass did not differ between the HC users and no-users of HC (data not shown). However, given the sample size of 23 non-HC users and 52 users our statistical power to detect a 5% difference between groups in lumbar spine BMD ($2\alpha = 0.05$ and $\beta = 0.20$) was only approximately 60%.

When all data were pooled, the plasma concentrations of 25OHD was significantly and positively correlated with VDBP ($r_s = 0.26$, $p = 0.03$) (Figure 1A) and further with 1,25(OH)$_2$D ($r_s = 0.43$, $p < 0.01$).

Figure 1. (A) Scatter plot of linear relations between plasma 25OHD and VDBP in 75 healthy Caucasian women stratified by use of hormonal contraceptives; **(B)** Scatter plot of linear relations between plasma 1,25OH$_2$D and VDBP in 75 healthy Caucasian women stratified by use of hormonal contraceptives.

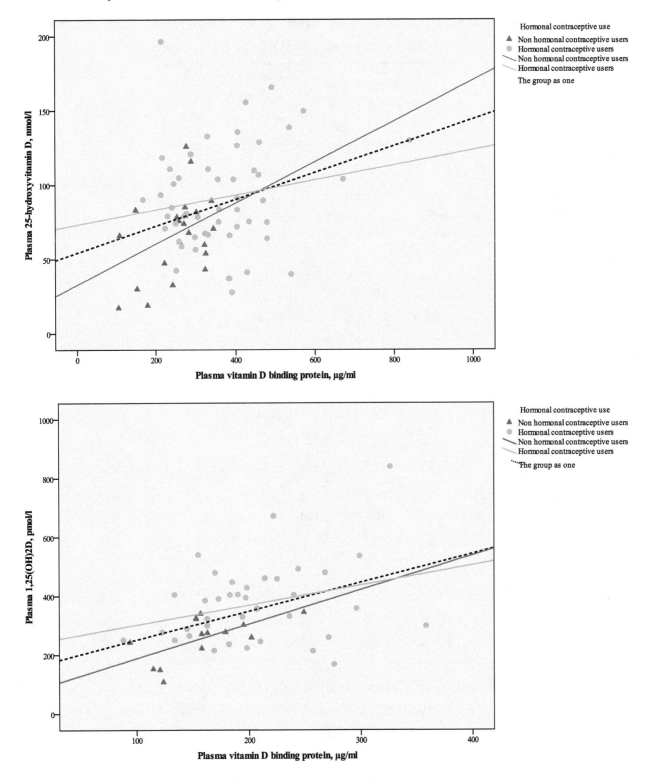

Plasma 1,25(OH)$_2$D was significantly and positively correlated with VDBP concentrations (r_s = 0.39, p < 0.01) when data for all women (HC users and non users) were pooled (Figure 1B).

3.1. The Effect of Use of Hormonal Contraceptives on P-25OHD, P-1,25OH₂D, and P-VDBP Concentrations

Table 2 details the biochemical indices measured as stratified by whether studied women used HC.

Table 2. Biochemical characteristics as stratified by use of hormonal contraceptives. Data are presented as Median with interquartile (p25; p75) ranges unless otherwise indicated.

	All, $n = 75$	Users of hormonal contraceptive users ($n = 52$)	Non-users of hormonal contraceptives ($n = 23$)	p value [1]
Plasma vitamin D binding protein, μg/mL	305 (251; 404)	358 (260; 432)	271 (179; 302)	<0.001
Plasma 25-hydroxyvitamin D, nmol/L	79 (64; 104)	84 (67; 111)	70 (47; 83)	0.01
Free index 25-hydroxyvitamin D ($\times 10^{-3}$)	14 (10; 19)	14 (10; 19)	15 (10; 17)	0.84
Plasma 1,25-dihydroxyvitamin D, pmol/L	185 (156; 224)	198 (163; 241)	158 (123; 183)	0.01
Free index 1,25-dihydroxyvitamin D ($\times 10^{-6}$)	31 (26; 41)	29 (25; 41)	36 (27; 43)	0.10
Vitamin D status, N (%)				
<50 nmol/L	12 (16)	6 (12)	6 (50)	
50–75 nmol/L	19 (25)	12 (23)	7 (37)	0.15 [2]
>75 nmol/L	44 (59)	34 (65)	10 (23)	
Plasma PTH, pmol/L	3.6 (2.9; 4.6)	3.3 (2.5; 4.3)	3.8 (3.4; 4.6)	0.36
Plasma calcium total, albumin adjusted, mmol/L	2.45 (2.42; 2.52)	2.46 (2.43; 2.51)	2.45 (2.40; 2.53)	0.94
Plasma phosphate, mmol/L	1.00 (0.93; 1.12)	0.97 (0.89; 1.09)	1.03 (0.95; 1.21)	0.05
Plasma creatinine, μmol/L	64 (57; 72)	65 (57; 73)	61 (58; 69)	0.22
Plasma calcitonin, pmol/L	10 (9; 12)	10 (9; 12)	9 (8; 11)	0.21
Plasma bone specific alkaline phosphatase, U/L	17.9 (14.8; 23.0)	16.5 (14.6; 21.0)	21.1 (14.8; 23.8)	0.22
Plasma osteocalcin, μg/L	26.9 (19.3; 30.9)	25.9 (19.0; 29.6)	29.6 (20.6; 39.2)	0.07
Urine NTx/creatinine ratio (mmol/mmol)	42.6 (30.9; 53.0)	39.3 (29.5; 50.8)	48.7 (38.8; 57.8)	0.11
Urine calcium/creatinine-ratio (mmol/mmol)	0.2 (0.1; 0.4)	0.2 (0.1; 0.4)	0.3 (0.1; 0.4)	0.52

[1] Independent-Samples Mann-Whitney U Test; [2] Chi-Square Tests.

Compared with the non-users, HC users has a significantly higher plasma concentrations of 25OHD, 1,25(OH)₂D, and VDBP ($p < 0.01$). The median plasma concentrations of 25OHD, 1,25(OH)₂D, and VDBP were respectively 16%, 13%, and 25%, higher in users compared to non-users of HC. However, FI-25OHD and FI-1,25(OH)₂D did not differ between groups.

Adjustment for between group differences in body weight did not change results.

The prevalence of a 25OHD concentration below 50 nmol/L was equal between groups, whereas there were three times as many users with a 25OHD concentration above 75.1 nmol/L as non-users of HC (Table 2).

The correlation between the plasma concentration of 25OHD and 1,25(OH)₂D was near significant in both users of HC ($r_s = 0.31$, $p = 0.06$) and in non-users of HC ($r = 0.49$, $p = 0.07$).

However, 25OHD and VDBP concentrations were not significantly correlated when groups were analyzed separately (in HC users: $r_s = 0.15$, $p = 0.29$ and in non-users: $r_s = 0.29$, $p = 0.18$). Plasma

$1,25(OH)_2D$ tended to be positively correlated with VDBP in non-users of HC ($r_s = 0.52$, $p = 0.06$), but not in HC users ($r_s = 0.21$, $p = 0.21$) (Figure 1B).

3.2. The Effect of Use of Hormonal Contraceptives on Calcium Homeostasis and Bone Turnover

As shown in Table 2, plasma concentrations of phosphate and osteocalcin were borderline significant lower in users-compared with non-users of HC; whereas no other measured indices differed between groups.

4. Discussion

We have studied a group of healthy young Danish women among whom 52 used HC and 23 did not. Our analyses showed significantly higher plasma concentrations of 25OHD, $1,25(OH)_2D$ and VDBP in users compared with non-users of HC, FI-25OHD and FI-1,25OH$_2$D were however not different between groups.

Our findings of increased VDBP concentrations in users of HC agrees with the findings in postmenopausal women receiving postmenopausal hormone substitution. In an earlier study from our group, initiation of postmenopausal oestrogen therapy caused a significant 8% increase in VDBP concentrations [19]. Similar results have been reported in pregnancy, during which an increase in VDBP concentration is observed [10,18].

Plasma $1,25(OH)_2D$ is known to suppress the secretion of PTH, stimulate the synthesis of osteocalcin and enhance intestinal absorption of calcium and phosphate [27,28]. The latter may be reflected in an increase renal excretion of these minerals [27]. Despite a significant increase in plasma $1,25(OH)_2D$ our data did not show any significant effect of HC on indices of calcium and phosphate homeostasis or bone metabolism. These findings may support the notion of the free hormone hypothesis, *i.e.*, that only the free fraction of the hormone has biological effects [29].

We assume based on our results and previous reports [5,10,15,18,19] that the estrogen component of HC may increase VDBP synthesis or decrease its catabolism. The concomitant increase in the total plasma $1,25(OH)_2D$ concentration may mirror a compensatory adjustment to maintain an unaltered concentration of the free fraction [10,16,18].

VDBP binding protects vitamin D metabolites from hydroxylase-mediated catabolism; an increase in VDBP may therefore reduce further metabolism of vitamin D metabolites, increasing their half-life. An alternative explanation is that, in parallel with the up regulation of the $1,25(OH)_2D$ concentration, the total 25OHD concentration is unregulated via unknown mechanisms, to maintain the free concentration of 25OHD, available to tissues. This may potentially explain the higher plasma concentration of the largely unregulated plasma concentration of 25OHD in HC users, however, this needs further investigation.

An important limitation of our study is the relative small sample size and the fact that women were healthy and all had plasma 25OHD concentrations over 25 nmol/L. This may have limited our ability to detect further potential effects of HC on calcium homeostasis and bone metabolism through variations in VDBP, 25OHD, and $1,25(OH)_2D$ in vitamin D deficiency (25OHD < 25 nmol/L). Further studies should therefore aim to investigate effects of HC in women with vitamin D deficiency.

Moreover, investigations in larger groups are needed to assess the effects of HC on vitamin D metabolites and its effect on muscle and bone, as well as other health outcomes.

5. Conclusions

In conclusion, use of HC is associated with an elevated plasma concentration of VDBP and concomitant higher plasma 25OHD and 1,25(OH)$_2$D. The free-indices of these vitamin D metabolites are however similar to non-users of HC. The point of emphasis: the use of HC should be considered in the interpretation of 25OHD and 1,25(OH)$_2$D vitamin D concentrations in women. Further studies should aim to clarify whether also in women with a low vitamin D supply, an HC induced increase in VDBP is accompanied by an increase in plasma 25OHD to maintain the free 25OHD level. Further research is also required to assess whether the free 25OHD index is a better marker of 25OHD tissue availability and has a higher correlation with indices of calcium homeostasis and bone metabolism than total 25OHD levels.

Acknowledgements

We are grateful for the financial support provided to the project from: The Danish Agency for Science, Technology and Innovation, The Aarhus University Research Foundation, AP Moeller Foundation for the Advancement of Medical Science, Svend Fældings Humanitære Fond, The Lundbeck Foundation, Aarhus University Fellowship, and Helga and Peter Kornings Foundation. Inez Schoenmakers and Shailja Nigdikar are supported through the core programme of the Nutrition and Bone Research group at MRC Human Nutrition Research funded by UK MRC (grant code U105960371).

Conflicts of Interest

The authors are not aware of any affiliations, memberships, funding, or financial holdings that might be perceived as affecting the objectivity of this study.

References

1. Holick, M.F. Vitamin D status: Measurement, interpretation, and clinical application. *Ann. Epidemiol.* **2009**, *19*, 73–78.
2. Mosekilde, L. Vitamin D and the elderly. *Clin. Endocrinol.* **2005**, *62*, 265–281.
3. Holick, M.F. Resurrection of vitamin D deficiency and rickets. *J. Clin. Investig.* **2006**, *116*, 2062–2072.
4. Hewison, M.; Burke, F.; Evans, K.N.; Lammas, D.A.; Sansom, D.M.; Liu, P.; Modlin, R.L.; Adams, J.S. Extra-renal 25-hydroxyvitamin D3–1alpha-hydroxylase in human health and disease. *J. Steroid Biochem. Mol. Biol.* **2007**, *103*, 316–321.
5. Bikle, D.D.; Gee, E.; Halloran, B.; Kowalski, M.A.; Ryzen, E.; Haddad, J.G. Assessment of the free fraction of 25-hydroxyvitamin D in serum and its regulation by albumin and the vitamin D-binding protein. *J. Clin. Endocrinol. Metab.* **1986**, *63*, 954–959.

6. Bikle, D.D.; Siiteri, P.K.; Ryzen, E.; Haddad, J.G. Serum protein binding of 1,25-dihydroxyvitamin D: A reevaluation by direct measurement of free metabolite levels. *J. Clin. Endocrinol. Metab.* **1985**, *61*, 969–975.

7. Holick, M.F.; Chen, T.C. Vitamin D deficiency: A worldwide problem with health consequences. *Am. J. Clin. Nutr.* **2008**, *87*, 1080S–1086S.

8. Chan, J.; Jaceldo-Siegl, K.; Fraser, G.E. Determinants of serum 25 hydroxyvitamin D levels in a nationwide cohort of blacks and non-Hispanic whites. *Cancer Causes Control* **2010**, *21*, 501–511.

9. Nesby-O'Dell, S.; Scanlon, K.S.; Cogswell, M.E.; Gillespie, C.; Hollis, B.W.; Looker, A.C.; Allen, C.; Doughertly, C.; Gunter, E.W.; Bowman, B.A. Hypovitaminosis D prevalence and determinants among African American and white women of reproductive age: Third National Health and Nutrition Examination Survey, 1988–1994. *Am. J. Clin. Nutr.* **2002**, *76*, 187–192.

10. Bouillon, R.; van Assche, F.A.; van Baelen, H.; Heyns, W.; de Moor, P. Influence of the vitamin D-binding protein on the serum concentration of 1,25-dihydroxyvitamin D3. Significance of the free 1,25-dihydroxyvitamin D3 concentration. *J. Clin. Investig.* **1981**, *67*, 589–596.

11. Haddad, J.G., Jr.; Walgate, J. Radioimmunoassay of the binding protein for vitamin D and its metabolites in human serum: Concentrations in normal subjects and patients with disorders of mineral homeostasis. *J. Clin. Investig.* **1976**, *58*, 1217–1222.

12. Møller, U.; Streym, S.; Heickendorff, L.; Mosekilde, L.; Rejnmark, L. Effects of 25OHD concentrations on chances of pregnancy and pregnancy outcomes. A cohort study in healthy Danish women. *Eur. J. Clin. Nutr.* **2012**, *66*, 862–868.

13. Cross, N.A.; Hillman, L.S.; Allen, S.H.; Krause, G.F. Changes in bone mineral density and markers of bone remodeling during lactation and postweaning in women consuming high amounts of calcium. *J. Bone Miner. Res.* **1995**, *10*, 1312–1320.

14. Ritchie, L.D.; Fung, E.B.; Halloran, B.P.; Turnlund, J.R.; van Loan, M.D.; Cann, C.E.; King, J.C. A longitudinal study of calcium homeostasis during human pregnancy and lactation and after resumption of menses. *Am. J. Clin. Nutr.* **1998**, *67*, 693–701.

15. Aarskog, D.; Aksnes, L.; Markestad, T.; Rodland, O. Effect of estrogen on vitamin D metabolism in tall girls. *J. Clin. Endocrinol. Metab.* **1983**, *57*, 1155–1158.

16. Harris, S.S.; Dawson-Hughes, B. The association of oral contraceptive use with plasma 25-hydroxyvitamin D levels. *J. Am. Coll. Nutr.* **1998**, *17*, 282–284.

17. Gagnon, C.; Baillargeon, J.P.; Desmarais, G.; Fink, G.D. Prevalence and predictors of vitamin D insufficiency in women of reproductive age living in northern latitude. *Eur. J. Endocrinol.* **2010**, *163*, 819–824.

18. Van Hoof, H.J.; de Sevaux, R.G.; van Baelen, H.; Swinkels, L.M.; Klipping, C.; Ross, H.A.; Sweep, C.G. Relationship between free and total 1,25-dihydroxyvitamin D in conditions of modified binding. *Eur. J. Endocrinol.* **2001**, *144*, 391–396.

19. Rejnmark, L.; Lauridsen, A.L.; Brot, C.; Vestergaard, P.; Heickendorff, L.; Nexo, E.; Mosekilde, L. Vitamin D and its binding protein Gc: Long-term variability in peri- and postmenopausal women with and without hormone replacement therapy. *Scand. J. Clin. Lab. Investig.* **2006**, *66*, 227–238.

20. Gravholt, C.H.; Leth-Larsen, R.; Lauridsen, A.L.; Thiel, S.; Hansen, T.K.; Holmskov, U.; Naeraa, R.W.; Christiansen, J.S. The effects of GH and hormone replacement therapy on serum concentrations of mannan-binding lectin, surfactant protein D and vitamin D binding protein in Turner syndrome. *Eur. J. Endocrinol.* **2004**, *150*, 355–362.

21. Moller, U.K.; við Streym, S.; Mosekilde, L.; Rejnmark, L. Changes in bone mineral density and body composition during pregnancy and postpartum. A controlled cohort study. *Osteoporos. Int.* **2012**, *23*, 1213–1223.

22. Hermann, A.P.; Thomsen, J.; Vestergaard, P.; Mosekilde, L.; Charles, P. Assessment of kalcium intake. A quick method comparerd to a 7 days food diary. *Calcif. Tissue Int.* **1999**, *64*, S82.

23. Maunsell, Z.; Wright, D.J.; Rainbow, S.J. Routine isotope-dilution liquid chromatography-tandem mass spectrometry assay for simultaneous measurement of the 25-hydroxy metabolites of vitamins D2 and D3. *Clin. Chem.* **2005**, *51*, 1683–1690.

24. Hojskov, C.S.; Heickendorff, L.; Moller, H.J. High-throughput liquid-liquid extraction and LCMSMS assay for determination of circulating 25(OH) vitamin D3 and D2 in the routine clinical laboratory. *Clin. Chim. Acta* **2010**, *411*, 114–116.

25. Schifter, S. A new highly sensitive radioimmunoassay for human calcitonin useful for physiological studies. *Clin. Chim. Acta* **1993**, *215*, 99–109.

26. Mosekilde, L. Vitamin D requirement and setting recommendation levels: Long-term perspectives. *Nutr. Rev.* **2008**, *66*, S170–S177.

27. Favus, M. *Primer on the Metabolic Bone Diseases and Disorders of Mineral Metabolism*, 6th ed.; Bikle, D.D., Christakos, S., Goldring, S.R., Guise, T.H., Holick, M.F., Jan de Beur, S., Kaplan, F.S., Kleerekoper, M., Langman, C.B., Lian, J.B., *et al.*, Eds.; American Society for Bone and Mineral Research: Washington, DC, USA, 2006; pp. 50–132.

28. Henry, H.L.; Norman, A.W. Vitamin D: Metabolism and biological actions. *Annu. Rev. Nutr.* **1984**, *4*, 493–520.

29. Mendel, C.M. The free hormone hypothesis: A physiologically based mathematical model. *Endocr. Rev.* **1989**, *10*, 232–274.

Permissions

The contributors of this book come from diverse backgrounds, making this book a truly international effort. This book will bring forth new frontiers with its revolutionizing research information and detailed analysis of the nascent developments around the world.

We would like to thank all the contributing authors for lending their expertise to make the book truly unique. They have played a crucial role in the development of this book. Without their invaluable contributions this book wouldn't have been possible. They have made vital efforts to compile up to date information on the varied aspects of this subject to make this book a valuable addition to the collection of many professionals and students.

This book was conceptualized with the vision of imparting up-to-date information and advanced data in this field. To ensure the same, a matchless editorial board was set up. Every individual on the board went through rigorous rounds of assessment to prove their worth. After which they invested a large part of their time researching and compiling the most relevant data for our readers.

The editorial board has been involved in producing this book since its inception. They have spent rigorous hours researching and exploring the diverse topics which have resulted in the successful publishing of this book. They have passed on their knowledge of decades through this book. To expedite this challenging task, the publisher supported the team at every step. A small team of assistant editors was also appointed to further simplify the editing procedure and attain best results for the readers.

Apart from the editorial board, the designing team has also invested a significant amount of their time in understanding the subject and creating the most relevant covers. They scrutinized every image to scout for the most suitable representation of the subject and create an appropriate cover for the book.

The publishing team has been an ardent support to the editorial, designing and production team. Their endless efforts to recruit the best for this project, has resulted in the accomplishment of this book. They are a veteran in the field of academics and their pool of knowledge is as vast as their experience in printing. Their expertise and guidance has proved useful at every step. Their uncompromising quality standards have made this book an exceptional effort. Their encouragement from time to time has been an inspiration for everyone.

The publisher and the editorial board hope that this book will prove to be a valuable piece of knowledge for researchers, students, practitioners and scholars across the globe.

List of Contributors

Laila Abdel-Wareth, Afrozul Haq, Andrew Turner, Arwa Salem, Faten Mustafa, Nafiz Hussein, Fasila Pallinalakam, Louisa Grundy and Gemma Patras
Pathology & Laboratory Medicine Institute, Sheikh Khalifa Medical City, Abu Dhabi 51900, UAE

Shoukat Khan
Pathology & Laboratory Medicine Department, Military Hospital, Riyadh 11159, Kingdom of Saudi Arabia

Jaishen Rajah
Pediatric Institute, Sheikh Khalifa Medical City, Abu Dhabi 51900, UAE

Daniel E. Roth and Robert E. Black
Department of International Health, The Johns Hopkins Bloomberg School of Public Health, 615 North Wolfe Street, Baltimore, MD 21205, USA

Abdullah Al Mahmud, Rubhana Raqib and Evana Akhtar
International Center for Diarrhoeal Disease Research, Bangladesh (ICDDR,B), GPO Box 128, Dhaka 1000, Bangladesh

Abdullah H. Baqui
Department of International Health, The Johns Hopkins Bloomberg School of Public Health, 615 North Wolfe Street, Baltimore, MD 21205, USA
International Center for Diarrhoeal Disease Research, Bangladesh (ICDDR,B), GPO Box 128, Dhaka 1000, Bangladesh

Matthias Wacker and Michael F. Holick
Vitamin D, Skin and Bone Research Laboratory, Section of Endocrinology, Nutrition, and Diabetes, Department of Medicine, Boston University Medical Center, 85 East Newton Street, M-1013, Boston, MA 02118, USA

Anna J. Jovanovich, Kristen Jablonski and Michel Chonchol
Division of Renal Diseases and Hypertension, University of Colorado Denver, Denver, CO 80045 USA

Adit A. Ginde
Department of Emergency Medicine, University of Colorado Denver, Denver, CO 80045 USA

John Holmen
Intermountain Healthcare, Salt Lake City, UT 84157, USA

Rebecca L. Allyn
Denver Health Medical Center, Denver, CO 80204, USA

Jessica Kendrick
Division of Renal Diseases and Hypertension, University of Colorado Denver, Denver, CO 80045 USA
Denver Health Medical Center, Denver, CO 80204, USA

Hassanali Vatanparast
Division of Nutrition and Dietetics, College of Pharmacy and Nutrition, University of Saskatchewan, Saskatoon, SK S7N 5A2, Canada
School of Public Health, University of Saskatchewan, Saskatoon, SK S7N 5A2, Canada

Christine Nisbet
Division of Nutrition and Dietetics, College of Pharmacy and Nutrition, University of Saskatchewan, Saskatoon, SK S7N 5A2, Canada

Brian Gushulak
Migration Health Consultants, Qualicum Beach, British Columbia, V9K 1S9, Canada

Ursula Thiem, Bartosz Olbramski and Kyra Borchhardt
Division of Nephrology and Dialysis, Department of Internal Medicine III, Medical University of Vienna, Spitalgasse 23, Vienna 1090, Austria

Lynda Thyer, Emma Ward and Rodney Smith
Macro Innovations Ltd., CB4 0DS Cambridge, UK

Maria Giulia Fiore and Marco Ruggiero
Department of Experimental and Clinical Biomedical Sciences, University of Firenze, 50134 Firenze, Italy

Stefano Magherini, Jacopo J. V. Branca, Gabriele Morucci, Massimo Gulisano and Stefania Pacini
Department of Experimental and Clinical Medicine, University of Firenze, 50134 Firenze, Italy

Fahad Alshahrani
Department of Medicine, King Abdulaziz Medical City, Riyadh 14611, Saudi Arabia

Naji Aljohani
Specialized Diabetes and Endocrine Center, King Fahad Medical City, Riyadh 59046, Saudi Arabia
Faculty of Medicine, King Saud bin Abdulaziz University for Health Sciences, Riyadh 22490, Saudi Arabia
Prince Mutaib Chair for Biomarkers of Osteoporosis, College of Science, King Saud University, Riyadh 11451, Saudi Arabia

Bo Mi Song
Department of Public Health, Yonsei University Graduate School, Seoul 120-752, Korea
Cardiovascular and Metabolic Disease Etiology Research Center, Yonsei University College of Medicine, Seoul 120-752, Korea

Young Mi Yoon
Cardiovascular and Metabolic Disease Etiology Research Center, Yonsei University College of Medicine, Seoul 120-752, Korea

Yumie Rhee, Chang Oh Kim and Eun Young Lee
Department of Internal Medicine, Yonsei University College of Medicine, Seoul 120-752, Korea

Yoosik Youm
Department of Sociology, Yonsei University College of Social Sciences, Seoul 120-752, Korea

Kyoung Min Kim
Department of Internal Medicine, Seoul National University Bundang Hospital, Seongnam 463-707, Korea

Ju-Mi Lee and Hyeon Chang Kim
Cardiovascular and Metabolic Disease Etiology Research Center, Yonsei University College of Medicine, Seoul 120-752, Korea
Department of Preventive Medicine, Yonsei University College of Medicine, Seoul 120-752, Korea

Dana Ogan and Kelly Pritchett
Department of Nutrition, Exercise and Health Science, Central Washington University, 400 E. University Way, Ellensburg, WA 98926, USA

Paloma Reguera-Leal
Unit of Public Health, Hygiene and Environmental Health, Department of Preventive Medicine and Public Health, Food Science, Toxicology and Legal Medicine, University of Valencia, 46100 Valencia, Spain

Maria Morales Suárez-Varela, Nuria Rubio-López and Agustín Llopis-González
Unit of Public Health, Hygiene and Environmental Health, Department of Preventive Medicine and Public Health, Food Science, Toxicology and Legal Medicine, University of Valencia, 46100 Valencia, Spain
CIBER Epidemiología y Salud Pública (CIBERESP), 28029 Madrid, Spain
Center for Advanced Research in Public Health (CSISP-FISABIO), 46010 Valencia, Spain

William B. Grant
Sunlight, Nutrition and Health Research Center, P.O. Box 641603, San Francisco, CA 94164, USA

Patricia G. Weyland and Jill Howie-Esquivel
Department of Physiological Nursing, School of Nursing, University of California, San Francisco (UCSF), #2 Koret Way Box 0610, San Francisco, CA 94143, USA

Billie Bonevski
Priority Research Centre for Translational Neuroscience and Mental Health, Level 5 McAuley Building, Mater Hospital, Cnr Edith & Platt Streets, Waratah, NSW, 2298, Australia

Jamie Bryant
Priority Research Centre in Health Behaviour, School of Medicine and Public Health, University of Newcastle, Hunter Medical Research Institute, Newcastle, 2305, Australia

Sylvie Lambert
Translational Cancer Research Unit, Ingham Institute for Applied Medical Research, South Western Sydney Clinical School, UNSW Medicine, The University of New South Wales, Sydney, 2170, Australia

Irena Brozek and Vanessa Rock
Cancer Council NSW, PO Box 572 Kings Cross, NSW, 1340, Australia

Ulla K. Møller, Susanna við Streym, Leif Mosekilde and Lars Rejnmark
Department of Endocrinology and Internal Medicine, THG, Aarhus University Hospital, Tage Hansens Gade 2, DK, Aarhus 8000, Denmark

Lars T. Jensen
Department of Clinical Physiology, Glostrup University Hospital, Copenhagen DK-2900, Denmark

Inez Schoenmakers and Shailja Nigdikar
MRC Human Nutrition Research, Cambridge CB1 9NL, UK

Index